the portable pediatrician

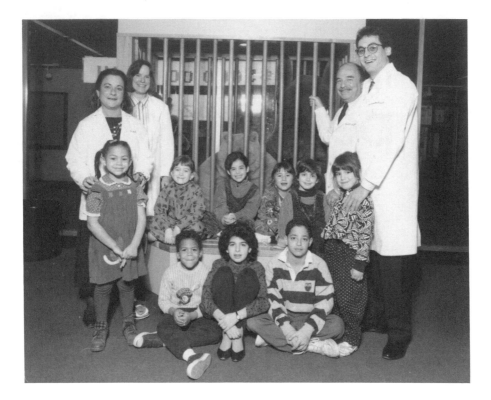

The authors (the big people in white coats, left to right: JAO, JAM, FAO, HM)
and friends in the lobby of The Johns Hopkins Children's Center.

the portable
pediatrician

Howard Markel, M.D.
Harriet Lane Home Research Fellow
Department of Pediatrics
The Johns Hopkins Children's Center;
Fellow, Institute of the History of Medicine
The Johns Hopkins University School of Medicine
Baltimore, Maryland

Jane A. Oski, M.D.
Department of Pediatrics
The Johns Hopkins Children's Center;
Clinical Fellow in Pediatrics
The Johns Hopkins University School of Medicine
Baltimore, Maryland

Frank A. Oski, M.D.
Director and Pediatrician-in-Chief
The Johns Hopkins Children's Center;
Given Professor and Chairman
Department of Pediatrics
The Johns Hopkins University School of Medicine
Baltimore, Maryland

Julia A. McMillan, M.D.
Deputy Director
The Johns Hopkins Children's Center;
Associate Professor and Deputy Chairman
Department of Pediatrics
The Johns Hopkins University School of Medicine
Baltimore, Maryland

HANLEY & BELFUS, INC./Philadelphia
MOSBY-YEAR BOOK, INC./St. Louis • Baltimore • Boston • Chicago • London
Philadelphia • Sydney • Toronto

Publisher: HANLEY & BELFUS, INC.
210 South 13th Street
Philadelphia, PA 19107
(215) 546-7293

North American and Worldwide sales and distribution:

MOSBY–YEAR BOOK, INC.
11830 Westline Industrial Drive
St. Louis, MO 63146

In Canada: MOSBY–YEAR BOOK, INC.
5240 Finch Avenue East
Unit 1
Scarborough, Ontario M1S 5A2
Canada

The Portable Pediatrician   ISBN 1-56053-007-3

Library of Congress catalog card number 91-58777

Last digit is the print number: 9 8 7 6 5 4 3 2

DEDICATION

We dedicate this book to our parents:
Bernice and Samuel Markel
Barbara and Frank Oski
Sara and Aram Oski
and
Dorothy and Robert McMillan,

and to all children, past, present, and future.

CONTENTS

PREFACE

The Portable Pediatrician is intended to instruct, enlighten, and entertain those who are studying or providing for the health care needs of children and adolescents. Although this book is clearly not meant to be an all-encompassing textbook of pediatrics, it is the authors' hope that the busy practitioner, house officer, medical student, or nurse can turn to these pages in the quest for an important bit of information that solves an immediate problem or to replenish his or her reservoir of knowledge in pediatrics.

We have arranged this book in a dictionary format so that the reader can look up in alphabetical order the subject or key word at hand for quick and ready reference. A more complete index is available at the end of the volume. References on which the individual entries have been based are also provided so that the reader can perform a more extensive search on the topic in question.

As in any endeavor, there are acknowledgements to be made. We would like to express our thanks to Lori Waugh, who patiently transcribed our handwritten notes into a typewritten manuscript; to Laurel Blewett, formerly Research Librarian for the Department of Pediatrics, The Johns Hopkins Hospital; to John J. Hanley and Linda C. Belfus, our editors and publishers; to the many interns, residents, and medical students on whom we tried out much of this material in the form of clinical rounds and teaching sessions; and, of course, to the children who are our patients and who make coming to work each morning such a joyful experience.

Howard Markel, M.D.
Jane A. Oski, M.D.
Frank A. Oski, M.D.
Julia A. McMillan, M.D.
Baltimore, Maryland

SIGNS AND SYMPTOMS—THE DIFFERENTIAL DIAGNOSIS

On some of the pages that follow are listed major signs and symptoms and their causes. The causes are classified as **COMMON, UNCOMMON** or **RARE**. The COMMON category contains those diseases that, in the aggregate, are responsible for approximately 90% of the patients who have that particular sign or symptom. The term is not meant to suggest that the entity itself is common. The designation UNCOMMON indicates that 1% to 10% of patients with the symptom or sign will be found in that category, whereas the designation RARE indicates the diseases that are responsible for less than 1% of the symptom or sign under discussion. It is common sense, when confronted with any given sign or symptom, to consider the COMMON causes first. (These entries are adapted from Dietz HC, Oski FA: Presenting signs and symptoms. In Oski FA, DeAngelis CD, Feigin FD, Warshaw JB (eds): Principles and Practice of Pediatrics. Philadelphia, Lippincott, 1990, pp 2023–2053.)

A

ABDOMINAL MASSES

Common Causes

Appendiceal abscess
Bladder distention
Fecal collection
Hepatomegaly (any cause)
Hydronephrosis
Multicystic dysplastic kidney
Neuroblastoma

Polycystic kidney disease
   (± liver involvement)
Pregnancy (± ectopic location)
Pyloric stenosis
Splenomegaly (any cause)
Wilms' tumor

Uncommon Causes

Adrenal hemorrhage
Hernia (± incarceration)
Intestinal duplications
Intussusception
Leukemia

Lymphoma
Ovarian cyst
Renal vein thrombosis
Teratoma (abdominal/ovarian)

Rare Causes

Abscess
Anterior meningocele
Aortic aneurysm
Benign cystic causes
   Urachal cyst
   Mesenteric cyst
   Omental cyst
   Pancreatic cyst/pseudocyst
Bezoar
Hepatobiliary causes
   Cholecystitis/ascending
      cholangitis
   Choledochal cyst
   Hemangioendothelioma
   Hydrops of the gallbladder
Hydrometrocolpos

Intestinal causes
   Intestinal atresia (proximal
      dilatation)
   Malrotation with volvulus
   Meconium plug/ileus
   Regional enteritis
Retroperitoneal lymphangioma
Solid tumors
   Granuloma-thecal cell tumor
Hepatoblastoma
   Hepatocellular carcinoma
   Lymphoma
   Mesoblastic nephroma
   Nephroblastomatosis
   Rhabdomyosarcoma

Reference: Oski FA, et al: Principles and Practice of Pediatrics. Philadelphia, J.B. Lippincott, 1990.

ABDOMINAL PAIN

ACUTE

Common Causes

Appendicitis
Bacterial enterocolitis
  Campylobacter
  Salmonella
  Shigella
  Yersinia

Dietary indiscretion
Food poisoning
Mesenteric lymphadenitis
Pharyngitis
Urinary tract infection
Viral gastroenteritis

Uncommon Causes

Cholecystitis/cholelithiasis
Diabetes mellitus
Hepatitis
Herpes zoster
Incarcerated hernia
Infectious mononucleosis
Intussusception
Meckel's diverticulum
Obstruction (adhesions)
Pelvic inflammatory disease
Peritonitis
  Post-trauma/instrumentation
  Spontaneous

Pneumonia
Pregnancy ($\pm$ ectopic location)
Sepsis
Trauma
  Bowel perforation
  Intramural hematoma
  Intraperitoneal blood
  Liver/spleen laceration
    or hematoma
  Musculocutaneous injury
  Pancreatic pseudocyst
Volvulus

Rare Causes

Abdominal abscess
Acute arrhythmia
Acute rheumatic fever
Adynamic ileus
  Drugs
  Metabolic
  Postsurgery/trauma
Ascites
Eosinophilic gastroenteritis
Glomerulonephritis
Hemolysis
Malignancy
  Leukemia/lymphoma

Solid tumor ($\pm$ rupture/hemorrhage)
Mesenteric arterial insufficiency/
  occlusion
Nephrolithiasis
Nephrotic syndrome
Obstructive nephropathy
Pancreatitis
Testicular torsion
Vasculitis
  Henoch-Schönlein purpura
  Kawasaki's disease
  Polyarteritis nodosa
  Systemic lupus erythematosus

RECURRENT

Common Causes

"Psychophysiologic"
    Conversion hysteria
    Depression
    Idiopathic recurrent pain
    Reaction anxiety
    Secondary gain
    Task-induced phobia (e.g., school, sports)

Uncommon Causes

Aerophagia
Constipation
Drugs
    Antibiotics
    Anticonvulsants
    Aspirin
    Bronchodilators
Dysmenorrhea
Enzymatic deficiency
    (e.g., lactose intolerance)
Food allergy
Hepatosplenomegaly (any etiology)

Hiatal hernia
Inflammatory bowel disease
Irritable bowel syndrome
Mittelschmerz syndrome
Parasitic infection
    Ascariasis
    Giardiasis
    Strongyloidiasis
    Trichinelliasis
Peptic ulcerative disease
Sickle-cell anemia
Urinary tract infection

Rare Causes

Abdominal epilepsy
Abdominal masses/malignancies
    Lymphoma
    Neuroblastoma
    Ovarian lesions
    Wilms' tumor
Abdominal migraine equivalent
Acute intermittent porphyria
Addison's disease
Angioneurotic edema
Bowel anomaly with obstruction
    Duplication
    Malrotation
    Stenosis
    Web
Choledochal cyst
Collagen vascular disease
Cystic fibrosis (meconium plug/ileus
    equivalent)

Endometriosis
Familial Mediterranean fever
Heavy metal intoxication
Hematocolpos
Hirschsprung's disease
Hyperlipoproteinemia
Hyperthyroidism
Hypoperfusion states
    Coarctation of the aorta
    Familial dysautonomia
    Superior mesenteric artery syndrome
Mesenteric cyst
Neurologic
    CNS mass lesion
    Radiculopathy
    Spinal cord injury/tumor
Recurrent/chronic arrhythmia
Recurrent pancreatitis
Wegener's granulomatosis

Reference: Oski FA, et al: Principles and Practice of Pediatrics. Philadelphia, J.B. Lippincott, 1990.

The Differential Diagnosis of Acute Lower Abdominal Pain in Adolescent Women

The complaint of lower abdominal pain in a sexually active adolescent female frequently points toward the work-up for acute pelvic inflammatory disease (PID). Symptoms that often accompany lower abdominal pain include urinary symptoms, nausea, vomiting, fever, malaise, and dyspareunia. Unfortunately these findings are seen in other pathologic processes involving the reproductive tract, as well as disease entities of the gastrointestinal tract and urinary tract. It is obvious, therefore, that one needs to consider a great many problems when evaluating the adolescent female complaining of lower abdominal pain.

Urinary Tract
Cystitis
Pyelonephritis
Urethritis
Other

Gastrointestinal Tract
Appendicitis
Constipation
Diverticulitis
Gastroenteritis
Inflammatory bowel disease
Irritable bowel syndrome
Other

Reproductive Tract
Acute pelvic inflammatory disease
Cervicitis
Dysmenorrhea (primary/secondary)
Ectopic pregnancy
Endometriosis
Endometritis
Mittelschmerz

Ovarian cyst (torsion/rupture)
Pregnancy (intrauterine/ectopic)
Ruptured follicle
Septic abortion
Threatened abortion
Torsion of adnexa
Tubo-ovarian abscess

The Closed-eyes Sign in Separating Nonspecific Abdominal Pain from the Acute Abdomen

The child presenting with an acute onset of abdominal pain is frequently a frustrating problem for the pediatrician. Indeed, more than 90% of these children have no organic source of pain that would be amenable to surgical intervention, and they are diagnosed as having "nonspecific abdominal pain." A group of three surgeons at the Radcliffe Hospital of Oxford University looked for the presence or absence of the "closed eyes" sign during abdominal palpation. Specifically, the surgeons hypothesized that patients with nonspecific abdominal pain were more likely to keep their eyes closed when an examiner palpates the abdomen, whereas patients with abdominal pain of an organic source usually kept their eyes open. The surgeons reasoned that patients with genuine abdominal tenderness are more likely to keep their eyes open in order to watch the examining physician carefully and to avoid unnecessary pain. The Oxonians studied 158 consecutive patients presenting to the emergency room with a complaint of abdominal pain. The data presented below support a new version of an old adage; the *eyes* have it.

Numbers of Patients Who Closed Their Eyes During Abdominal Palpation

	NO. OF PATIENTS OBSERVED			NO. (%) WHO CLOSED THEIR EYES		
DIAGNOSIS	TOTAL	MALE	FEMALE	TOTAL	MALE	FEMALE
Appendicitis	53	31	22	2 (4)	2	—
Other disease	38	20	18	4 (11)		4
Non specific abdominal pain	67	25	42	22 (33)	3	19

Gray DWR, Dixon JM, Collin J: The closed eyes sign: An aid to diagnosing nonspecific abdominal pain. Br Med J 297:837, 1988.

ACID-BASE

Acid-Base Imbalance in Childhood, Which Can Lead to Coma

Imbalances in a child's acid-base state can progress to severe metabolic derangement and coma. Systemic acidosis or alkalosis generally results from either a primary metabolic process or respiratory abnormalities; the specific causes of these derangements are many. Listed below are the more frequently occurring conditions that can alter a child's acid-base status and progress to coma.

1. **Metabolic acidosis** (increased anion gap)
   a. Lactic acidosis (e.g., hypoxic-ischemic insult; septic shock)
   b. Diabetic ketoacidosis
   c. Renal failure and uremia
   d. Organic acidurias
   e. Ingestions (e.g., methanol, paraldehyde, ethylene glycol, acetone, etc.)
   f. Salicylate poisoning (late)
   g. Severe diarrhea

2. **Respiratory acidosis** (apena or hypoventilation)
   a. Supratentorial or infratentorial lesions
   b. Ingestions (e.g., narcotics, barbiturates, sedatives, clonidine)
   c. Respiratory muscle fatigue; neuromuscular disease
   d. Metabolic encephalopathies
   e. Generalized seizure activity

3. **Respiratory alkalosis** (hyperventilation)
   a. Intracranial hypertension
   b. Septic shock (early)
   c. Hepatic failure
   d. Salicylate poisoning (early)
   e. Reye's syndrome
   f. Brainstem dysfunction

Reference: James HE: Neurologic evaluation and support in the child with an acute brain insult. Pediatr Ann 15:16–22, 1986.

Relationship of pH to Pa_{CO_2} and Base Change

A rapid calculation will often be of great help in interpreting the significance of blood gas values. When the child is very sick, every second saved can be of enormous importance. Listed below are two useful facts that can enable you to interpret the carbon dioxide and the pH results.

1. A change of Pa_{CO_2} of 10 torr is associated with a decrease or increase in pH of 0.08 units:

    Pa_{CO_2} 10 torr ↑ or ↓ pH 0.08

    For example:

    Pa_{CO_2} 40 torr—pH 7.40—Normal
    Pa_{CO_2} 50 torr—pH 7.32—Respiratory Acidosis—Hypoventilation
    Pa_{CO_2} 30 torr—pH 7.48—Respiratory Alkalosis—Hyperventilation

2. A base change (base excess or base deficit) of 10 mEq/L is associated with a pH change of 0.15.

    For example:

    Pa_{CO_2} 40 torr—pH 7.25
       Normal Pa_{CO_2}—No respiratory component
       Calculated pH 7.40
       Measured pH 7.25
       pH difference—0.15
       Base deficit = 10 mEq/L—Metabolic acidosis
    No respiratory component—Metabolic acidosis only

Modified from McMillan JA, et al: The Whole Pediatrician Catalog, Vol 3. Philadelphia, W.B. Saunders, 1982.

ALOPECIA

Common Causes

Alopecia areata
Distal trichorrhexis nodosa
Physiologic (newborns)
   Temporal recession at puberty

Tinea capitis
Traction alopecia
Trichotillomania (also *trichologia*)

Uncommon Causes

Acute bacterial infections
   Cellulitis
   Folliculitis decalvans
   Pyoderma
Burns
Cancer therapy
   Antimetabolites
   Radiation

Chemical injury
Kerion
Proximal trichorrhexis nodosa
Psoriasis
Seborrhea
Viral infections
   Herpes simplex
   Varicella

Rare Causes

Circumscribed alopecia
  Androgenic alopecia
  Aplasia cutis
  Conradi's disease (autosomal dominant chondrodysplasia punctata)
  Epidermal nevi-organoid
  Follicular aplasia
  Goltz's syndrome (focal dermal hypoplasia)
  Hair follicle hamartoma
  Incontinentia pigmenti
  Infections
  Tuberculosis
  Inflammatory etiologies
    Keratosis follicularis
    Lichen planus
    Morphea
    Porokeratosis of Mibelli
    Sarcoid
    Systemic lupus erythematosus
  Myotonic dystrophy
Diffuse alopecia
  Anagen effluvium
    Cytostatic agents in plant
      Mimosine
      Selemocystothionine
    Radium
    Thallium
  Anhidrotic ecterodermal dysplasia
  Atrichia congenita
  Cartilage-hair hypoplasia
  Chondroectodermal dysplasia
  Crouzon's syndrome (craniofacial dystosis)
  Hair shaft deformities
    Monilethrix

Diffuse alopecia *(Cont.)*
  Pili torti
    Classic form
    Trichopoliodystrophy (Menkes syndrome)
    Trichorrhexis invaginata
    Trichorrhexis nodosa
      Argininosuccinic aciduria
  Hallermann-Streiff syndrome (mandibulo-oculofacial syndrome)
  Hidrotic ectodermal dysplasia
  Langer-Giedion syndrome (trichorhinophalangeal syndrome type II)
  Marinesco-Sjögren syndrome
  Oculodentodigital dysplasia
  Progeria
  Rothmund-Thomson syndrome (congenital poikiloderma)
  Telogen effluvium
    Childbirth
    Chronic infection/illness
    Drugs
      Anticoagulants
      Anticonvulsants
      Antikeratinizing drugs
      Antithyroid drugs
      Heavy metals
      Hormones
    Excessive dieting
    High fever
    Hypothyroidism
    Stress
    Surgery

Reference: Oski FA, et al: Principles and Practice of Pediatrics. Philadelphia, J.B. Lippincott, 1990.

ALPHA-FETOPROTEIN

Maternal Serum—α-fetoprotein Screening

Maternal serum α-fetoprotein (MSAFP) screening has been quite successful in identifying neural tube defects in pregnancy. Approximately 80 to 85% of all open neural tube defects can be detected by this method. There also may be a relationship of the MSAFP to other birth defects such as Down syndrome and various chromosomal abnormalities.

1. **Findings associated with elevated MSAFP**

   More advanced gestational age
   Multiple gestation
   Fetal death
   Neural tube defects
   Ventral wall defects
   Congenital nephrosis

   Other fetal malformations
   Oligohydraminos
   Placental anomalies or insufficiency
   Fetomaternal transfusion
   Maternal liver disease or malignancy
   Normal pregnancy

2. **Adverse outcomes of pregnancy associated with unexplained MSAFP elevations**

   Spontaneous abortion
   Stillbirth
   Prematurity

   Intrauterine growth retardation
   Congenital anomalies
   Possibly pre-eclampsia

3. **Findings associated with low MSAFP**

   Less advanced gestational age
   Missed abortion
   Hydatidiform mole
   Non-pregnancy

   Fetal chromosomal anomalies
   (e.g., Down syndrome, trisomies
   13 and 18, Turner syndrome)
   Normal pregnancy

Reference: Burton BK: Maternal serum α-fetoprotein screening. Pediatr Ann 18:687–697, 1989.

AMENORRHEA

Amenorrhea in the Adolescent

Amenorrhea is defined as the absence of normal, spontaneous menstrual periods in a woman of reproductive age. It is typically separated into two forms: primary amenorrhea (the adolescent female who has never achieved menarche), and secondary amenorrhea (the cessation of menstrual cycles, once menarche has occurred, for 3 to 6 months). The most common cause of amenorrhea is pregnancy (including missed abortion and ectopic pregnancy). It is vital to consider amenorrhea, whether primary or secondary, as a symptom and not a disease process in and of itself. Although there is a large number of disease entities that can yield amenorrhea, the basic disease process generally involves one of the following dysfunctions: (1) inadequate hormonal stimulation of the endometrium; (2) an inability of the endometrium to respond to hormonal stimulation; or (3) an obstruction to the outflow of endometrial sloughing. The following table outlines the major causes of amenorrhea.

Etiology of Amenorrhea

I. CENTRAL NERVOUS SYSTEM (GENERAL)	B. Neoplasm (*Cont.*)
A. Infection	2. Glioma
1. Encephalitis	3. Pineal tumor
2. Meningitis	C. Congenital anomalies
B. Neoplasm	1. Hydrocephaly
1. Craniopharyngioma	2. Sellar malformation

Table continued on next page.

Etiology of Amenorrhea (Cont.)

II. HYPOTHALAMIC
  A. Infection
    1. Tuberculosis (granuloma)
    2. Syphilis (gumma)
  B. Inflammatory
    1. Sarcoidosis (granuloma)
  C. Neoplasm
    1. Craniopharyngioma
    2. Midline teratoma
  D. Syndrome
    1. Kallmann's
    2. Fröhlich's
    3. Laurence-Moon-Bardet-Biedl
  E. Tumor
    1. Hamartoma
    2. Hand-Schüller-Christian disease
  F. Congenital anomaly
    1. Idiopathic hypogonadotropic hypogonadism
  G. Constitutional delay
  H. Hypothalamic hyperprolactinemia

III. PITUITARY
  A. Neoplasm
    1. Adenoma
      a. Lactotrophic
      b. Cushing's disease
      c. Acromegaly
      d. Chromophobe
    2. Carcinoma
  B. Idiopathic—congenital
    1. Hypopituitarism—partial or complete
  C. Space occupying lesion
    1. Arterial aneurysm
    2. Empty sella
  D. Inflammatory
    1. Sarcoidosis
  E. Infiltrative
    1. Hemachromatosis
      a. Idiopathic
      b. Congenital anemia (e.g., thalassemia)
  F. Trauma

IV. GONADAL
  A. Gonadal dysgenesis
    1. Turner's syndrome
    2. Pure gonadal dysgenesis
    3. Mixed gonadal dysgenesis
    4. XX gonadal dysgenesis
    5. XY gonadal dysgenesis (Swyer's syndrome)
  B. Insensitive ovary
    1. Resistant ovary—Savage's syndrome
    2. Afollicular ovary
      a. Idiopathic—premature aging
      b. Injury (e.g., radiation, chemotherapy)
      c. Autoimmune disease
      d. Infection (e.g., mumps oophoritis)
      e. Infiltrative/mucopolysaccharidosis

  C. Gonadal agenesis
    1. Anorchia (early, late)
    2. Ovarian agenesis
      a. Idiopathic
      b. Surgical
  D. Ovarian tumor
    1. Androgen-producing
  E. True hermaphroditism

V. UTERINE-VAGINAL
  A. Müllerian agenesis (Rokitansky's syndrome)
  B. Vaginal agenesis—isolated
  C. Cervical agenesis—isolated
  D. Vaginal septum—transverse
  E. Imperforate hymen
  F. Asherman's syndrome—infectious

VI. GENERAL CONDITIONS
  A. Endocrinopathy
    1. Thyroid disease
      a. Hypothyroidism
      b. Hyperthyroidism
    2. Adrenal disease
      a. Cushing's syndrome
      b. Congenital adrenal hyperplasia
      c. Adrenal androgen tumor
    3. Androgen excess syndrome
      a. Polycystic ovarian disease
      b. Exogenous androgen therapy
    4. Male pseudohermaphroditism
      a. Androgen insensitivity syndromes
      b. Androgen biosynthetic defects
    5. Estrogen biosynthetic defects
    6. Diabetes
  B. Systemic disease (severe)
    1. Examples
      a. Crohn's disease
      b. Hepatic failure
      c. Glomerulonephritis
      d. Systemic lupus erythematosus
  C. Nutritional problem
    1. Generalized malnutrition (moderate to severe)
    2. Weight fluctuations—acute
  D. Psychiatric disease
    1. Anorexia nervosa
    2. Psychosis
  E. Miscellaneous conditions
    1. Exercise-induced
    2. Stress-related
  F. Pregnancy (including missed abortions and ectopic pregnancies)

Reference: Soules MR: Adolescent amenorrhea. Pediatr Clin North Am 34:1083–1103, 1987.

ANDROGENS

Clinical Causes of Androgen Excess in Adolescence

Hirsutism, the increase of sexually stimulated (i.e., androgen-mediated) terminal hair located in the midline of the body and including the face, often accompanies the other tribulations of puberty and adolescence. The presence of excessive facial hair is an unfortunate stigmata to the adolescent woman and is rife with social and psychological implications. Most commonly, hirsutism is confused with hypertrichosis, a generalized increase of vellus or lanugo hair, particularly on the limbs (lanugo on the fetus is replaced by vellus on the infant, which is then replaced by terminal hair). Excessive hair growth that is felt to be androgen-mediated warrants evaluation in order to identify those hirsute girls with Cushing's syndrome, congenital adrenal hyperplasia, or an androgen-producing neoplasm.

In evaluating the hirsute adolescent female, careful attention to the history and physical are necessary, specifically the progression and pattern of hair growth. A detailed menstrual history, appearance of secondary sexual characteristics, body habitus, and weight are also valuable. Laboratory measurements of serum testosterone (which reflects adrenal and ovarian secretion of androgens in addition to peripheral conversion of 4-androstenedione) and DHEA-sulfate (an androgen that is almost exclusively adrenal in origin) should be obtained. A pelvic examination and, depending upon one's findings, and abdominal and pelvic CT scan are useful in delineating ovarian or adrenal tumors. Finally, if congenital adrenal hyperplasia is suggested in the young patient by strong family history of hirsuitism, androgen excess, or hypertension, ACTH stimulation testing and serum 17-OH progesterone measurements are indicated.

Listed below are common causes of androgen excess in adolescence.

1. **Ovarian causes**
   a. Polycystic ovarian syndrome
   b. Neoplasms.

2. **Adrenal causes**
   a. Congenital adrenal hyperplasia
      i. 21-hydroxylase deficiency
      ii. 11 β-hydroxylase deficiency
      iii. 3β-01-dehydrogenase deficiency
   b. Neoplasm
   c. Nodular hyperplasia
   d. Cushing's syndrome

3. **Idiopathic** (altered sensitivity and/or metabolism of androgens in the pilosebaceous unit)

4. **Iatrogenic**
   a. Phenytoin
   b. Danazol
   c. Androgenic steroids

5. **Genetic**
   a. Incomplete forms of testicular feminization
   b. Mosaic forms of gonadal dysgenesis

6. **Miscellaneous**
   a. Acromegaly
   b. Porphyria

Adapted from: Kustin J, Rebar RW: Hirsutism in young adolescent girls. Pediatr Ann 15:522–528, 1986.

ANEMIAS

Rule of 34s

The sequence of numbers 34 applies to several values in pediatric hematology. These include:

34   mg bilirubin produced/gm Hb

3.4   mg iron/gm Hb

3.42   nuclear lobes/neutrophil, the upper limit of normal when averaging 100 or more neutrophils

1.34   cubic centimeters of oxygen carried by each gram of hemoglobin (if you don't mind stretching the rule of 34s a little)

Reference: Sills R: Personal communication, 1977.

Anemia in Early Infancy

During the first months of life there are many causes of anemia. Anemia during the first 3 months of life is rarely a result of nutritional iron deficiency. The accompanying table is intended to call your attention to the more likely causes of anemia that occur at birth and at 2 or 3 months of age, as well as to provide you with leads to establishing the diagnosis.

Common Causes of Anemia in Early Infancy

AGE	DIAGNOSIS	SUPPORTING DATA
At birth	Hemorrhage	
	Obstetric accidents (placenta previa, abruptio placentae, incision of placenta, rupture of cord, rupture of anomalous placental vessel)	History and visual inspection of placenta and cord
	Occult hemorrhage	
	Fetomaternal	Demonstration of fetal cells in maternal circulation
	Twin-to-twin	Demonstration of significant difference in hemoglobin values of identical twins
	Internal hemorrhage (intracranial, retroperitoneal, intrahepatic, intrasplenic, cephalhematoma)	Physical examination
	Isoimmunization	Blood groups of mother and infant; evidence of antibody on infant's red cells

Table continued on next page.

Common Causes of Anemia in Early Infancy (Cont.)

AGE	DIAGNOSIS	SUPPORTING DATA
At birth (Cont.)	Inherited defect of red cell (includes G-6-PD deficiency, pyruvate kinase deficiency, hereditary spherocytosis, elliptocytosis, stomatocytosis, etc.)	Red cell morphology, family history, and appropriate screening tests
	Acquired defect (generally in association with hypoxemia, acidosis, or infection)	Physical findings, red cell morphology, coagulation disturbance, blood and urine cultures, and serologic studies and gamma-M determination
	Red cell hypoplasia (Blackfan-Diamond syndrome, congenital leukemia, osteopetrosis)	Rare disorders; bone marrow aspirate
2–3 months	Iron deficiency as a consequence of previous hemorrhage	Obstetric history when available
	Late manifestation of previous isoimmunization	Blood types of mother and infant; maternal antibody titers
	Hereditary defects of the red cell	Persistence of hemolytic anemia; red cell morphology and laboratory tests
	Thalassemia major	Red cell morphology, splenomegaly, persistence of fetal hemoglobin elevation, family studies
	Sickle cell anemia	Red cell morphology, hemoglobin electrophoresis
	Vitamin E deficiency	Infant of low birth weight; red cell morphology, low serum E level, positive hydrogen peroxide hemolysis test
	Folic acid deficiency	Premature infant, history of infections or diarrhea, red cell and marrow morphology, response to folic acid
	Persistent infection	Elevated titers to rubella, cytomegalovirus, toxoplasmosis
	Renal tubular acidosis	Acidosis, hypochloremia, mild azotemia, urine pH of 6.0 or greater in presence of acidosis

From McMillan JA, et al: The Whole Pediatrician Catalog. Philadelphia, W.B. Saunders, 1977, with permission.

Anemias Associated with a Low MCV*

98% of anemias with low MCV:
Iron deficiency
α-thalassemia
β-thalassemia

Others:
Lead poisoning†
Protein-calorie malnutrition
Copper deficiency
Sideroblastic anemia

*MCV = mean cell volume.
† Microcytosis most commonly results from associated iron deficiency.

ANION GAP

In these days of automated laboratory procedures, most sick patients will have their serum electrolytes measured. Obvious abnormalities are easily recognized. Hidden clues to diagnosis are also present in these numbers. Interpretation of the "anion gap" provides such a clue.

The principle of electroneutrality is always working and dictates that the sum of the positive charges, i.e., the mEq/L of cations, be exactly counterbalanced by the number of negative charges, i.e., the mEq/L of anions.

The principal cations in the plasma include sodium, potassium, calcium, and magnesium. The principal anions are chloride, bicarbonate, carbonic acid, dissolved carbon dioxide, albumin, globulin, sulfate, phosphate, and the organic acids, lactic and pyruvic acid.

Measurement of all the anions and cations is not required for interpretation of the patient's status. The serum sodium and potassium are representative of the extracellular fluid cations, and, in fact, account for 95% of the cations present. Chloride and bicarbonate account for 85% of the anions. Thus, the sum of the usually measured anions does not fully counterbalance the sum of the measured cations. Their difference is termed the anion gap. Because of potassium's relatively low and stable serum concentration, it has only a minor influence on the anion gap. Therefore the anion gap equation can be simplified to read as follows:

$$\text{Anion gap} = \text{sodium} - (\text{chloride} + \text{bicarbonate})$$

The normal value for the anion gap is approximately 12.0 ± 2.0. The normal range for the anion gap is thus 8 to 16 mEq/L.

Causes of a high anion gap include:

Metabolic acidosis
Dehydration
Therapy with sodium salts of
    strong acids

Therapy with certain antibiotics
Carbenicillin, large doses
    of sodium penicillin
Alkalosis

Specific causes of *high anion gap* metabolic *acidosis* include:

Uremia
Ketoacidosis

Lactic acidosis
Salicylate intoxication

Methanol intoxication
Paraldehyde toxicity

Specific causes of *normal anion gap* metabolic *acidosis* include:

Gastrointestinal bicarbonate loss
    Diarrhea or pancreatic fistula
Ureterenterostomy
Drugs
    Acetazolamide
    Sulfamylon
    Cholestyramine
    Acidifying agents (ammonium chloride, oral calcium chloride, arginine,
        hydrochloride, lysine hydrochloride)
    Rapid intravenous hydration
    Hyperalimentation
    Posthypocapnia
    Renal tubular acidosis

Causes of a *low anion gap* include:

Reduced concentration of unmeasured anions	Systematic overestimation of serum chloride
Dilution	Bromism
Hypoalbuminemia	Retained nonsodium cations
Systematic underestimation of serum sodium	Paraproteinemia
Severe hypernatremia	Hypercalcemia
Hyperviscosity	Hypermagnesemia

Reference: Emmett M, Narins RG: Clinical use of the anion gap. Medicine 56:38, 1977. From McMillan JA, et al: The Whole Pediatrician Catalog, Vol 2. Philadelphia, W.B. Saunders, 1979, pp 104–105, with permission.

ANOREXIA

Common Causes

Acute infection
Apparent anorexia
    Dieting/fear of obesity
    Manipulative behavior
    Unrealistic expectations of caretakers

Uncommon Causes

Chronic infection
Drugs
    Aminophylline
    Amphetamines
    Anticonvulsants
    Antihistamines
    Antimetabolites
    Digitalis
    Narcotics
Esophagitis/gastroesophageal reflux
Food aversion in athletes
Iron deficiency

Irritable bowel syndrome
Pregnancy
Psychosocial deprivation
    (neglect/abuse)
Psychosocial factors
    Chronic mental/environmental stress
      Anxiety
      Fear
      Loneliness/boredom
    Depression
    Grief
    Mania

Rare Causes

Acquired immunodeficiency
    syndrome (AIDS)
Adrenogenital syndrome
Alcohol/drug abuse
Anorexia nervosa
Chronic disease
Collagen vascular disease
Congestive heart failure

Cyanotic heart disease
Electrolyte disturbances
    Hypochloremia
    Hypokalemia
Endocrine disease
    Addison's disease
    Diabetes insipidus
    Hyperparathyroidism

Endocrine Disease *(Cont.)*
  Hypothyroidism
  Panhypopituitarism
Hypervitaminosis A
Inborn errors of metabolism
Kwashiorkor
Lead poisoning
Liver failure
Neurologic
  Congenital degenerative disease
  Diencephalic syndrome
  Hypothalamic lesions
  Increased intracranial pressure
  Mental retardation/cerebral palsy
Pain avoidance
  Appendicitis
  Constipation
  Gastrointestinal obstruction
  Inflammatory bowel disease
  Pancreatitis
  Superior mesenteric syndrome
Polycythemia
Postsurgical outcome
Pulmonary insufficiency
Renal failure
Renal tubular acidosis
Schizophrenia
Zinc deficiency

Reference: Oski FA, et al: Principles and Practice of Pediatrics. Philadelphia, J.B. Lippincott, 1990.

Anorexia Nervosa and Bulimia

Anorexia nervosa is characterized by excessive weight loss due to a self-inflicted starvation and a morbid, and often unrealistic, fear of becoming too fat. Amenorrhea frequently accompanies this disorder in women; a decreased libido has been noted in anorexic men. A related eating disorder, bulimia, is compulsive overeating followed by drastic attempts to avoid gaining weight as a result of the eating binge, e.g., self-induced vomiting, the ingestion of self-prescribed laxatives or diuretics, and strenuous exercise. These two eating disorders share many features and can actually evolve from one into the other; classically, anorexia nervosa evolves into bulimia. They also have distinctive features that can distinguish one from the other.

Comparison of Anorexia Nervosa (Food-Restricting) and Bulimia

ANOREXIA NERVOSA (FOOD-RESTRICTING)	BULIMIA
Similar Features	
1. Psychological	
a. Fear of fatness	d. Variable degree of distortion of body size
b. Active pursuit of weight loss	
c. Fear of loss of control of eating	e. Family history of affective disorder
2. Medical	
a. Orthostatic hypotension	f. Constipation
b. Return to prepubertal breast development	g. Acrocyanosis
	h. Lanugo hair
c. Amenorrhea	i. Pedal edema
d. Bradycardia	j. Loss of subcutaneous lipid layer
e. Lowered core temperature	and decreased muscle mass
(All of the above medical complications are the result of starvation.)	

Table continued on next page.

Comparison of Anorexia Nervosa (Food-Restricting) and Bulimia (Cont.)

ANOREXIA NERVOSA (FOOD-RESTRICTING)	BULIMIA
Contrasting Features	
1. Food intake severely restricted	1. Control of intake is lost resulting in binges
2. Less vomiting, diuretic, or laxative abuse	2. Self-induced vomiting, laxative and diuretic abuse
3. Younger	3. Older
4. More obsessional, perfectionistic characteristics	4. More histrionic, antisocial features with loss of impulse control
5. Denies hunger	5. Experiences hunger
6. Severe weight loss	6. Less severe but variable weight loss
7. Most of the medical complications stem from chronic starvation	7. Many medical complications may stem from starvation but there also exist a number of gastrointestinal complaints that result from self-induced vomiting and laxative and diuretic abuse (e.g., loss of dental enamel, paratoid gland swelling, dry mouth, esophagitis, gastric dysrhythmia, irritable bowel syndrome, and constipation). Renal problems, hypokalemic alkalosis, cardiac arrhythmias, and tetany can also result from laxative and diuretic abuse. Scars on the dorsum of the hand from frequent, self-induced vomiting.
8. Eating behavior is a source of pride	8. Eating behavior is a source of shame
9. Less sexually active	9. More sexually active
10. Amenorrhea or loss of sex drive	10. Variable amenorrhea and change in sex drive
11. Death from starvation acutely; chronically from starvation or suicide	11. Death from hypokalemia acutely; chronically from suicide
12. Patient is described as a "model" child	12. Patient often exhibits behavioral abnormalities

Adapted from: Andersen AE: Anorexia nervosa and bulimia: Biological, psychological, and sociocultural aspects. In Galler JR (ed): Nutrition and Behavior. New York, Plenum Publishing, 1984, pp 305–338.

ANTIBIOTICS

Tasteful Antibiotics, or "Just a Spoonful of Sugar Helps the Medicine Go Down"

These days, the successful marketing of antibiotic suspensions for children is as competitive as any other industry. Creating an effective and safe antibiotic is simply not enough. It also has to taste good! Listed below are the flavors, sugar content, and availability of some of the most commonly prescribed antibiotics in general pediatric practice:

Antimicrobial Suspensions Tested

SUSPENSION TRADE NAME	GENERIC NAME	PRODUCER	STRENGTH (mg/5 ml)	COLOR	FLAVOR	PRIMARY SWEETNER(S)
Augmentin	Amoxicillin/ clavulanate	Beecham	250 mg	Cream	Orange	Saccharin
Trimox	Amoxicillin	Squibb	250 mg	Pink	Cherry	Sucrose
Ceclor	Cefaclor	Lilly	250 mg	Pink	Strawberry	Sucrose
Suprax	Cefixime	Lederle	100 mg	Cream	Strawberry	Sucrose
Keflex	Cephalexin	Dista	250 mg	Orange	Bubble gum	Sucrose
Dynapen	Dicloxacillin	Bristol	62.5 mg	Pink	Orange/ pineapple	Saccharin/ sucrose
Pediazole	Erythromycin ES/sulfisoxazole	Ross	200 mg/ 600 mg	White	Strawberry/ banana	Sucrose
Erythromycin ES	Erythromycin ethylsuccinate	Barr	200 mg	Pink	Cherry	Sucrose
Ilosone	Erythromycin estolate	Dista	250 mg	Red	Cherry	Sucrose
Grifulvin V	Griseofulvin microsize	Ortho	125 mg	Peach	Raspberry	Saccharin/ sucrose
VeeTids	Penicillin VK	Squibb	250 mg	Red	Berry-like	Saccharin/ sucrose
Gantrisin	Sulfisoxazole	Roche	500 mg	White	Raspberry	Sucrose
Achromycin-V	Tetracycline	Lederle	25 mg	Red	Cherry	Sucrose
Sulfatrim	Trimethoprim/ sulfamethoxazole	Barre	40 mg/ 200 mg	Pink	Cherry	Saccharin/ sucrose

Reference: Ruff ME, et al: Antimicrobial drug suspensions: A blind comparison of taste of 14 common pediatric drugs. Pediatr Infect Dis J 10:30–33, 1991, with permission.

ANTICONVULSANTS

The anticonvulsants often produce side-effects. The commonly used anticonvulsants and their commonly produced side-effects are described in the table below.

Side-effects of Commonly Used Anticonvulsants

ANTICONVULSANT	PREDICTABLE	IDIOSYNCRATIC
Carbamazepine	Diplopia Dizziness Drowsiness Headache Nausea Hyponatremia Hypocalcemia Orofacial dyskinesia Cardiac arrhythmia	Agranulocytosis Aplastic anemia Hepatotoxicity Photosensitivity Stevens-Johnson syndrome Lupus-like syndrome Morbilliform rash Thrombocytopenia Pseudolymphoma

Table continued on next page.

Side-effects of Commonly Used Anticonvulsants (Cont.)

ANTICONVULSANT	PREDICTABLE		IDIOSYNCRATIC
Sodium valproate	Anorexia Dyspepsia Nausea Vomiting Hair loss Rash	Peripheral edema Weight gain Drowsiness Tremor	Acute pancreatitis Hepatotoxicity Thrombocytopenia Hyperammonemia Stupor Encephalopathy Teratogenicity

Phenytoin	Anorexia
	Dyspepsia
	Nausea
	Vomiting
	Aggression
	Ataxia
	Cognitive
	  impairment
	Depression
	Drowsiness
	Headache
	Nystagmus
		Paradoxical
		  seizures
		Gum hypertrophy
		Coarse facies
		Hirsutism
		Megaloblastic
		  anemia
		Hyperglycemia
		Hypocalcemia
		Osteomalacia
		Neonatal
		  hemorrhage
			Blood dyscrasias
			Lupus-like syndrome
			Reduced serum IgA
			Pseudolymphoma
			Peripheral neuropathy
			Rash
			Stevens-Johnson syndrome
			Dupuytren's contracture
			Hepatotoxicity
			Teratogenicity

Phenobarbitone	Fatigue
	Listlessness
	Tiredness
	Depression
	Insomnia*
	Distractability*
	Aggression*
	Poor memory
		Decreased libido
		Impotence
		Folate
		  deficiency
		Neonatal
		  hemorrhage
		Hypocalcemia
		Osteomalacia
			Macropapular rash
			Exfoliation
			Toxic epidermal
			  necrolysis
			Hepatotoxicity
			Dupuytren's contracture
			Frozen shoulder
			Teratogenicity

Primadone	Nausea
	Vomiting
	Drowsiness
	Weakness
	Dizziness
	Diplopia
	Nystagmus
	Ataxia
	Personality
	  change
		Psychosis
		Neonatal
		  hemorrhage
		Decreased libido
		Impotence
		Hypocalcemia
		Osteomalacia
		Megaloblastic anemia
		Neonatal
		  hemorrhage
			Rash
			Agranulocytosis
			Thrombocytopenia
			Lupus-like syndrome
			Teratogenicity

Ethosuximide	Anorexia Nausea Vomiting Agitation Drowsiness	Headache Lethargy Parkinsonism Psychosis	Rash Erythema multiforme Stevens-Johnson syndrome Lupus-like syndrome Agranulocytosis Aplastic anemia
Clonazepam/ clobazam	Fatigue Dizziness Drowsiness Ataxia Irritability* Aggression*	Hyperkinesia* Hypersalivation* Bronchorrhea* Weight gain Muscle weakness Psychosis	Rash Thrombocytopenia

*In children
Adapted from Brodie MJ: Anticonvulsants. Lancet 336:350–354, 1990, with permission.

APNEA

Common Causes

Breathholding spells
Bronchiolitis
Extrinsic suffocation
Gastroesophageal reflux/aspiration

Idiopathic (? CNS immaturity)
Prematurity
Seizure

Uncommon Causes

Asthma
Bronchopulmonary dysplasia "spells
CNS hypoperfusion
CNS trauma/bleed
Congenital airway anomaly
Hypoglycemia
Hypoxemia/hypercarbia (severe)
Infection
   Croup
   Meningitis/encephalitis

Infection *(Cont.)*
   Epiglottitis
   Pertussis
   Pneumonia
   Sepsis
Laryngospasm
Lyaryngo-tracheo-bronchomalacia
Obstructive sleep apnea
SIDS
Toxins/drugs

Rare Causes

Anemia
Arrhythmia
Glossoptosis
Guillain-Barré syndrome
Hypocalcemia
Increased intracranial pressure
Infantile botulism
Intraventricular hemorrhage
Macroglossia
Metabolic disease
   Hyperammonemia

Metabolic disease *(Cont.)*
   Inborn errors
   Metabolic alkalosis
Micrognathia
Ondine's curse
Spinal cord injury
   Cervical spine instability
   Down syndrome
   Dwarfism
   Trauma
Tumor (CNS, airway)

Reference: Oski FA, et al: Principles and Practice of Pediatrics. Philadelphia, J.B. Lippincott, 1990.

Sleep Apnea

The child with unrecognized sleep apnea may present to the pediatrician with any number of chief complaints: cardiovascular abnormalities, failure to thrive, pulmonary abnormalities, obesity, apparent mental retardation, and recurrent respiratory infections. An inadequate history may fail to reveal the culprit.

Sleep apnea can occur in infants, children and adults of any age, although the incidence is known to increase with age and be more prevalent among males than females. The diagnosis depends upon an eye for the predisposing factors and an ear for the symptoms.

Sleep apnea: Predisposing factors

Enlarged tonsils or adenoids
Upper airway or maxillofacial
  abnormalities
Hyperthyroidism
Obesity-Pickwickian syndrome

Down syndrome
Hypotonic cerebral palsy
Congenital myopathies
Pharyngeal "sphincter"
Dysautonomia

Symptoms of sleep apnea patients	% of patients
Snoring—usually all night every night; worse with respiratory infections	91
Apnea—observed by parents	81
Restless sleep and abnormal sleep positions	70
Awakenings from sleep at night	60
Nocturnal enuresis (children > 4 years of age)	33
Daytime somnolence	31
Irritability, hyperactivity	22
Cardiomegaly	6

The most common cause of sleep apnea in infancy and childhood is tonsillar and adenoidal hypertrophy, which may require surgical intervention. Beware the symptoms and predispositions. You may avert congestive heart failure or cor pulmonale!

References: Oski FA, et al: Principles and Practice of Pediatrics. Philadelphia, J.B. Lippincott, 1990.
Tunnessen WW: Pediatric puzzler: A sound clue to FTT. Contemp Peds, Sept. 1:83–85, 1984.

THE ARGYLL ROBERTSON PUPIL

Its Clinical Significance

The Argyll Robertson pupil as a sign of tabes dorsalis or neurosyphilis was described in 1868 by the eye surgeon Douglas Moray Cooper Lamb Argyll Robertson (1837–1909) of Edinburgh, Scotland. It is a miotic pupil that accommodates but fails to react to direct light. The sign is caused by lesions to the area immediately rostral to the Edinger-Westphal nucleus of the midbrain and can be found in a number of conditions that affect this area (see figure). For example, Charles Dickens, in his 1855 novel *Little Dorrit*, described a young girl named Maggy who was severely afflicted with "brain fever" or encephalitis and whose eyes were "very little affected by light" and stood "unnaturally still." More important to the present day clinician is the association of the Argyll Robertson pupil with Bannwarth's lymphocytic meningoradiculitis, a syndrome of radicular pain, cranial nerve palsies, and sensory and motor impairment secondary to infection with *Borrelia burgdorferi* or Lyme disease.

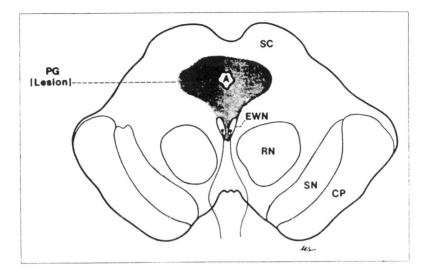

Lesions in the shaded area (periaqueductal gray [PG]) interrupt descending pathways from the oculomotor complex to the Edinger-Westphal nucleus (EWN). SC = superior colliculus; A = aqueduct; RN = red nucleus; SN = substantia nigra; CP = cerebral peduncle. (From Dasco CC, Bortz DL, Am J Med 86:199–202, 1989, with permission.)

Listed below are reported non-syphilitic causes of the Argyll Robertson pupil.

1. Diabetes mellitus
2. Multiple sclerosis
3. Wernicke's encephalopathy
4. Dejerine-Sottas progressive hypertrophic neuritis
5. Charcot-Marie-Tooth disease (peroneal muscular atrophy)
6. Tumors and hemorrhage affecting the Edinger-Westphal nucleus (e.g., midbrain tumors such as pinealomas, third ventricle gliomas, and pituitary stalk tumors)
7. Herpes zoster
8. Lyme disease (Bannwarth's syndrome)
9. Sarcoidosis
10. von Economo's disease (encephalitis secondary to influenza)

References: Dasco CC, Bortz DL: Significance of the Argyll Robertson pupil in clinical medicine. Am J Med 86:199–202, 1989.

Markel H: The childhood suffering of Charles Dickens and his literary children. Pharos 48:5–8, 1985.

ARTHRITIS

Differential Diagnosis of Childhood Arthritis

Arthritis in childhood represents a special problem to the pediatrician, because both the types and etiologies cover a broad spectrum. In the child with suspected septic arthritis, an early diagnosis is especially important for the prevention of deformities and/or functional impairment.

Clinical Criteria for Diagnosis of Childhood Arthritis

1. Swelling of a joint
2. Limitation of motion with heat, pain, or tenderness

DIAGNOSIS	DEFINITION
Juvenile rheumatoid arthritis	See JRA entries
Enteroarthritis	Antecedent enterobacterial infection (*Yersinia, Salmonella, Shigella,* or *Campylobacter* species) verified by stool culture or agglutination titer $\geq$ 1:160.
Septic arthritis	Positive bacterial culture from synovial fluid
Transient synovitis of the hip (TSH)	Acute hip effusion verified by ultrasonography, roentgenography, synovial fluid aspirate, or clinical findings
Henoch-Schönlein purpura	Typical clinical picture with petechial rash and normal platelet count
Serum sickness	Acute urticaria 5–12 days after vaccination
Acute transient arthritis	Disease duration < 3 months; diagnosis of exclusion
Arthralgia	Joint pain without trauma; no physical signs of arthritis
Orthopedic disease	Arthroscopically or radiologically verified bone disease, or internal derangement of joint, especially knee
Others: mixed connective tissue disease, systemic lupus erythematosus, polymyositis, acute lymphocytic leukemia	

Laboratory Tests in the Differential Diagnosis of Juvenile Arthritis

PATIENT GROUP	TEST	SIGNIFICANCE
All children with joint symptoms	C reactive protein (CRP), erythrocyte sedimentation rate (ESR), CBC, platelet count, urinalysis, bacterial culture of throat smear	CRP > 20, ESR > 20, WBC > 1500, and T° > 38.5°C suggest septic or enteroarthritis. Low CRP and absence of fever with acute limp and hip pain suggest TSH. An ESR 20 in the presence of a low CRP and no fever suggests JRA or other connective tissue disease and necessitates further immunologic workup. JRA may also present as FUO.
Arthritis lasting longer than 2 weeks	Anti-nuclear antibodies, serum immunoglobulins, *Yersinia* antibiodies, *Salmonella* antibodies, stool bacterial culture	Elevated in JRA and other CT diseases. IgG elevated in JRA. Yersinia and/or salmonella Ab's are thought to be valid indicators of enteroarthritis as are positive stool cultures. EA onset generally acute while JRA normally insidious.

Table continued on next page.

Laboratory Tests in the Differential Diagnosis of Juvenile Arthritis (Cont.)

PATIENT GROUP	TEST	SIGNIFICANCE
Special indications	Rheumatoid factor, antistreptolysin O (ASO)	Rarely indicated in child < 8 years of age. Both tests for suspected ARF.
	Viral antibodies	Indicated when systemic onset JRA suspected.
	Chlamydia antibodies	Rare in childhood reactive arthritis. More commonly seen in adults.

Reference: Kunnamo I, et al: Clinical Signs and laboratory tests in the differential diagnosis of arthritis in children. Am J Dis Child 141:34–40, 1987.

The Three Modes of Onset of Juvenile Rheumatoid Arthritis

Juvenile rheumatoid arthritis (JRA) differs from rheumatoid arthritis in adults in several ways, including types of onset. The three forms of onset of JRA are: (1) the acute febrile onset (systemic disease), (2) the monoarticular or pauciarticular onset (oligoarthritis), and (3) polyarticular onset (polyarthritis).

Systemic disease is manifested by spiking fevers on a daily basis plus the appearance of a characteristic rash.

Oligoarthritis is defined as onset in four or fewer joints, often only one, usually the knee.

Polyarthritis is defined as onset in five or more joints.

All three forms can mimic other diseases and the diagnosis is often one of exclusion. It is important to be intimately familiar with the clinical signs and symptoms of each type of onset to avoid the serious consequences of misdiagnosis.

Approximately 5% of all cases of JRA begin in childhood (by definition before 16 years, usually between 1 and 3 years). It is the most common pediatric connective tissue disease, and about a quarter of a million children in the U.S. are affected.

Three Modes of Onset of Juvenile Rheumatoid Arthritis

	ACUTE FEBRILE ONSET	MONOARTICULAR ONSET	POLYARTICULAR ONSET
Per cent	20	30	50
Joint Manifestations	One-half have no joint swelling at onset. The other one-half have only arthralgia. Pain may be inferred from the flexed-knee position in which these children tend to lie.	The knee is most common site of onset. Other sites are ankle, elbow, wrist and finger joints. Swelling, stiffness, and pain are usually minimal. Painful tendinitis or bursitis, especially of the heel, may be the presenting symptom.	Four or more joints are involved. May have abrupt onset with painful swelling of knees, ankles, feet, and hands. May have insidious onset with no complaint of pain. Joint involvement must be inferred from guarding movements and knee-flexed position.

Table continued on next page.

Three Modes of Onset of Juvenile Rheumatoid Arthritis (Cont.)

	ACUTE FEBRILE ONSET	MONOARTICULAR ONSET	POLYARTICULAR ONSET
Joint Manifestations *(Cont.)*		In early stages, the arthritis may be asymmetrical and migrating.	Arthritis may be migratory at first. Cervical spine may be involved. Subcutaneous nodules are not present.
Fever	Daily spikes to 105° F or higher with temperature falling sometimes to subnormal levels. Fever may precede arthritis by weeks, months, or years.	There may be low-grade daily fever spikes.	Low-grade fever with daily spikes.
Rash	90% have macular or slightly maculopapular rash usually on the trunk and extremities, occasionally on the neck and face. Rash is rarely pruritic, is usually fleeting with macules appearing for a few hours during the day or week, usually in conjunction with fever. Rash is more florid when the skin is rubbed or scratched (Köbner phenomenon).	Rash is sometimes present, but is rarely of diagnostic help.	Maculopapular rash is sometimes present.
Iridocyclitis	Rarely occurs in patients presenting in this way.	This group is most susceptible to ocular disease. It is often asymptomatic and may smolder for weeks or months. It may be the first manifestation of the disease. If undetected and untreated, it may lead to blindness from band keratopathy and cataracts. Diagnosis may be made only by slit lamp examination.	Rarely occurs in patients presenting in this way.
Lymphadenopathy	May be generalized. Splenomegaly may be present. Enlarged mesenteric nodes may lead to abdominal pain and vomiting. Lymphadenopathy may suggest lymphoma or leukemia.	Infrequent.	Infrequent.
Cardiac manifestations	10% have pericarditis clinically. Pericarditis may last 2 to 12 weeks and may recur years later. Myocarditis and resulting heart failure may occur.	—	Infrequent.

Table continued on next page.

Three Modes of Onset of Juvenile Rheumatoid Arthritis (Cont.)

	ACUTE FEBRILE ONSET	MONOARTICULAR ONSET	POLYARTICULAR ONSET
General appearance	Patient is usually irritable, listless, anorectic, and suffers from weight loss.	May have generalized symptoms.	Patient is usually listless, anorectic, and under-weight.
Laboratory	Neutrophilic leuko-cytosis with WBC of 15,000 to 50,000/mm³ There may be a moderate normocytic, normochromic anemia The ESR is usually elevated.	CBC and ESR may be normal. X-ray examination may reveal accelerated matu-ration or early closure of epiphyses, periosteal pro-liferation, metaphyseal overgrowth of long bones, especially about the knee. Synovial fluid aspiration reveals clear to opalescent fluid with good to poor mucin clot, 15,000 to 25,000 WBC/mm³ with 50 to 90% neutrophils. Glucose of synovial fluid is about 25 mg/100 ml less than the serum glucose.	WBC may be elevated, but is rarely higher than 20,000. ESR is elevated, usually corresponding roughly to the intensity of the arthritis.
Differential diagnosis	Must be differentiated from other connective tissue diseases by absence of antinuclear antibody, difference in the nature of the rash, and age of onset (peak onset of JRA is 1 to 3 years of age, while SLE is rare in children under 5 years of age).	Must be differentiated from traumatic injury and from infectious arthritis by synovial fluid analysis. (Onset of symptoms commonly follows trauma.)	Must be differentiated from rheumatic fever by difference in fever pattern (fever of rheumatic fever is remittent or sustained), by x-ray findings, and by arthritis persisting longer than a few weeks. Differentiation from the arthritis somctimcs accompanying rubella is made by detection of an increase in the HI anti-body to rubella in acute and convalescent sera. The synovial fluid of rubella arthritis has a predominance of mononuclear cells.

Reference: Calabro JJ: Hospital Practice, February 1974, p 61.

ATAXIA

Ataxia, Muscle Weakness, Extrapyramidal Disorders

The following tables cover a broad range of neuromuscular disorders that comprise an area of difficult differential diagnosis for the clinician. A child with ataxia, muscle weakness, or extrapyramidal signs and symptoms should be examined with particular care because identification of the clinical disorder can often indicate the site of the lesion.

Differential Diagnosis of Chronic Progressive Ataxia

CLINICAL DISORDER	PRECEDING HISTORY	USUAL YEAR OF ONSET IN CHILDREN	EXAMINATION	USUAL LABORATORY EXAMINATION	USUAL PROGNOSIS
Arnold-Chiari malformation	Headache, dysphagia		Palatal and tongue weakness, pyramidal signs, ataxia	May have hydrocephalus, spina bifida	Slowly progressive; stationary after surgery
Hereditary spinocerebellar ataxia	Stumbling, dizziness, familial incidence	7–10	Ataxia, loss of position sense, extensor plantar responses, kyphoscoliosis, pes cavus	Frequent associated ECG changes	Progressive, with death usually by 30 years of age
Abetalipoproteinemia	Fatty diarrhea at 6 weeks to 2 years of age	2–17	Cerebellar ataxia, posterior column signs, retinitis pigmentosa, scoliosis, pes cavus	Acanthocytosis, lack of β-lipoprotein in serum	Slowly progressive
Dentate cerebellar ataxia	Myoclonus, convulsions	7–17	Ataxia with severe intention tremor		Slowly progressive
Hereditary cerebellar ataxia	Familial incidence	3–17	Ataxia, optic atrophy, occasionally associated posterior column and pyramidal tract signs	Pneumoencephalogram: small cerebellar folia	Slowly progressive
Ataxia telangiectasia	Recurrent sinopulmonary infections in two-thirds of cases; familial incidence	1–3	Oculocutaneous telangiectasia at 4 to 6 years; ataxia, choreoathetosis, dysarthria	Chest roentgenogram: bronchiectasis; absence of IgA in serum	Death before 25 years of age
Cerebellar tumors	Headache, vomiting		Papilledema, ataxia, nystagmus	Skull roentgenogram: separation of sutures	Progressive until operated
Heredopathia atactica polyneuritiformis	Anorexia, failing vision, unsteady, familial incidence	4–7	Retinitis pigmentosa, ataxia, deafness, polyneuropathy, ichthyosis	Elevated phytanic acid in blood, increased spinal fluid protein	Slowly progressive with death
Multiple sclerosis	Preceding neurologic symptoms	14–17	Optic neuritis; brain stem, cerebellar, pyramidal, or sensory signs	Spinal fluid may reveal increased cells, protein, or γ-globin	Exacerbations and remissions
Spinal cord tumor	May have numbness or bladder disorder		Ataxia with weakness or sensory loss	Defect on myelography	Progressive until operated

Differential Diagnosis of Acute Ataxia

CLINICAL DISORDER	PRECEDING HISTORY	EXAMINATION	LABORATORY EXAMINATION	USUAL PROGNOSIS
Acute cerebellar ataxia	Half have had a prodromal systemic illness, occasionally exanthems	Cerebellar ataxia	Spinal fluid usually normal	Recovery
Dilantin intoxication	Convulsions treated with phenytoin	Cerebellar ataxia, nystagmus	High serum phenytoin level	Recovery
Cerebellar tumor or abscess	Headache, vomiting	Papilledema, ataxia, nystagmus	Separation of cranial sutures	Progressive until operated
Hartnup syndrome	Skin eruptions on exposure to sun; familial incidence	Skin lesions, ataxia, nystagmus, mental disturbances	Aminoaciduria, increased indole in urine	Recurrent ataxia
Multiple sclerosis	Preceding neurologic symptoms	Optic neuritis; brain stem, cerebellar, pyramidal or sensory signs	Spinal fluid may reveal increased cells, protein or γ-globulin	Exacerbations and remissions
Encephalitides	Headache, stiff neck, fever	Cerebral and brain stem signs; also may have ataxia	Spinal fluid: lymphocytosis; possible virus isolation or rise in antibody titer	May be fatal, or slow recovery with or without residual
Spinal cord tumor	May have numbness or bladder disorder	Ataxia with weakness or sensory loss	Defect on myelography	Progressive until operated
Infectious polyneuropathy	Half have a prodromal systemic illness	Ataxia with motor and sensory loss	Spinal fluid: normal cells, increased protein	May be fatal, but recovery usually complete

Differential Diagnosis of Disorders of Muscle, Anterior Horn Cell, and Peripheral Nerves

CLINICAL AND LABORATORY FEATURES	MUSCLE	ANTERIOR HORN CELL	PERIPHERAL NERVES
Site of predisposition	Usually proximal and axial musculature	Proximal and/or distal extremity musculature	Usually distal extremity musculature
Deep tendon reflexes	Preserved until late in course	Reduced to absent early in course	Reduced to absent early in course
Sensation deficit	Rarely observed	Not observed	Usually present
Fasciculations	Usually absent	Frequently present	Occasionally present

Table continued on next page.

*Differential Diagnosis of Disorders of Muscle, Anterior Horn Cell,
and Peripheral Nerves (Cont.)*

CLINICAL AND LABORATORY FEATURES	MUSCLE	ANTERIOR HORN CELL	PERIPHERAL NERVES
CSF protein	Normal	Normal or elevated	Elevated or normal
Electromyography Interference pattern	Normal until late in disease	Reduced	Reduced
Fibrillation potentials	Not usually present	Usually present	Present
Action potentials	Short duration	Prolonged with occasional giant potentials	Prolonged with normal or polyphasic potentials
Evoked sensory and mixed nerve potentials	Normal	Normal	Absent, diminished amplitude, or prolonged conduction time

Differential Diagnosis of Extrapyramidal Disorders

DISORDER	FAMILIAL	SIGNS	ASSOCIATED FINDINGS
Hepatolenticular degeneration	Autosomal recessive	Rigidity, tremor, dystonia, dementia, corneal ring, jaundice	Increased urinary and hepatic copper, low serum ceruloplasmin
Juvenile parkinsonism	Rarely	Resting tremor, rigidity, bradykinesia	Decreased dopamine level in substantia nigra
Kernicterus	No	Athetosis, deafness, occasional intellectual impairment	Neonatal hyperbilirubinemia
Huntington's disease	Autosomal dominant	Rigidity, chorea, convulsions, dementia	
Torsion dystonia	Autosomal dominant or recessive	Dystonia, involuntary movements, normal intellect	
Chorea minor (Sydenham's)	No	Involuntary choreic movements, possible carditis	Group A streptococcal infections
Absence of hypoxanthine-guanine phosphoribosyl transferase (Lesch-Nyhan syndrome)	X-linked recessive	Choreoathetosis, mental retardation, self-mutilation	Increased urinary and blood uric acid

Reference: Farmer TW (ed): Pediatric Neurology, New York, Harper & Row, 1975, pp 400, 403, 411, and 466, with permission.

B

BACK PAIN

Common Causes

Mechanical derangement (muscle strain or poor posture)
Scheuermann's kyphosis

Scoliosis
Spondylolysis/spondylolisthesis

Uncommon Causes

Disc space infection (discitis)
Rheumatic disorders
Sacroiliac joint infections
Spina bifida occulta

Spinal cord tumors (lipomas, teratomas)
Vertebral osteomyelitis

Rare Causes

Aneurysmal bone cyst
Aseptic necrosis of vertebrae
Benign osteoblastoma
Eosinophilic granuloma of vertebrae
Hemangioma of bone
Herniated nucleus pulposus
Malignancy involving bone (neuroblastoma, leukemia)

Osteomalacia of the spine
Paraspinal tumor or infection
Secondary hyperparathyroidism
Tuberculosis of the spine
Vertebral osteoid osteoma

A Pain in the Back

The differential diagnosis of back pain in infants and children may not be as lengthy as that of chest pain, but the possibilities are equally perplexing. Unlike back pain in adults, which frequently defies identification of an etiology, nearly 75% of children with back pain have a definable cause. Because the presentation can be variable, an understanding of the potential etiologies and a rational approach to the work-up can save time and money in needless examinations and tests.

When a child presents with sudden-onset refusal to walk (or sit), irritability, elevated temperature, abdominal pain and/or nausea, vomiting, and anorexia—and laboratory studies consistent with inflammation—the physician must immediately differentiate between infectious and noninfectious etiologies. Although the distinction between the generally benign entity of discitis and inevitably destructive osteomyelitis is relatively simple (see table), one must also consider meningitis, appendicitis, peritonitis, septic arthritis, and urinary tract infections. With the help of the flow chart and tables below, differentiation will be simpler and the oftentimes delayed diagnosis of discitis will not evade the pediatrician.

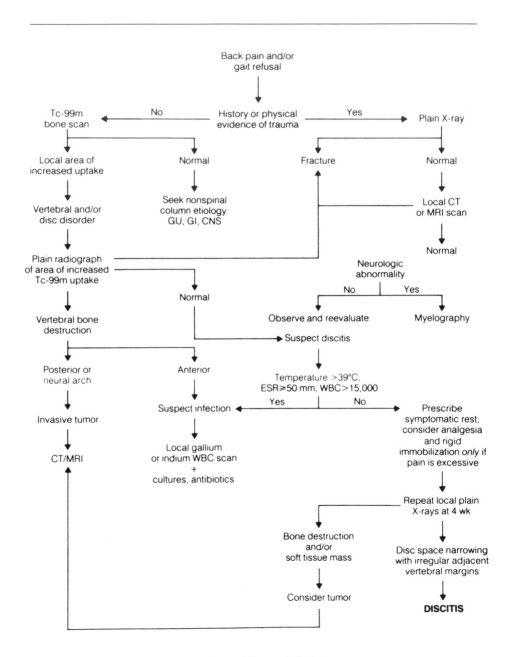

Problem solving and discitis.

Discitis vs. Intervertebral Infection

	DISCITIS	INFECTIOUS VERTEBRAL OSTEOMYELITIS
Mean age	4 yr	9.8 yr
Sex (M:F)	0.6:1	2.4:1
Complaint cited most often	Gait refusal	Severe pain, even at rest
History of trauma	20%	4%
Vertebral site	Lumbar	Thoracic or lumbar
Mean maximum temperature	$< 100°$ F	$> 101°$ F
Mean maximum WBC count	$< 8,000/\mu$L	$> 15,000/\mu$L
Mean maximum ESR	< 35 mm	> 50 mm
Plain radiographs		
At outset	Normal	Normal
At 4 wk	Disc space narrowing	Bony destruction
Tc-99m bone scan at outset	Positive	Positive
Gallium scan at outset	Negative	Positive
Indium-labeled WBC scan at outset	Negative	Positive
Blood or local tissue culture	2% positive	60% positive
Fate of disc	Regenerates; often narrow	Destroyed
Fate of vertebral body	Unaffected	Destroyed
Fate of neural arch	Unaffected	Often destroyed
Fatality	0%	6%
Chronic persistent illness	0%	8%
Clinical duration	2–5 wk; always < 12 wk	Many months

Vertebral Disorders in Children

ENTITY	USUAL SITE	ETIOLOGY	PEAK AGE	BEST TEST	LABS
Infection	Thoracic or lumbar spine	Staphylococcus, TB or abscess formation	8 yr	Plain x-ray; look for vertebral destruction	Blood and tissue culture for ↑ WBC, ↑ ESR and ↑ platelets
Tumors					
Malignant	Low back, pelvis	Pelvic invasion with marrow tumors or chondrosarcoma	Adolescence	Plain x-ray; look for bony lesion w/soft tissue mass	Histology
Nonmalignant	Neural arches	Osteoblastoma	Adolescence	Plain x-ray	None
	Posterior	Osteoid	Adolescence	Look for sclerotic nidus w/ lucent halo	

Table continued on next page.

Vertebral Disorders in Children (Cont.)

ENTITY	USUAL SITE	ETIOLOGY	PEAK AGE	BEST TEST	LABS
Discitis	Lumbar anterior aspect	Avascular necrosis of epiphyseal end plates and discs	4 yr	Early: Tc-99m uptake. After 4 wk: disc-space narrowing on plain x-ray	None
Spondylolysis	L–4, L–5 vertebrae	Traumatic defect in posterior aspect of pars articularis	Early teens	Oblique plain x-ray	None
Spondylolisthesis	L–5, S–1 vertebrae	Forward slippage (L–5 moves anterior to S–1) in pt w/spondylolysis	During growth spurt	Standing lateral plain x-ray	None
Scheuermann's kyphosis	Lower thoracic vertebrae	Osteochondrosis w/herniation of disc into vertebral bodies; w/anterior narrowing of disc space; disc walled off in vertebra (Schmorl's node)	Adolescence	Standing lateral plain x-ray shows Schmorl's node	Node

References: Sills EM: What's causing the back pain? Contemp Pediatr Nov:85–96, 1988. Leahy AL, et al: Discitis as a cause of abdominal pain in children. Surgery April:412–414, 1984.

BACTERIAL ENDOCARDITIS

Extracardiac Manifestations of Bacterial Endocarditis

The patient with bacterial endocarditis presents both a diagnostic and a therapeutic challenge. The myriad manifestations of the disease result from the hemodynamic, embolic, and immunologic sequelae of the endovascular infection.

The following review of the more common extracardiac manifestations may serve as an aid in diagnosis and management of this disease.

Extracardiac Manifestations of Bacterial Endocarditis

MANIFESTATION	COMMENT
I. Renal 1. Microscopic hematuria and proteinuria 2. Occasionally azotemia 3. Abnormalities usually resolve with effective antimicrobial therapy	1. Biopsy a. Focal glomerulonephritis *or* b. Diffuse proliferative glomerulonephritis

Table continued on next page.

Extracardiac Manifestations of Bacterial Endocarditis (Cont.)

MANIFESTATION	COMMENT
II. Neurologic	
1. Major neurologic complications are:	1. Neurologic complications occur in 25–40% of patients with bacterial endocarditis
a. Cerebral infarction in region of middle cerebral arteries secondary to emboli (most common neurologic complication)	2. The mortality of patients with neurologic complications is > 50%
b. Meningeal signs and symptoms	3. Embolic phenomenon are usually seen in endocarditis due to *S. aureus, Pneumococcus, Enterobacteriaceae,* and anaerobic streptococci
c. Seizures	
d. Intracranial hemorrhage	4. *Mitral* valve endocarditis produces major cerebral emboli more frequently than *aortic* valve endocarditis
e. Large macroscopic brain abscesses are uncommon	
f. Microscopic brain abscesses are common and reflect multiple microemboli	5. Mycotic aneurysms occur more frequently in the *early* course of *acute* endocarditis than *late* in the course of *subacute* endocarditis
	6. CSF exam tends to reflect the nature of the infecting organisms; i.e. virulent organisms are more likely to produce meningitis with a purulent CSF than are less virulent organisms, which are likely to produce a sterile "aseptic" CSF
III. Musculoskeletal	
1. Arthralgia—usually in shoulder, knee, hip	1. Musculoskeletal findings are seen in approximately 44% of patients with bacterial endocarditis
2. True synovitis	
a. Ankle, knee, wrist most frequent	
b. Usually sterile	
c. Biopsy shows acute inflammatory changes	
3. Low back pain	
a. Often severe	
b. Often demonstrates spinal tenderness and decreased range of motion	
c. X-rays usually normal	
d. Usually not secondary to disc space infection	
4. Myalgias—often localized to thighs and calves	
5. Miscellaneous	
a. Clubbing of the digits	
b. Hypertrophic osteoarthropathy	
c. Avascular necrosis of hip	
IV. Skin	
1. Petechiae	
2. Osler's nodes	
3. Janeway lesions	
4. Periungual erythema	
5. Subungual "splinter" hemorrhages	

Table continued on next page.

Extracardiac Manifestations of Bacterial Endocarditis (Cont.)

MANIFESTATION	COMMENT
V. *Hematologic*	
1. Anemia	
2. Thrombocytopenia (in the absence of disseminated intravascular coagulation)	
3. Monocytosis	
4. Splenomegaly	
5. Plasmacytosis of bone marrow	
6. Disseminated intravascular coagulation	
VI. *Serologic*	
1. Elevated ESR	1. Titers of circulating immune
2. Elevated serum gamma globulins	complexes highest in patients with:
3. Positive rheumatoid factor	a. Right-sided endocarditis
4. Positive antinuclear antibody	b. Extravascular manifestations
5. Circulating immune complexes	c. Signs of infection for more than
6. Presence in serum of cryoglobulins	4 weeks
7. Low serum complement	

References: Pruitt AA, Rubin RH, Karchmer AW, Duncan GW: Medicine 57:329, 1978. Churchill MA, Geraci JE, Hunder GG: Ann Intern Med 87:754, 1977. Bajer AS, Theofilopoulos AN, Eisenberg R, et al: N Engl J Med 295:1500, 1976.

From McMillan JA, et al: The Whole Pediatrician Catalog, Vol. 3. Philadelphia, W.B. Saunders, 1982, pp 294–297, with permission.

BASAL SKULL FRACTURE

Recognition of Basal Skull Fractures

Basal fractures through the floor of the skull are usually linear. They are difficult to recognize in x-ray studies and are diagnosed clinically. The clues to the diagnosis include:

1. Bleeding from nose, eyes, or ears, or discoloration in the mastoid area (ecchymosis behind the ear, or Battle's sign). The "racoon eye" may be seen, with a hematoma in the upper lid.
2. Blood and CSF behind the eardrum, causing a bulging of the membrane. Otorrhea occurs when the tympanic membrane is ruptured.
3. Cerebrospinal rhinorrhea. Some believe that testing the nasal discharge for the presence of glucose is an indication of CSF leak. However, approximately 75 to 90% of normal children will give a positive glucose oxidase test strip in their nasal secretions, which makes the use of such a test for CSF leak valueless.
4. Cranial nerve palsies, involving cranial nerves I, III, and VIII.
5. Appearance of "sinusitis."
6. Presence of pneumocephaly.

A basal skull fracture can lead to meningitis by spread of organisms from the nose or ear, and prophylactic use of penicillins is justifiable.

Reference: Hull HF, Morrow G III: Glucorrhea revisited. JAMA, 234:1052, 1975.

BEHAVIOR

Behavioral Concerns of Parents

If you were to provide a behavioral checklist to middle-class parents of children 1.5 to 6 years of age, which behaviors would they note as being of greatest concern to them? Listed below are these behaviors listed in order of frequency.

Are you prepared to discuss these topics with parents?

Behavioral Concerns of Parents

BEHAVIOR	PERCENTAGE
Stubbornness	29%
Poor appetite	23%
Getting child to sleep	22%
Effects of both parents working	22%
Day care	19%
Restless sleep	18%
Temper tantrums	16%
Feelings hurt too easily	16%
Problems at meals	15%
"High strung"/easily upset	15%
Wanting too much attention	12%
Disobedient	12%
Hyperactive	12%
New sibling	11%
Moving	10%

Reference: Triggs EG, Perrin EC: Listening carefully: Improving communication about behavior and development. Clin Pediatr 28:185–192, 1989.

BLADDER

Bladder Capacity in Children

Bladder capacity correlates linearly with age from birth to the 11th year. *The bladder capacity in ounces equals age in years plus 2, with a standard deviation of 2 ounces.* Knowledge of the functional bladder capacity, with a detailed history, may suggest a diagnosis of large or small bladder capacity. Children with infrequent voiding tend to have larger bladder capacities, whereas those with frequency or enuresis have smaller than predicted capacities.

Reference: Berger RM, et al: Bladder capacity (ounces) equals age (years) plus 2 predicts normal bladder capacity and aids in diagnosis of abnormal voiding patterns. J Urol 129:347–349, 1983.

BLISTERING

Neonatal Blistering Disorders

A number of disorders can give rise to neonatal blisters, ranging from the benign suction blister (which is presumably caused by thumb, finger, or distal forearm sucking in utero) to epidermolysis bullosa, a heterogeneous group of inherited skin disorders notable for marked skin fragility. Listed below is the differential diagnosis for blistering disorders of the neonate.

Differential Diagnosis for Blistering Disorders

CONDITION	ONSET	PATHOLOGIC FEATURES	CLINICAL FEATURES
Epidermolysis bullosa (EB)			
1. EB simplex (usually autosomal dominant inheritance)	Usually at birth	Intraepidermal blisters	Trauma causes blisters; patients have mild involvement without scarring in the absence of infection. Mucous membranes are usually spared. Teeth develop normally. Typically a benign course with normal life-span and no significant functional impairment.
2. Junctional EB (autosomal recessive inheritance)	At birth	Blistering occurs in the lamina lucida between the epidermis and dermis	Trauma causes extensive blistering on the skin and any mucosal membrane. In one type (junctional EB letalis of Herlitz-Pearson), GI involvement is frequent, leading to perforation, sepsis, and death in early infancy. In other subtypes, patients follow a more indolent course and survive to adulthood, although nonhealing cutaneous wounds yield significant morbidity.
3. Dystrophic EB (there exist both autosomal recessive and autosomal dominant forms)	At birth	Blistering occurs in the dermis, below the lamina densa	Lesions heal with milia formation and marked scarring that can lead to crippling deformities.
Bullous congenital ichthyosiform erythroderma (autosomal dominant)	At birth	Vacuolization of cells of granular and upper spinous layers	Red scaly skin; secondary bacterial infection; thick, grayish brown scales after age 3 mo.

Table continued on next page.

Differential Diagnosis for Blistering Disorders (Cont.)

CONDITION	ONSET	PATHOLOGIC FEATURES	CLINICAL FEATURES
Congenital herpes simplex virus infection	In first 20 days; mean = 6 days	Intraepidermal blisters with multiple thin-walled vesicles on an erythematous base	Blisters and bullae; positive Tzanck smear and viral culture; fever, poor feeding, hypothermia, and lethargy.
Aplasia cutis congenita (usually autosomal dominant, but autosomal recessive also reported)	At birth	Ulcer down to subcutaneous tissue	Absence of skin on scalp; similar cutaneous defects may be present elsewhere; limb abnormalities; some cases associated with epidermolysis bullosa.
Staphylococcal scalded skin syndrome	2–30 days	Blisters below or within granular layer	Abrupt onset of erythema, followed by blistering and exfoliation; responds to antibiotics.
Suction blisters	At birth	—	One or two blisters on thumb, finger, radial aspect of forearm, presumably due to sucking in utero; spontaneous resolution.

Reference: Lin AN, Carter DM: Epidermolysis bullosa: When the skin falls apart. J Pediatr 114:349–355, 1989.

Bullous Eruptions in the Newborn

Eruptions of vesicles (raised, fluid-filled lesions < 1 cm) and bullae (raised, fluid-filled lesions > 1 cm) in the neonatal period are due to a variety of mostly unrelated conditions, with different treatments and prognoses in each category. The following table lists the principal criteria for the differential diagnosis of bullous eruptions in the nursery.

Principal Criteria for Differential Diagnosis of Bullous Eruptions

DISEASE OR CONDITION	CHARACTER OF LESIONS	DISTRI-BUTION	MUCOSAL INVOLVE-MENT	OTHER ECTODERMAL DEFECTS	SCARRING	COURSE
Epidermolysis bullosa	Clear blisters; sometimes hemorrhagic noninflammatory base	Sites of trauma or friction	Yes	Yes	Yes or no	Chronic or fatal
Bullous impetigo	Blisters, clear, opaque, purulent	General, particularly flexures	Possible	No	Yes	Short
Congenital syphilis	Bullae and maculo-papules	Palms, soles, trunk, and limbs	Yes	Yes	No (other than rhagades)	Short

Table continued on next page.

Principal Criteria for Differential Diagnosis of Bullous Eruptions (Cont.)

DISEASE OR CONDITION	CHARACTER OF LESIONS	DISTRI- BUTION	MUCOSAL INVOLVE- MENT	OTHER ECTODERMAL DEFECTS	SCARRING	COURSE
Dermatitis herpetiformis	Vesicles and bullae in crops; also urticarial lesions	In infants face and limbs chiefly involved	Some- times	No	Minimal in long- standing cases	One-third curable. Chronic or recurrent
Burns	Erythema, bullae, des- quamation	Anywhere	No	No	Yes, if deep	Depends on type, depth, and therapy
Congenital porphyria	Red urine, photosen- sitivity of skin, erythe- ma, bullae	Areas exposed to sunlight	No	Pigmented teeth	Pig- mented scars	Chronic
Erythema multiforme bullosa	Dusky red circinate plaques, papules, bullae	Trunk, limbs, face	Yes	No	No	Short or recurrent
Dermatitis medica- mentosa	May be vesicular	No particular site	No	No	No	Short
Papular urticaria	Papules, bullae, vesicles, pustules	Trunk only or limbs	No	No	No	Short or recurrent
Chickenpox		Trunk, face, limbs	Yes	No	Yes	Short
Smallpox	Vesicles, pustules	Limbs, trunk, face	Yes	No	Yes	Short
Kaposi's varicelliform eruption	Vesicles, pustules	Exposed parts	No	Pre-existing skin disease of infantile eczema or Besnier's prurigo	No	May be fatal
Herpes zoster	Vesicles	Classical girdle	No	No	Yes	Short
Bullous erysipelas	Raised tender ery- thema, bullae	Perium- bilical, limbs, face, trunk	Rarely	Nil	Nil	Short with therapy
Benign familial pemphigus (Hailey's disease)	Vesicles and bullae	Anywhere	No	No	Nil	Benign chronic

Table continued on next page.

Principal Criteria for Differential Diagnosis of Bullous Eruptions (Cont.)

DISEASE OR CONDITION	CHARACTER OF LESIONS	DISTRI-BUTION	MUCOSAL INVOLVE-MENT	OTHER ECTODERMAL DEFECTS	SCARRING	COURSE
Contact dermatitis	Often vesicles and bullae	Anywhere	No	No	No	Short
Phytophoto-dermatitis	Vesicles and bullae	Areas exposed to sunlight	No	No	No	Short
Acrodermatitis enteropathica	Crops scaling, vesiculo-bullous	Near orifices, around eyes, elbows, knees, hands, feet	Yes	Hair scanty	No	May be fatal

Reference: Lewis IC, Steven EM, Farquhar JW: Epidermolysis bullosa in the newborn. Arch Dis Child 30:277, 1955, with permission.

BLOOD CULTURES

Changing the Needle When Inoculating Blood Cultures: A No-Benefit and High-Risk Procedure

For some time now, in response to the high prevalence of HIV and hepatitis B infections, the U.S. Centers for Disease Control has recommended that needles should never be recapped in order to prevent unnecessary needle-stick injuries. Yet, many phlebotomists and physicians routinely recap and change needles before blood-culture inoculation. A group of pediatricians and pathologists at the University of Virginia were concerned about this clinical paradigm and designed a study to compare the extrinsic contamination rate in blood cultures when the needle was and was not changed.

The investigators had 108 medical students obtain 182 blood specimens from each other using standard methods. Each blood sample was inoculated into two culture bottles. The first bottle was inoculated with the needle used for phlebotomy, and the second was inoculated after a needle change. Of the 182 culture bottles, 4 (2.2%) were contaminated when the needle was not changed and 1 (0.6%) was contaminated when the needle was changed. This small difference was found to be statistically insignificant, and the possibility of having failed to detect a 5% difference in contamination rate was small.

The conclusion of this study, therefore, was that the risk of needle-stick injury incurred by changing the needle before inoculation of blood culture bottles seems to be *unjustified*.

Reference: Leisure MK, Moore DM, Schwartzman JD, et al: Changing the needle when inoculating blood cultures. A no-benefit and high risk procedure. JAMA 264:2111–2112, 1990.

BODY TEMPERATURE

A Comparison of Rectal, Axillary, and Inguinal Temperatures in Full-Term Newborn Infants

What is the mean temperature in the various sites commonly employed for the measurement of a newborn's temperature? In the study described below, rectal thermometers were inserted 2.5 cm into the rectum. Inguinal temperatures were measured by abducting the infant's leg, locating the femoral pulse, placing the bulb of the thermometer lateral to the pulse site, and adducting the leg to create a seal. Readings were recorded every 30 seconds after placement and were discontinued when no change occurred for 90 seconds.

Mean and Maximal Temperatures and Ranges
for Rectal, Axillary, and Inguinal Sites

SITE	MEAN TEMPERATURE (°F)	RANGE (°F)
Rectal	98.7	97.6–100.4
Axillary	98.5	97.2–100.2
Inguinal	97.9	96.4– 99.2

Reference: Bliss-Holtz: J Nursing Research 38:85–87, 1989.

BONE MARROW EXAMINATIONS

Is There a Role for Bone Marrow Examinations in the Child with Prolonged Fever?

When evaluating a child with prolonged fever, the question of whether or not to perform a bone marrow examination is often posed. Bone marrow examinations have been shown to be of great use for aid in the diagnosis of malignancy, but their usefulness for detecting occult infections has been the source of a long and, excuse the pun, heated debate. Recently, a group of physicians at the Texas Children's Hospital reviewed 414 cases of children with prolonged fevers in order to assess this situation.

In their retrospective series, noninfectious causes of prolonged fever were revealed by the bone marrow examination in 34 (8.2%) of the 414 study patients (e.g., malignant conditions such as acute leukemia, both newly diagnosed and relapsed, lymphoma, solid tumors, and chronic myelocytic leukemia, in addition to nonmalignant illness such as virus-associated hemophagocytic syndrome, histiocytosis, and hypoplastic anemia). In the majority of these cases, a diagnosis of myelopthisis was clinically suspected before the bone marrow was obtained.

An infectious etiology of prolonged fever was uncovered in 15 (3.6%) of the febrile episodes. It should be noted that only one patient of the 414 children studied had a positive marrow culture (for *Salmonella*, group D) without concurrent positive cultures from any other source. In patients who were immunocompetent, the yield of positive marrow cultures was rather low (1.9%), whereas in immunocompromised children (particularly those with AIDS) the yield was 8.7%.

With these data in mind, the following conclusions were reached.
1. Bone marrow examination *is* indicated in the child with prolonged fever and clinical or laboratory evidence consistent with malignancy.
2. Bone marrow examination may be helpful in ascertaining the diagnosis of opportunistic infection in the febrile, immunocompromised patient, especially a child with AIDS.
3. Bone marrow examination in the child with prolonged fever but no findings suggestive of malignancy or immunodeficiency is probably not warranted as a means of detecting occult infection.

Reference: Hayani A, Mahoney DH, Fernbach DJ: Role of bone marrow examination in the child with prolonged fever. J Pediatr 116:919–920, 1990.

BREAST MASSES

Breast Masses and Lesions in the Infant, Child, and Adolescent

Lesions and masses of the breast generate a great deal of concern upon discovery. This holds particularly true for such lesions among the pediatric age group, despite the fact that the overwhelming majority of lesions in this population are benign. There do, however, exist some lesions that require immediate attention (e.g., mastitis in the newborn or developing breast and the rarely occurring malignancy). Clinicians, therefore, need to be able to recognize and assess these lesions in order to offer appropriate treatment and reassurance to their patients. As each age group seen in pediatrics (i.e., neonatal, prepubertal, and adolescent) has its own set of breast masses or lesions, we present the differential diagnosis in a chronologic manner:

Infancy

1. **Neonatal hypertrophy** presents as a palpable, tender mass with or without a milky nipple secretion ("witch's milk"), which is most likely due to a low prolactin level in a premature infant that rises postnatally to that of a normal-term infant. The milky discharge should abate within 4 to 6 weeks of life, although it may take up to 1 year for the breast enlargement to recede.
2. **Mastitis and resultant abscess** present as a tender, erythematous breast mass, usually with fever. This is, perhaps, the only breast lesion in the pediatric population that requires immediate intervention. Mastitis and resultant abscesses tend to occur in the infant aged 2 weeks to 6 months, but can occur at any time. Both gram-positive organisms (e.g., *Staphylococcus aureus*) and gram negative organisms (e.g., *E. coli*) are common culprits; antibiotic therapy, therefore, should be broad in its spectrum. Warm compresses are also useful. Septicemia is a concern in the young infant. Increased pressure and inflammation from the infection itself and surgical drainage by an overzealous surgeon can result in future deformity of the breast in an infant or prepubertal girl.

3. **Polythelia** is the presence of one or more supernumerary nipples along the "milk-line," which extends from the axilla to the symphysis pubis. About 50% of the patients with polythelia have some other congenital anomaly; renal anomalies lead the list.

Prepubertal

1. **Premature thelarche** refers to the onset of bilateral or unilateral breast development before the age of 7½. It is most likely a disorder of hypothalamic hormone receptor sensitivity, as opposed to hypothalamic-pituitary tract tumors or primary ovarian neoplasms.
2. **Precocious puberty**
3. **Unsustained puberty**
4. **Pseudopuberty**
5. **Gynecomastia** (breast enlargement in males)
6. **Polythelia/polymastia** (the presence of more than 2 breasts)

Adolescence

1. **Thelarche:** normal development of the female breast which may begin as early as age 8 but, on average, occurs at age 11.
2. **Gynecomastia**
3. **Fibroadenoma** is the most common breast lesion of adolescent females. It presents as a unilateral, mobile, slowly growing, isolated, rubbery mass (1–8 cm in size). These lesions are benign.
4. **Juvenile giant fibroadenoma** is a rapidly growing fibroadenoma seen most commonly in adolescent black females. It is a benign tumor usually treated by surgical excision.
5. **Cystosarcoma phylloides** is a rapidly growing, large breast mass seen commonly in adolescent black females. It is firm to palpation, has discrete mass borders, and can cause skin or nipple retraction, necrosis, and discharge. Conversion to a malignant tumor has been reported and surgical excision is recommended.
6. **Cystic breast disease** involves cystic lesions in the breast that become painful during the perimenstrual period. Because the disease is self-limiting and usually resolves at the close of adolescence, hormonal manipulation is ill-advised.
7. **Intraductal papilloma** is a benign, subareolar, cylindrical mass with or without a brown to frankly bloody discharge.
8. **Virginal breast hypertrophy** refers to the symmetric enlargement of all breast tissue after puberty. No specific hormonal imbalance has been identified. The breasts can be quite painful and their size embarrassing.
9. **Trauma-induced mass** (fat necrosis) can result in subsequent scarring with a firm, palpable nodular mass.
10. **Polythelia/polymastia**
11. **Carcinoma**
12. **Metastatic sarcoma**

Reference: Dudgeon DL: Pediatric breast lesions: Take the conservative approach. Contemp Pediatr 2:61–73, 1985.

BREATHHOLDING

Breathholding Spell or Idiopathic Epilepsy?

Breathholding is a common occurrence in infants and children 6 months to 4 years of age, with about 5% having at least one breathholding spell and some losing consciousness during a prolonged attack. The onset is always with crying, and the characteristic picture of crying and breathholding distinguishes benign episodes from convulsions. The behavior almost always disappears before school age. Some advise parents to leave the room during breathholding to discourage the behavior, but this may be difficult to carry out.

Features of breathholding that distinguish it from grand mal seizures are shown in the accompanying table.

Distinguishing Features of Breathholding and Grand Mal Seizures

	GRAND MAL (IDIOPATHIC EPILEPSY)	ANOXIC CONVULSION (BREATHHOLDING SPELL)
Age of onset	Rarely in infancy	Often begins in infancy
Family history	None or positive for epilepsy	Often positive for breath-holding spell or fainting
Precipitating factors	Usually absent (or specific sensory stimuli or nonspecific stresses)	Usually present (specific emotional or nociceptive stimuli)
Occurrence during sleep	Common	Never
Posture	Variable	Usually erect
Sequence and patterns	Single cry (may be absent) with loss of consciousness → tonic → clonic phases, cyanosis may occur later in attack; flushed at first, pale after attack	Long crying or single gasp, cyanosis or pallor → loss of consciousness → limpness → clonic jerks → opisthotonos → clonic jerks
Perspiration	Warm sweat	Cold sweat
Heart rate	Markedly increased	Decreased, asystole, or slightly increased
Duration	Usually > 1 minute	Usually 1 minute or less
Incontinence and tongue biting	Common	Uncommon (but may occur)
Postictal state	Confusion and sleep common	No confusion. Fatigue common
Interictal EEG	Usually bilateral discharges	Usually normal
Oculocardiac activation	No response or bradycardia; 7% may have asystole of less than 4 seconds; asymptomatic	About 50% have asystole > 2 seconds, usually > 4 seconds; attack may be precipated
Ictal EEG	Generalized, high-voltage polyspike discharges, gradually subsiding into slow waves and depression for several minutes	Isoelectric pattern preceded and followed by diffuse high-voltage delta waves, promptly reverting to normal pattern upon recovery of consciousness

References: Lombroso CT, Lerman P: Breathholding spells (cyanotic and palid infantile syncope). Pediatrics 39:563, 1967.
  Dimario FJ: Breath-holding spells in childhood. Am J Dis Child 146:125–131, 1992.

BUGS

Bugs in the Band-Aid Box

Wide-eyed and frightened, they appear with white knuckles clutching the metal Band-Aid box. Their gaze is intense and expectant.

You suspect what is in the box without having them tell.

"Is it alive?" you ask phlegmatically.

Frequently, residents of the Band-Aid box include the following:

Crab Lice *(Phthirus pubis)*

This small (1 mm), round, reddish-brown louse causes itching. Transmission is by close personal contact. On close examination, the crab louse is found in the pubic area with its head buried in a hair follicle or clutching two adjacent hairs. The dark nits are frequently difficult to find. Crabs may infest the chest and axillary hair *as well as the eyelashes. Treatment:* 25 per cent benzyl benzoate or gamma benzene hexachloride on two successive days. Infested eyelashes are treated with daily application of yellow oxide of mercury.

Crab louse *(Phthirus pubis)*

Scalp Lice *(Pediculus humanus var. capitis)*

This long (up to 4 mm), slender, white louse causes pruritus and excoriations with frequent secondary infection. The densest involvement is posteriorly, behind the ears. There may be tender occipital nodes as well as excoriated bites on the neck and shoulders. You may not find the adult louse, but the small white nits glued to hair shafts are obvious. Nits fluoresce under Wood's light. *Treatment:* Gamma benzene hexachloride shampoo for two days, repeated in a week. Comb out nits with a fine-toothed comb.

Body Lice *(Pediculus humanus var. corporis)*

The adult louse is 1 to 4 mm long and lives, loves, and lays eggs (nits) in the seams of clothing. This louse feeds on the body, leaving an urticarial wheal with a hemorrhagic central punctum.

Examination of the skin reveals parallel linear excoriations that often are secondarily infected. *Treatment:* Thorough laundering of clothes and bedding. Iron all seams. Bedding and clothing may be dusted with 10 per cent DDT powder. 1 per cent gamma benzene hexachloride may be applied topically once.

Head or body louse *(Pediculus humanus* var. *capitis* or *corporis)*

Pinworms *(Enterobius vermicularis)*

The patient may find small, white worms at the anal orifice in the early morning hours. Infestation produces intense perianal pruritus, which leads to excoriations, lichenification, and infection. Bruxism and nightmares are common. The diagnosis is usually made by identifying ova on transparent tape that has been pressed to perianal skin at bedtime. *Treatment:* The Medical Letter has recommended pyrantel pamoate (Banminth) (11 mg/kg) as a single oral dose. Mebendazole, 100 × one dose, regardless of weight, may also be used. The treatment should be repeated in two weeks.

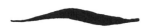

Female pinworm (*E. vermicularis*)

Maggots (Fly Larvae)

Rarely, maggots will be picked from an open sore, the nose, the ear canal, or from the stool.

Maggot

Fish Tapeworm *(Diphyllobothrium latum)*

This is a very large cestode that produces enormous numbers of yellowish eggs. It has been an occupational disease of Jewish housewives who taste raw ground fish to check seasoning when making gefilte fish. Thus, its incidence may be decreasing (at least in this population). Immobile, white, flat segments may be found in the stool. Treatment is with niclosamide, 1 gm for children under 35 kg and 1.5 gm for children over 35 kg. The tablets should be chewed thoroughly.

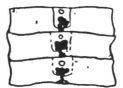

Fish tapeworm (*D. latum*)

Beef Tapeworm *(Taenia saginata)*

Gravid, white, mobile segments of this worm may be passed in the stool. *Treatment:* Quinacrine, 200 mg every 5–10 min for four dosages, on an empty stomach, followed by a magnesium sulfate purge 2 to 4 hr later. Niclosamide may also be employed in the same dose as for fish tapeworm.

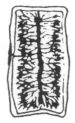

Beef tapeworm (*T. saginata*)

Roundworm *(Ascaris lumbricoides)*

Ascaris lumbricoides is characterized by an elongated, cylindric, nonsegmented, translucent, flesh-colored body 15–35 cm long. A cosmopolitan worm, ascaris infects 25 per cent of the world's population. One or more worms may be passed in the stool or, less frequently, vomited. Worms have been known to crawl out of the nose, ear, and umbilical fissures! *Treatment:* Piperazine citrate syrup 75 mg/kg daily × 2. Pyrantel pamoate may also be employed as a single-dose therapy (11 mg/kg with a 1-gm maximal dose).

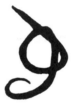

Roundworm (*A. lumbricoides*)

Debris

Vegetable particles, such as seeds (corn), stems, and celery, and other debris, like dirt, gravel, stringy fuzz, and cellophane, can be swollen and discolored by passage through the alimentary canal. Even a normal person would be alarmed, and the person with parasitophobia will be in panic. *Treatment:* Show the patient the characteristics of the debris by hand lens or dissecting microscope.

Miscellaneous

Products of conception, menstrual blood clots thought to be products of conception, "grape-like bodies" of hydatidiform mole, fragments of tampons, and clotted mucus and blood from cystitis have all made it to the Band-Aid box.

Reference: Gottlieb AJ, Zamkoff KW, Jastremski MS, Scalzo A, Imboden KJ: The Band-Aid box. In The Whole Internist Catalog. Philadelphia, W.B. Saunders Company, 1980, pp 497–499, with permission.

Keeping Bugs at Bay

For those of you who hate bugs of all kinds, including mosquitoes, chiggers, flies, and ticks, the following advice from *The New York Times* ought to come in handy. We hope this makes your summer more pleasant and a bit less itchy.

Keeping Bugs at Bay *(Cont.)*

Entomologists predict clouds of mosquitos this summer, a result of heavy spring rains. Drain all stagnant water on roofs and in yards. Chiggers, flies and other insects will also be out looking for food. Here are ways to keep flying pests, particularly mosquitoes, from assaulting you.

Repellents	Repellents containing DEET are most effective, but apply with care. Do not apply to hands or face or use in concentrations stronger than 50 percent; 15 percent is recommended.
Clothing	Don't look like a flower. Many bugs are attracted to bright colors.
Perspiration	Wash off perspiration. Sweat produces a scent that attracts bugs.
Chlorine	Add a capful or two of chlorinated bleach to your bath water or take a swim in a chlorinated pool. The smell repels most insects.
Sun oil	Oily sun screens make skin too slippery for insects to get a grip.
Food and fragrance	Avoid alcohol and foods high in serotonin, like bananas and nuts. Mosquitoes are attracted to those scents. Avoid perfume, cologne and hair spray.

Sources: Dr. Roger Grothaus, Raid Center for Insect Control, Racine, Wis., and Dr. Jeffrey D. Bernhart, New York City Department of Health.

From Guidepost: Keeping bugs at bay. *The New York Times*, 1991, with permission.

Oh, for boyhood's painless play,
Sleep that wakes in laughing day,
Health that mocks the doctor's rules,
Knowledge never learned of schools,
Of the wild bee's morning chase,
Of the wild flower's time and place,
Flight of fowl and habitude
Of the tenants of the wood;
How the tortoise bears his shell,
How the woodchuck digs his cell,
And the groundmole sinks his well;
How the robin feeds her young,
How the oriole's nest is hung,
Where the whitest lilies blow,
Where the freshest berries grow,
Where the ground-nut trails its vine,
Where the wood-grape's clusters shine,
Of the black wasp's cunning way,—
Mason of his walls of clay,—
And the architectural plans
Of gray-hornet artisans!—
For, eschewing books and tasks,
Nature answers all he asks,
Hand in hand with her he walks,
Face to face with her he talks,
Part and parcel of her joy,—
Blessings on the barefoot boy!

John Greenleaf Whittier
The Barefoot Boy

C

CALCIUM

Idiopathic Hypercalciuria in Childhood

The most common metabolic cause of renal calculi in adults is idiopathic hypercalciuria (IH). Children with IH have been noted with increasing frequency to present with a myriad of lower urinary tract signs and symptoms, including calculi, renal colic, hematuria (gross and microscopic), dysuria, frequency-urgency syndrome, pyuria, proteinuria (<100 mg/day), enuresis, osteopenia, failure to thrive, and recurrent urinary tract infections. Given the rather significant manifestations of IH in childhood, the potential that these children will become stone-formers in adult life, and the well-known morbidity of urolithiasis in adults, the following review of idiopathic hypercalciuria in childhood is offered.

1. **Definition:** Hypercalciuria is an abnormally high urine calcium excretion rate (>2 mg/kg body weight/day) and is either primary (idiopathic) or secondary to a variety of pathologic entities. Investigators have identified two types of IH: *absorptive IH*, which involves a defect of the intestinal absorption of dietary calcium; and *renal leak IH*, which is related to a defect of incomplete renal tubular reabsorption of filtered calcium.

2. **Disorders Associated with Hypercalciuria**

   Immobilization*
   Diuretic therapy (e.g., furosemide)*
   Corticosteroid therapy*
   Type I renal tubular acidosis
   High dietary calcium
   Sarcoidosis
   Syndrome of inappropriate ADH
      secretion

   Hyperparathyroidism
   Cushing's syndrome
   Medullary sponge kidney
   Lead poisoning
   Tubular dysfunction
      (e.g., Fanconi's syndrome,
      Wilson's disease)
   Juvenile rheumatoid arthritis

3. **Factors Affecting Renal Calcium Excretion**

   Glomerular filtration rate
   Extracellular volume
   Serum calcium
   Serum phosphate
   Blood acid-base status
   Dietary intake of calcium
      and sodium

   Vitamin D metabolism (both at the
      intestinal and renal tubular levels)
   Parathyroid hormone
   Calcitonin
   Glucocorticoids
   Mineralocorticoids
   Diuretics (e.g., furosemide)

---

*The most common causes of hypercalciuria in childhood are indicated by the asterisk.

49

4. **The laboratory approach to evaluating a child with suspected hypercalciuria**

   Random urine calcium/creatinine ratio
   a. If the urine calcium/creatinine ratio is <0.18 mg/mg, quantify with a 24-hour urine
   b. If the 24-hour urine [Ca] > 2 mg/kg body weight, RULE OUT:
      i. Secondary causes of hypercalciuria (obtain serum calcium, phosphate, magnesium, bicarbonate, alkaline phosphatase, and blood pH
      ii. Urinary tract infections (perform urine culture).

5. **Therapeutic approaches to children with noncalculi urinary tract disorders due to IH.**

   a. **General treatment measures** include a fluid intake large enough to allow a high urine flow rate but not large enough to complicate disorders such as enuresis. Excess salt intake should be avoided because increased dietary sodium and the subsequent increased renal filtered sodium load can lead to hypercalciuria. Dietary oxalate (e.g., fruit juices, chocolate, tea) should be avoided because urinary oxalate can serve as the nidus for early urinary calcium crystalization.

   b. **Dietary calcium.** Although restricting dietary calcium in adults with renal stones secondary to IH is frequently recommended, such restriction is usually not indicated in the growing child. A positive calcium balance is optimal for normal development and bone and tissue growth. However, the restriction of dietary calcium is probably indicated in children who develop kidney stones due to absorptive IH and are at risk for destructive renal disease—but, again, the dietary calcium restriction should be limited as much as possible. Children who experience recurrent gross hematuria and severe frequency-urgency syndrome due to absorptive IH are the only patients who should be prescribed moderate-to-severe dietary calcium restrictions.

   c. **Pharmacologic therapy.** The physician should carefully weigh the risks of the disease's morbidity against the potential side-effects of pharmacologic agents. Children presenting with recurrent gross hematuria, debilitation or severe frequency-urgency syndrome, severe dysuria, persistent urinary incontinence, severe abdominal pain, or recurrent urinary tract infections are all possible candidates for drug intervention.

   Thiazides are the most commonly prescribed agent for IH. These drugs presumably enhance calcium reabsorption in the ascending loop of Henle.

Reference: Heiliczer JD, Canonigo BB, Bishof NA, Moore ES: Noncalculi urinary tract disorders secondary to idiopathic hypercalciuria in children. Pediatr Clin North Am 34:711–718, 1987.

Nondairy Foods Rich in Calcium

Consider caring for a lactase-deficient child who required a high dietary calcium intake. Which calcium-rich foods could you use rather than resorting to medicinal calcium supplements? A few examples of other-than-cow-in-origin calcium are as follows:

CALCIUM: mg
PER AVERAGE SERVING

Cereals
Barley cereal, Gerbers, 1 cup .. 231
Oatmeal, ¾ cup 153
Pablum barley cereal,
   ¾ cup, cooked 2210
Pablum cereal, mixed,
   ¾ cup, cooked 2210

Cereal Flours
Cornmeal, whole grain, 1 cup 354
Soy flour, low-fat, 1 cup 263
Wheat flour, self-rising,
   enriched, 1 cup 303

Fish
Herring, canned, solids
   and liquids, 3½ oz 147
Mackerel, canned, 3½ oz 260
Sardines, Atlantic, canned
   in oil, 3½ oz 354
Smelt, Atlantic, canned,
   3½ oz 358

Fruits
Figs, dried, 3½ oz 126
Oranges, 1 large 96

CALCIUM: mg
PER AVERAGE SERVING

Nuts
Almonds, unblanched, 3½ oz .. 254
Brazil nuts, 3½ oz 186

Legumes and Seeds
Soybean curd (Tofu), 4 oz 154
Beans, common, dried,
   ½ cup 144
Garbanzo beans, dried,
   ½ cup 150
Sunflower seed kernels,
   3½ oz 120

Syrups and Sugars
Molasses, cane, third extraction,
   blackstrap, 3½ oz 579
Maple sugar, 3½ oz 180

Vegetables
Broccoli, cooked, 1 cup 132
Spoon cabbage, raw, 3½ oz ... 165
Collards, cooked, ½ cup 152
Dandelion greens, cooked,
   ½ cup 140
Lamb's-quarters, cooked,
   ½ cup 258

Reference: American Academy of Pediatrics: Pediatric Nutrition Handbook, 2nd ed. Elk Grove Village, IL, American Academy of Pediatrics, 1985, p 372.

CANDIDAL INFECTION

Penile Plaque—An Early Sign of Neonatal *Candida* Infection

Systemic candidal infections occur in immunosuppressed and immunocompromised patients, particularly those whose normal bacterial flora are suppressed by the use of broad-spectrum antibiotics. Diagnosis of candidal infection is often delayed by the failure to suspect fungal disease as well as by delayed growth of yeast from patient specimens.

The premature neonate is both immunodeficient and likely to be treated with multiple antibiotics. The use of indwelling catheters provides an additional risk factor for the development of candidal infection.

The development of a white plaque adherent to the tip of the penis but beneath the foreskin of male premature infants may provide early evidence of candiduria and disseminated candidal infection. Urine, blood, and cerebrospinal fluid and/or endotracheal aspirate cultures should be used to confirm the suspicion provoked by this finding. The detection of the penile plaque allows early initiation of antifungal therapy. It is hypothesized that the plaque is formed by *Candida* that originates in the perineum or the urine and then forms visible growth in the moist area underlying the foreskin.

Careful examination of the genitalia is important even in the intensive care nursery.

Reference: Ruderman JW: A clue (tip-off) to urinary infection with *Candida.* Pediatr Infect Dis J 9:586–588, 1990.

CAROTENEMIA

Carotenemia or, Better Expressed, Hypercarotenemia

Carotenemia is a common condition characterized by a yellow-orange discoloration of the skin and concomitant elevated serum carotene levels. The majority of these cases are harmless and due to the ingestion of large amounts of carotene-rich foods over a long period of time (e.g., carrots, sweet potatoes, squash). The syndrome is associated rarely with disease entities such as diabetes mellitus and hypothyroidism.

Conditions Associated with Carotenemia

Excessive dietary intake (the most common cause of carotenemia)
Diabetes mellitus
Hypothyroidism
Simmonds' disease (panhypopituitarism)
Hypothalamic amenorrhea
Anorexia nervosa
Human castrates

Liver disease
Renal disease (e.g., chronic glomerulonephritis and nephrotic syndrome)
Inborn errors of metabolism
Familial conditions
Malaria

Clinical Manifestations

1. Yellow pigmentation of the skin, most prominently on palms, soles, and naso-labial folds
2. Carotene is excreted by the sebaceous sweat glands; thus, the discoloration of the skin is most prominent where sweating is most profuse.
3. It gradually extends over the body.
4. Sclera are always spared from carotene staining. (Corneum of the skin has a high lipid content with an affinity for carotene; the mucosa has no affinity to carotene.)
5. Elevated serum carotene level.
6. Patients rarely complain of constitutional symptoms, such as loss of appetite, malaise, itching, and right upper quadrant abdominal pain.

Differential Diagnosis

Jaundice
Lycopenemia (orange-reddish discoloration of the skin due to an increased consumption of lycopene-rich foods, especially tomatoes)
Excessive ingestion or percutaneous absorption of chemicals such as quinacrine, mepacrine, dinitrophenol, saffron, picric acid, and canthaxanthin, the major coloring constituent in "tanning capsules."

Treatment

Avoid carotene-rich foods but consume a well-balanced diet. The yellow discoloration resolves over several weeks to months, although serum carotene levels drop severely after only 1 week of a carotene-poor diet. If carotenemia does not resolve or an underlying etiology is suspected, an appropriate investigation should ensue.

Foods High in Carotene Content

Vegetables		Fruits	Other
Alfalfa	Rutabagas	Apples	Butter
Asparagus	Spinach	Apricots	Egg yolks
Beans	Squash	Berries	Milk
Beet greens	Sweet potatoes	Cantaloupes	Palm Oil
Broccoli	Yellow turnips	Figs	Yellow corn
Carrots	Watercress	Mangoes	Yellow fat
Chard		Oranges	
Collard greens		Papayas	
Cucumbers		Pawpaws	
Endive		Peaches	
Escarole		Pineapples	
Kale		Prunes	

Adapted from: Leung AKC: Carotenemia. Advances in Pediatrics 34:223–248, 1987.

CAT SCRATCH DISEASE

Diagnostic Criteria for Cat Scratch Disease

Cat scratch disease is a self-limited bacterial infection that is usually transmitted to humans by felines, although other animals have been implicated. It presents primarily in children with a single lymph node enlargement or regional lymphadenitis and an ocular, skin, or mucous membrane lesion in the region of the adenitis. Other manifestations include fever, malaise, headache, anorexia, rash, sore throat, splenomegaly, and, rarely, a severe, chronic, systemic form of the illness. The symptoms can last for weeks to months.

The most important historical information in confirming a diagnosis of cat scratch disease is whether or not the patient has had contact with a cat; 99% of cat scratch disease patients have had such contact, and 78% of that population have had contact with a kitten. An inoculation site is also vital to the diagnosis. Of the criteria listed below, at least 3 of the 4 noted are required for diagnosis of cat scratch disease. To these criteria most cat scratch afficianados would add pertinent laboratory data to rule out *other* causes of lymphadenopathy.

1. Single or regional lymphadenopathy.
2. Animal contact, with a scratch or inoculation lesion.
3. Positive cat scratch skin test.
4. Node or inoculum site with compatible histopathology or Warthin-Starry stain positive organisms.

Differential Diagnosis

Other infections causing adenopathy:

Infectious mononucleosis	Streptococcal infection	Toxoplasmosis
Mycobacterial infection	Tularemia	Sporotrichosis
Staphylococcal infection	Syphilis	

Other fungi

Noninfectious disorders:

Lymphoma	Congenital cysts
Sarcoid	Kawasaki disease

Reference: Moriarty RA, Margileth AM. Cat scratch disease. Infect Dis Clin North Am 1:575–590, 1987.

Unusual Manifestations of Cat Scratch Disease

Common associated symptoms of cat scratch disease include fever, malaise, headache, and myalgia. One or more of these symptoms occur in approximately 50% of patients with the disease. In addition, approximately 50% of patients will have or recall a painless papule at the site of the scratch. The papule may progress to form a pustule or a vesicle, but it resolves spontaneously after 1 to 3 weeks and usually precedes the development of lymphadenopathy by several weeks.

A small number of patients with cat scratch disease may develop unusual manifestations, many of which suggest disseminated involvement. These unusual features include the following:

Encephalopathy	Erythema multiforme
Radiculitis	Pruritic, maculopapular rash
Oculoglandular syndrome	Atypical pneumonia
Thrombocytopenia	Osteolytic bone lesions
Erythema nodosum	Hepatic and splenic granulomas

Because it is now known that at least some of the above unusual manifestations of cat scratch disease may be seen in patients without associated lymphadenopathy, it is important to keep this diagnosis in mind when patients are seen with any of the problems listed.

References: Carithers HA: Cat-scratch disease: An overview based on a study of 1,200 patients. Am J Dis Child 139:1124–1133, 1985; Delahoussaye PM, Osborne BM: Cat-scratch disease presenting as abdominal visceral granulomas. J Infect Dis 161:71–78, 1990; Daye S, McHenry JA, Roscelli JD: Pruritic rash associated with cat scratch disease. Pediatrics 81:559–561, 1988; Malatack JJ, Altman HA, Nard JA: Cat-scratch disease without adenopathy. J Pediatr 114:101–104, 1989.

CERVICITIS

Cervicitis and Vulvovaginitis in the Adolescent

There exists much overlap in the clinical presentations of cervical, vaginal, uterine, fallopian tube, and urinary tract infections. Most of these entities share the same symptoms such as dysuria, vulvar pruritis, dyspareunia, and increased or altered vaginal discharge. It is essential, therefore, when evaluating adolescent women with such complaints to (1) exclude the diagnosis of upper tract disease, such as endometritis, salpingitis, and pyelonephritis; (2) differentiate among vaginitis, cervicitis, urethritis, and cystitis; and (3) identify the specific etiologic agent that is causing the infection so that the proper treatment can be prescribed. Listed below are the various causes of vulvovaginitis and cervicitis:

1. **Vulvovaginitis**

    a. Physiologic leukorrhea (normal vaginal discharge that increases in volume with estrogen stimulation)
    b. Candidiasis (e.g., *Candida albicans* and *Torulopsis glabrata*)
    c. Trichomoniasis (*Trichomonas vaginalis*)
    d. Bacterial vaginosis (this entity occurs in 30 to 50% of women with vaginitis, making it the most common cause of abnormal vaginal discharge. It is probably the result of an interplay between the overgrowth of *Gardnerella vaginalis* and various anaerobes, and the subsequent decrease in the presence of lactobacilli that normally inhabit the vagina)
    e. Foreign body (e.g., tampons, IUDs, etc.)
    f. Allergic or contact vulvovaginitis (e.g., contact with soaps and other cleaning agents, spermicides, lubricants, douches, sanitary napkins, nylon or rayon underwear, obesity, hot weather, poor hygiene, etc.)
    g. Allergic seminal vulvovaginitis
    h. Psychosomatic illness should be considered when an adolescent frequently presents with vaginal symptoms but without objective evidence of vulvar or vaginal inflammation or discharge.

2. **Other Causes of Vulvovaginal Complaints**

    a. Systemic conditions.
        i. Fistulas from the bladder or rectum (e.g. Crohn's disease, Stevens-Johnson syndrome, Behçet's syndrome)
        ii. Tropical ulcerations (e.g., amebiasis, filariasis, tuberculosis, schistosomiasis)
        iii. Systemic illnesses (e.g., typhoid, smallpox, varicella, measles, scarlet fever)
        iv. Dermatologic complaints (e.g., atopic dermatitis, seborrheic dermatitis, psoriasis, lichen sclerosus)
        v. Anatomic anomalies (e.g., aberrant urethral orifice, labial agglutination, urethral prolapse)

    b. Vulvar lesions
        i. Condyloma acuminatum
        ii. Genital herpes
        iii. Syphilis
        iv. Chancroid
        v. Lymphogranuloma venereum
        vi. Granuloma inguinale
        vii. Pediculosis
        viii. Scabies
        ix. Bartholinitis
        x. Skenitis
        xi. Tumors (e.g., carcinoma, sarcoma, botryoides, vaginal polyps)
        xii. Pemphigus
        xiii. Acute ulcerative vulvitis
        xiv. Lipschütz ulcer

3. Cervicitis

Whatever its etiology, cervicitis should be considered a sexually transmitted disease with great potential to spread to other sexual partners as well as to extend, in the case of contact, from the cervix to the endometrium and salpinx. Etiologies include:

   a. *Chlamydia trachomatis*
   b. *Neisseria gonorrhoeae*
   c. Herpes simplex virus
   d. Possible etiologic agents include *Mycoplasma hominis, Ureaplasma urealyticum*, and group B streptococci.

Reference: Rosenfeld WD, Clark J: Vulvovaginitis and cervicitis. Pediatr Clin North Am 36:489–511, 1989.

CHEST PAIN

Common Causes

Costochondritic
   Arthritis
   Infectious costochondritis
   Tietze's syndrome
Cough
Herpes zoster
Idiopathic
Indigestion (heartburn, esophagitis)

Mitral valve prolapse
Musculoskeletal (strain, occult trauma)
Pneumonitis
Psychogenic
Reactive airway disease
Sickle-cell disease
Trauma

Uncommon Causes

Arrhythmia
Congenital heart disease
Congestive heart failure
Esophageal (trauma associated
   with vomiting, foreign body)

Pleuritis/pleurisy
Pneumothorax
Precordial catch

Rare Causes

Cholecystitis
Diaphragmatic irritation
   Abscess
   Fitz-Hugh–Curtis syndrome
   Peritonitis
   Ruptured viscus
   Tumor
Endocarditis
Juvenile rheumatoid arthritis

Myocardial ischemia (e.g., anomalous
   coronary artery)
Myocarditis
Osteomyelitis (vertebrae, ribs)
Peptic ulcerative disease
Pericarditis
Pneumomediastinum
Pulmonary embolism
Rheumatic fever

CHOLESTEROL

Screening and Managing Cholesterol Levels in Children

The following table summarizes the American Academy of Pediatrics (AAP)/ American Heart Association's (AHA) and the National Cholesterol Education Program's (NCEP) recommendations for testing and managing cholesterol in children. The American Health Foundation's (AHF) recommended universal, population-based approach to cholesterol control is also presented in outline.

Recommendations for Screening and Managing Cholesterol in Children

High-risk, patient-based approach

	AAP/AHA RECOMMENDATIONS	NCEP RECOMMENDATIONS
Screening strategy	Screen children over 2 yr of age who have a family history of hyperlipidemia (parent, sibling, grand- parent, uncle, aunt) or early myocardial infarc- tion (males under 50 yr, females under 60 yr).	Screen children over 2 yr who have a *parental* history of hyperlipidemia ($>$240 mg/dl total cholesterol) or a family history of early CAD (under 55 yr for males and females).* Also *con- sider* screening if family history is not obtainable or patient has several risk factors for CAD inde- pendent of history (obesity, hypertension, smoking).
Screening method	Screen initially with fast- ing lipid profile. Repeat and average LDL-C. If elevated, exclude second- ary causes of hyperlipidemia.	If child has family history of early CAD, screen initially with two lipid profiles.[†] In other high-risk patients, screen initially with nonfasting total cholesterol. If total cholesterol is borderline (170–199 mg/dl), repeat and average results. If initial screening measurement is 200 mg/dl or more, or the average of two measure- ments is $>$170 mg/dl, perform two lipid profiles.[†]
Management		Total cholesterol is normal ($<$170 mg/dl): Rou- tine care, repeat cholesterol testing 5 yr later.
		Low risk lipid profile (LDL-C $<$110 mg/dl, less than 75th percentile): Routine care, repeat lipid profile every 5 yr.
		Moderate-risk lipid profile (LDL-C 110–129 mg/ dl, 75th to 95th percentile): Dietary counseling, follow-up lipid profile in 1 yr.
		High-risk lipid profile (LDL-C $\geq$130 mg/dl, 95th percentile): Dietary counseling, perform lipid profiles on parents, initiate step 1 diet. Repeat lipid profile in 6 wk. If unchanged, intensify step 1 diet and repeat lipid profile in 3 mo. If still unchanged, initiate step 2 diet and repeat lipid profile in 3 mo. Refer to lipid specialist if diet therapy ineffective.

* The NCEP defines a family history of early CAD as having parents or grand parents 55 yr of age or under who have had one or more of the following: coronary atherosclerosis diagnosed by coronary arteriography; balloon angioplasty or coronary artery bypass surgery; documented myocardial infarction, angina pectoris, peripheral vascular disease, cerebrovascular disease, or sudden cardiac death.

† A repeat nonfasting total cholesterol measurement or second fasting lipid profile should be done no sooner than 1 wk after initial test and no later than 8 wk after initial test. The second measurement is unacceptable if the total cholesterol or LDL-C level is within 30 mg/dl of the initial measurement. If unacceptable, obtain a third measurement.

Table continued on next page.

Recommendations for Screening and Managing Cholesterol in Children (Cont.)

Universal, population-based approach (recommended by AHF)

Screening strategy	Screen all children over 2 yr of age. Consider repeat screening every 5 yr thereafter.
Screening method	Screen initially with nonfasting total cholesterol, and proceed to fasting lipid profile if levels are elevated as described above under NCEP recommendations.
Management	See recommendations above.

Reference: Modified from Schuman AJ: A guide to office cholesterol testing. Contemp Pediatr October:17–42, 1991.

CLINICAL JUDGMENT

Quantifying Judgment in the Evaluation of Sick Children

We all use judgment and experience to distinguish the "sick" child from the "not-so-sick" child. No amount of wisdom and no laboratory test will make this distinction accurate in every case, but the scale below will help you quantify your judgment, or at least it will help you recognize how you reach your own conclusions.

*Six Observation Items and Their Scales**

OBSERVATION ITEM	1 NORMAL	3 MODERATE IMPAIRMENT	5 SEVERE IMPAIRMENT
Quality of cry	Strong with normal tone or content and not crying	Whimpering or sobbing	Weak or moaning or high pitched
Reaction to parental stimulation	Cries briefly then stops or content and not crying	Cries off and on	Continual cry or hardly responds
State variation	If aware, stays awake; or if asleep and stimulated, wakes up quickly	Eyes close briefly— awake; awakes with prolonged stimulation	Fails to sleep or will not rouse
Color	Pink	Pale extremities or acrocyanosis	Pale, cyanotic, mottled, or ashen
Hydration	Skin normal, eyes normal, and mucous membranes moist	Skin, eyes normal and mouth slightly dry	Skin doughy or tented, and dry mucous membranes and/or sunken eyes
Response (talk, smile) to social overtures	Smiles or alerts (≤2 mo)	Brief smile, alerts briefly (≤2 mo)	No smile; face anxious, dull, and expressionless or no alerting (≤2 mo)

* Source—see reference below; with permission.

To use this system, assign a score of 1–3 for each of the observation items. When the investigators used the scale to evaluate children less than 24 months of age who had fever of 38.3°C or more, only 2.7% of children with a score of less than 10 had a serious illness, whereas 92.3% of those with a score greater than or equal to 16 were seriously ill. Among those children with scores of 11 to 15, serious illness was found in 26.2%. A child was defined as having a serious illness if a bacterial pathogen was isolated from blood, CSF, urine, stool, joint fluid, or deep soft tissue aspirate, or if electrolyte abnormality, pulmonary infiltrates on chest x-ray, abnormal blood gases, or CSF pleocytosis was found.

It might be helpful to compare your own instincts to this scale to find out why you conclude what you do.

Reference: McCarthy PL, Sharpe MR, Spiesel SZ, et al: Observation scales to identify serious illness in febrile children. Pediatrics 70:802, 806 (table), 1982.

COCAINE

Differential Diagnosis of Cocaine Intoxication

The acute manifestations of severe cocaine ingestion are many. Manifestations may be divided systematically:

1. Autonomic nervous system overactivity
   a. Dilated pupils   c. Diaphoresis
   b. Tachycardia   d. Pallor secondary to vasoconstriction
2. Central nervous system
   a. Dysphoric agitation   b. Tremor   d. Coma
      or stimulation   c. Convulsions   e. Hyperthermia
3. Cardiovascular
   a. Small doses slow the heart rate
   b. High doses increase the heart rate and elevate the blood pressure
   c. Dysrhythmias
4. Respiratory (stimulation followed by depression of the respiratory center)

It is important when entertaining the diagnosis of cocaine intoxication to consider other clinical entities that may mimic it:

Medical differential of cocaine ingestion:

Thyroid storm	Sedative/hypnotic	Sepsis
Hypoglycemia	withdrawal	Pheochromocytoma
Thiamine deficiency	Seizure disorders	Head injury
Acute psychosis		

Chemical differential of cocaine ingestion:

Stimulants/sympathomimetics	Amphetamines	Cyclic antidepressants
Phenylpropanolamine	Anticholinergic agent	Strychnine
Phencyclidine (smoked)	Hallucinogens	

Reference: Mofenson HC, Caraccio TR: Cocaine. Pediatr Ann 16:864–873, 1987.

COMA

Common Causes

CNS trauma
  Cerebral edema
  Concussion
  Hemorrhage
    Epidural
    Subarachnoid
    Subdural
  Increased intra-
    cranial pressure

Drug intoxication
  Analgesics
  Anticonvulsants
  Antihistamines
  Benzodiazepines
  Digoxin
  Ethanol
  Heavy metals
  Hydrocarbons

Drug intoxication *(Cont.)*
  Hypnotics
    Barbiturates
  Insulin
  Lithium
  Organophosphates
  Phencyclidine
  Phenothiazines
  Salicylate
  Tricyclic antidepressants

Uncommon Causes

Cardiorespiratory
  Cardiopulmonary arrest
  Hypercapnea
  Hypotension/shock
  Hypoxemia
Infections
  Abscess
  Encephalitis
  Meningitis
Metabolic
  Hyper/hypocalcemia
  Hyper/hypomagnesemia

Metabolic *(Cont.)*
  Hypernatremia
  Hypoglycemia
  Hyponatremia
    Water intoxication
  Metabolic acidosis
  Metabolic alkalosis
Postictal state
Postoperative
  General anesthesia
  Hypotension/hypoxemia
Sepsis

Rare Causes

Cardiac
  Arrhythmia
  Hypertension
  Hypoperfusion
    Aortic stenosis
    Coarctation of the aorta
Cerebral tumors/metastases
Cerebrovascular
  Hemorrhage
  Thrombophlebitis
  Vasculitis
  Venous thrombosis
Dehydration
Diabetic ketoacidosis
Endocrine disorders
  Addison's disease
  Congenital adrenal hyperplasia
  Cushing's disease

Inborn errors of metabolism
  Hyperammonemia
  Hypoglycemia
Heat stroke
Hepatic failure
Hypothermia
Malignant hyperthermia
Porphyria
Postinfectious encephalomyelitis
  Measles
  Other viral infections
Psychiatric disturbances
  Fugue state
  Hysteria
Reye's syndrome
Sudden infant death syndrome (SIDS)
Uremia

Evaluation of the Comatose Child

There exist three important categories of central nervous system lesions that can cause alterations in one's level of consciousness: (1) supratentorial mass lesions, (2) infratentorial mass lesions, and (3) metabolic abnormalities. In evaluating the comatose child at the time of presentation, careful notice of the neurologic findings and determination of the type of CNS lesion incurred are very useful in dictating acute medical management.

1. **Supratentorial Mass Lesions**

    a. Important causes of supratentorial lesions that yield progressive deterioration in children:
        i. Cerebral hyperemia secondary to head trauma
        ii. Epidural and subdural hematomas
        iii. Intracerebral hemorrhages
        iv. Acute hydrocephalus
        v. Subdural hemorrhages
        vi. Severe systemic hypertension
        vii. Obstruction of an existing ventricular-peritoneal shunt
        viii. Bleeding arteriovenous malformation

    b. Neurologic findings of supratentorial lesions
        i. Initial signs and symptoms suggest focal hemispheric disease
        ii. Signs progress in a rostral to caudal direction
        iii. Pupillary reflexes are usually depressed
        iv. Motor signs are often symmetrical

2. **Infratentorial Mass Lesions (Posterior Fossa)**

    These lesions can yield coma either by destroying the ascending reticular activating system or by compression of that system by a mass or tumor.

    a. Important causes of infratentorial lesions:
        i. Brainstem contusions associated with trauma
        ii. Cerebellar hemorrhage or tumor with secondary hydrocephalus
        iii. Brainstem encephalitis
        iv. Basilar artery thrombosis

    b. Neurologic findings of infratentorial lesions
        i. Brainstem signs and symptoms are common.
        ii. Signs are not rostral to caudal in evolution.
        iii. Cranial nerve palsies are common.
        iv. Abnormalities of the respiratory pattern are common and appear at the onset of coma.

3. **Metabolic Disorders**

    Metabolic disorders make up the majority of nontraumatic processes that cause acute coma in the pediatric patient.

    a. Important causes of metabolic coma:
        i. Hypoxic-ischemic coma (e.g., respiratory failure, shock, severe anemia, apnea of infancy, carbon monoxide poisoning, cerebral vasculitis)

ii. Infections (e.g., encephalitis, meningitis, botulism)
iii. Postictal state
iv. Hypoglycemia
v. Nonendocrine organ failure (e.g., hepatic and renal)
vi. Endocrine organ failure (e.g., pancreas, adrenal, thyroid, pituitary)
vii. Poisonings (e.g., narcotics, barbiturates, sedatives, etc.)
viii. Miscellaneous (e.g., Reye's syndrome, electrolyte abnormalities, and hypothermia or hyperthermia)

b. Neurologic findings of metabolic lesions
i. Stupor or coma precede motor signs.
ii. Motor signs are usually symmetrically depressed.
iii. Pupillary reactions are preserved.
iv. Acid-base imbalance is common.
v. Seizures or abnormal motor movements are common findings.

Reference: James HE: Neurologic evaluation and support in the child with an acute brain insult. Pediatr Ann 15:16–22, 1986.

Ingestions and the Pupillary Examination in a Comatose Child

When confronted with a comatose child, the possibility of ingestion of a toxic or poisonous substance should always be considered. A history should be obtained addressing which medications and poisonous substances are at home, how they are kept separate from the child, and if there is any suspicion on the parents' part that the child may have ingested something. Modern advances in technology and pharmacology have made the serum and urine toxicologic screening tests most useful to the diagnosis of toxic ingestion. The examination of a comatose child's pupillary size and reactivity, however, remains a useful bedside exam that can be performed with a minimum of difficulty and time. Although the pupillary exam is not nearly as specific as the toxicologic screening tests, it can point the way toward considering a diagnosis of ingestion of poison.

The Pupillary Examination and Coma

MYDRIASIS (DILATION OF THE PUPIL)		MIOSIS (CONTRACTION OF THE PUPIL)	
Amphetamines	Cocaine	Opiates	Methadone
Antihistamines	Ephedrine	Barbiturates	Carbon monoxide
Atropine	Ethyl alcohol	Propoxyphen	Organophosphates
Botulism	Snake venom	Meperidine	Clonidine

Reference: James HE: Neurologic evaluation and support in the child with an acute brain insult. Pediatr Ann 15:16–22, 1986.

CONGENITAL HEART DISEASE

The First Manifestation of Congenital Heart Disease

Depending on the nature of the anatomic lesion, the first sign or symptom of congenital heart disease may vary. The table below is designed to serve as a guide to the most likely lesions, given the clinical presentation.

Marked Cyanosis	Congestive Heart Failure	Heart Murmur
Transposition of the great arteries	Aortic atresia	Patent ductus arteriosus
Pulmonary atresia and stenosis with intact ventricular septum	Coarctation of the aorta	Pulmonary stenosis
	Double outlet right ventricle syndrome	Aortic stenosis
Tetralogy of Fallot with severe pulmonary stenosis	Patent ductus arteriosus	Pulmonary artery stenosis
	Truncus arteriosus	Ventricular septal defect
Complex pulmonary atresias	Ventricular septal defect	
	Arteriovenous fistulas	Arteriovenous fistulas
Tricuspid atresia	**Abnormal Heart Rate**	Atrioventricular valve regurgitations
Ebstein's malformation of the tricuspid valve	Supraventricular tachycardia	
	Heart block	

References: Rowe R, Mehrizi A: The Neonate with Congenital Heart Disease. Philadelphia, W.B. Saunders Company, 1968, p 105; Fyler DC (ed): Nadas' Pediatric Cardiology. Philadelphia, Hanley & Belfus, 1992.

Recurrence Risks for Congenital Heart Disease

Congenital cardiac lesions are thought to recur in three patterns of inheritance:

1. As part of a single gene defect syndrome (2%).
2. Chromosomal abnormalities (4%).
3. Multifactorial inheritance (94%).

Some single gene syndromes that often include cardiac defects are listed in the following table.

Selected Single Mutant Gene Syndromes with Cardiovascular Disease Other than Coronary Artery

AUTOSOMAL DOMINANT	AUTOSOMAL RECESSIVE	X-LINKED
Apert	Adrenogenital syndrome	Incontinentia pigmenti
Crouzon	Alkaptonuria	Mucopolysaccharidosis II
Ehlers-Danlos	Carpenter	Muscular dystrophy
Forney	Conradi	
Holt-Oram	Cutis laxa	
IHSS (not strictly a syndrome)	Ellis-van Creveld	
	Friedreich's ataxis	
Leopard	Glycogenosis IIa, IIIa, IV	
Marfan	Jervell and Lange-Nielsen	
Myotonic dystrophy	Laurence-Moon-Biedl	
Neurofibromatosis	Mucolipidosis III	
Osteogenesis imperfecta	Mucopolysaccharidosis II, IV, V, VI	
	Osteogenesis imperfecta	
Romano-Ward	Refsum	
Treacher Collins	Seckel	
Tuberous sclerosis	Smith-Lemli-Opitz	
Ullrich-Noonan	Thrombocytopenia with absent radius (TAR)	
	Weill-Marchesani	

The recurrence risk for congenital heart disease in families in which one member has one of these syndromes depends on the recurrence risk for the syndrome (generally 25 to 50%) and the frequency with which congenital heart disease is encountered in the syndrome.

The recurrence risk for congenital heart disease due to a chromosomal abnormality depends on the risk of recurrence of the chromosomal defect. A familial tendency for nondisjunction and the presence of a translocation in the chromosomal pattern of one parent may increase the likelihood of recurrence. Some chromosomal defects are associated with particular cardiac abnormalities. The more common chromosomal aberrations and their associated cardiac defects are listed in the following table.

Congenital Heart Disease in Selected Chromosomal Aberrations

POPULATION STUDIED	PERCENTAGE INCIDENCE OF CHD	MOST COMMON LESIONS		
		1	2	3
General population	1	VSD	PDA	ASD
4p—	40	VSD	ASD	PDA
5p—(cri du chat)	25	VSD	PDA	ASD
C mosaic	50	VSD		
13 trisomy	90	VSD	PDA	Dex
13q—	50	VSD		
18 trisomy	90+	VSD	PDA	PS
18q—	50	VSD	AV	ASD
21 trisomy	50	VSD	AV canal	ASD
XO Turner	35	Coarc	AS	ASD
XXXXY	14	PDA	ASD	

VSD = Ventricular septal defect. PDA = Patent ductus arteriosis. ASD = Atrial septal defect. Dex = Dextrocardia. PS = Pulmonic stenosis. AV = Atrioventricular. Coarc = Coarctation of aorta. AS = Aortic stenosis.

The essential components of multifactorial inheritance of congenital heart defects include: (1) a genetic predisposition to cardiovascular maldevelopment, (2) a genetic predisposition to be adversely affected by environmental teratogens, and (3) an environmental insult occurring at a vulnerable period of cardiac development (i.e., very early in pregnancy). Since there is no method of quantitating the presence of these three risks for a given offspring, a few percentages may be kept in mind:

1. In general, the risk of recurrence of congenital heart disease in a given family is 1 to 5%.
2. The more common the heart defect in the affected family member, the more likely that defect is to recur.
3. The risk to subsequent offspring of two parents triples if two existing family members are affected. (For example, the risk of recurrence of a ventriculoseptal defect is about 5% if one previous sibling is affected; however, it increases to approximately 15% if one sibling and one parent or two siblings are affected.)
4. If the majority of family members have some form of congenital cardiac defect the risk to subsequent offspring approaches 100%. More specifically, if three first-degree family members are affected, the risk in future pregnancies is 60 to 100%.

Recurrence risks for siblings of family members with congenital heart defects are shown in the following table:

Recurrence Risks for Congenital Heart Defects in Siblings

DEFECT	PERCENT AT RISK	
	1 SIBLING AFFECTED	2 SIBLINGS AFFECTED
Ventricular septal defect	3	10
Patent ductus arteriosus	3	10
Atrial septal defect	2.5	8
Tetralogy of Fallot	2.5	8
Pulmonary stenosis	2	6
Coarctation of aorta	2	6
Aortic stenosis	2	6
Transposition	1.5	5
Endocardial cushion defects	3	10
Fibroelastosis	4	12
Hypoplastic left heart	2	6
Tricuspid atresia	1	3
Ebstein anomaly	1	3
Truncus arteriosus	1	3
Pulmonary atresia	1	3

Based on combined data published during two decades from European and North American populations. (From Nora JJ, Nora AH: Update on counseling the family with a first-degree relative with a congenital heart defect. Am J Med Genet 29:137–142, 1988, with permission.)

References: Nora JJ, Wolf RF: Recurrence risks in the family. In Kidd BSL, Rowe RD (eds): The Child with Congenital Heart Disease after Surgery. Mount Kisco, New York, Futura Publishing Company, 1976, pp 451–460; Fyler DC (ed): Nadas' Pediatric Cardiology. Philadelphia, Hanley & Belfus, 1992. Adapted from McMillan JA, et al: The Whole Pediatrician Catalog, Vol. 3 Philadelphia, W.B. Saunders, 1982, with permission.

CONSTIPATION

Common Causes

Appendicitis
Breastfeeding (begins
  around 6 weeks of age)
Cow's milk ingestion
Drugs
  Anticholinergics
  Antihistamines
  Narcotics
  Phenothiazines
Dysfunctional toilet
  training
Emotional disturbances
Functional ileus
Immobility

Inappropriate expectations of the caretaker
Intentional withholding
Intestinal abnormalities
  Atresia
  Hirschsprung's disease
  Microcolon
  Volvulus
  Web
Low dietary fiber
Meconium plug/ileus
Meningomyelocele
Mental retardation/cerebral palsy
Painful defecation (hemorrhoids, fissure,
  skin irritation)

Uncommon Causes

Diabetes mellitus
Electrolyte disturbances
   Hyper/hypocalcemia
   Hyperkalemia
Hypothyroidism
Imperforate anus/anal stenosis

Intestinal pseudo-obstruction
Lead poisoning
Salmonellosis
Spinal cord injury/tumor
Starvation

Rare Causes

Amyloidosis
Botulism
Dolichocolon
Myopathies/myotonias
Pheochromocytoma

Sacral malformations
Scleroderma
Tetanus
Tethered cord

CONTRACEPTION

Side Effects of Hormonal Contraception

The mnemonic ACHES for recalling the dangerous side-effecs of oral contraceptive use is well known (**A**: abdominal pain; **C**: chest pain, cough, and shortness of breath; **H**: headaches; **E**: eye problems such as blurred vision; **S**: severe leg pain in the calves and thighs). There exist, however, a great many other untoward effects from oral contraceptive use that may paly a role in an adolescent woman's decision not to comply with this method of birth control. Arranged in terms of the hormonal cause, these untoward effects are presented below:

Hormonal Side Effects of Oral Contraceptives

ESTROGEN EXCESS	PROGESTIN EXCESS	ESTROGEN DEFICIENCY	PROGESTIN DEFICIENCY
Nausea, vomiting Edema bloating Cyclic weight gain	Fatigue, depression Acne, oily skin, hirsutism	Irritability, nervousness Hot flashes, motor symptoms	Late breakthrough bleeding and spotting
Dysmenorrhea, uterine cramps	Alopecia Increased appetite, shortened menses	Early midcycle spotting Decreased amount of early menstrual flow	Heavy menstrual flow and clots Delayed onset of menses, dys-menorrhea, weight loss
Breast tenderness, increased breast size, vascular headaches	Decreased libido Headaches between pill packages	No withdrawal bleeding Dry vaginal mucosa, atrophic vaginitis	
Chloasma Lactation supression Irritability, depression	Dilated leg veins Cholestatic jaundice	Headaches Depression	

Adapted from Dickey RP: Medical approaches to reproductive regulation: The pill. In Managing Contraceptive Pill Patients, 4th ed. Oklahoma, Creative Informatics, Inc., 1984.

Reference: Shearin RB, Boehlke JR: Hormonal contraception. Pediatr Clin North Am 36:697–715, 1989.

CORTISOL

Cortisol Replacement During Febrile Episodes

Daily cortisol production rates among normal children have previously been estimated at 12 mg/m²/day. The detection of clinical evidence of cortisol excess among children with adrenal insufficiency treated with this dose suggests that it may be too high. A new study using recently developed, more accurate methods of determining cortisol production rates in normal children suggests that 7 mg/m²/day may be a more appropriate dose.

Whatever the baseline dose of cortisol used to treat patients with adrenal insufficiency, an increase in that dose is recommended during periods of stress. The most common form of generalized stress during childhood is febrile illness. The usual recommendation is that the daily dose of steroid should be increased 2- to 3-fold during febrile illnesses. In fact, when 105 normal children 1 month to 12 years of age were studied, those children with upper respiratory infection, streptococcal pharyngitis, and otitis media experienced serum cortisol increases of 2- to 3-fold, whereas those children with pneumonia, fever of unknown origin, and bacterial meningitis demonstrated a 5- to 6-fold rise. It seems prudent to attempt to reproduce these apparently physiologic stress levels of serum cortisol for children with inadequate intrinsic production during severe physiologic stress. It is also important to remember that oral replacement should be approximately twice the above recommendations because of poor oral absorption and hepatic biodegradation.

References: Nickels DA, Moore DC: Serum cortisol responses in febrile children. Pediatr Infect Dis J 8:16–19, 1989; Linder BL, Esteban NV, Yergey AL, et al: Cortisol production rate in childhood and adolescence. J Pediatr 117:892–896, 1990.

COUGH

Common Causes

Allergic disease
Aspiration (direct or indirect)
Atelectasis
Bacterial infection
  Bronchiectasis
  Bronchitis
  Pneumonia
  Sinusitis
  Tracheitis
Congestive heart failure
Environmental pollution
Foreign body
Gastroesophageal reflux

Infections, other
  Chlamydia
  Mycoplasma
  Pertussis
Postnasal drip
Reactive airway disease
Smoking/passive smoking
Viral infection
  Bronchiolitis
  Croup
  Pneumonitis
  Upper respiratory infection

Uncommon Causes

Cystic fibrosis
Malformation of the airway
Malignancy (primary or metastatic)
Mediastinal adenopathy
Psychogenic

Tracheobronchomalacia
Tracheoesophageal fistula
Tuberculosis
Vascular ring

Rare

Allergic bronchopulmonary aspergillosis
Auricular nerve stimulation
Bronchogenic cyst
Congenital lobar emphysema
Immotile cilia syndrome
Lymphocytic interstitial pneumonitis

Opportunistic infections (PCP, CMV, MAI, fungal)
Parasitic infection
Pulmonary embolism
Pulmonary hemosiderosis
Pulmonary sequestration
Sarcoidosis

Habit (Psychogenic) Cough

Habit cough is a transient tic disorder that may be seen in early adolescence, especially in puberty, and, by definition (*DSM-III-R*), lasts more than 1 month and less than 1 year. The behavior may be seen as part of Gilles de la Tourette syndrome but is usually an independent entity. The clinical features were described by Berman:

... persistent violent spasms of barky, harsh, nonproductive cough, occurring almost always during the waking hours and unaccompanied by systemic signs and symptoms of chronic disease; a paucity or complete absence of abnormal findings in the chest; lack of response to most potent cough preparations; and a cough that remains unchanged after exertion, laughter, infection, dampness, and extremes of temperature.

The diagnosis requires exclusion of organic causes. Habit cough usually disappears with sleep, which is not the case with most organic diseases.

Other motor tics include throat clearing, eye blinking, neck stretching, sniffing, grimacing, shrugging, and grunting. Hyper- and hypoventilation syndromes are also possibilities.

Reference: Berman BA: Habit cough in adolescent children. Ann Allergy 24:43–46, 1966.

CRAYONS

"Classic"Crayons

PHILADELPHIA, Oct. 2—This week Binney & Smith Inc., the manufacturer of Crayola crayons, brought back eight colors from retirement, albeit temporarily. Last year, with much hoopla, the company stopped using maize, violet blue, raw umber, orange yellow, blue gray, green blue, orange red and lemon yellow and replaced them with neon colors.

The crayons, now called "classics," will be packaged separately from a box of 64 in a special commemorative tin with notes about the crayons and their retirement, said J. O'Brien, a company spokesman. . . .

"The response has been amazing," said Mr. O'Brien, speaking of the withdrawal of the eight. "You just have to watch an adult open that box and sniff it. It's like a time machine."

For some, opening the green and yellow box is like Proust discovering 64 madeleines. Mr. O'Brien, 32 years old, said he gets the feeling each morning in Binney & Smith's headquarters in Easton, Pa. As he opens his car door, he smells a billion crayons melting. Some who protested the withdrawal of the eight said it was like removing a favorite baby blanket or toy.

Thousands were heartened by the crayons' temporary comeback. Others were not.

"It's a limited victory," said Kenneth E. Lang, the founder of Rumps, the Raw Umber and Maize Preservation Society. Mr. Lang, from Locust Valley, L.I., said he felt cheated.

"Raw umber and maize represent a bygone time in America," he said. "You can't draw a picture of Nebraska or Kansas or South Dakota without using these colors." . . .

From *The New York Times*, October 3, 1991, with permission.

CREAMATOCRIT

Now that more than 50% of women are initially breastfeeding their infants, questions commonly arise about the adequacy of the milk being produced. Abnormalities in milk composition are quite rare and are overdiagnosed. The misinterpretation of a spot creamatocrit to determine the percentage of milk fat contributes to this overdiagnosis. The creamatocrit can be a reliable reflection of milk fat content when a 24-hour sample or an entire expressed feeding from one or both breasts is used and when the procedure has been standardized by comparison with gravimetric tests of milk fat content.

The creamatocrit takes advantage of the fact that fat is the major determinant of the energy value of the milk sample.

A sample of human milk is placed in a hematocrit tube and spun in a microcentrifuge at full speed for 15 minutes. The fat rises to the top of the column. The cream layer, easily visible, is read from the hematocrit capillary tube, and, like a hematocrit, is expressed as a percentage of the milk column in the tube. This is the "creamatocrit."

This number can then be employed in a formula which will provide you with the energy content of the milk expressed as kcal per liter. The formula is:

$$kcal/liter = 290 + 66.8 \times creamatocrit$$

For example: A human milk sample is found to have a creamatocrit of 5%. Its caloric value is:

$$290 + 66.8 \times 5$$

or

$$625 \text{ calories per liter.}$$

Note: Creamatocrits should be read within one hour of centrifugation, because after that time the cream column begins to "unpack," and falsely elevated values are obtained.

Reference: Lemons JA, et al: Simple method for determining the caloric and fat content of human milk. Pediatrics 66:626–628, 1980.

CRYING

The Crying Infant

Unexplained, excessive crying in the afebrile infant usually achieves just what it is meant to achieve: every adult around wants to find its cause and make it stop. In investigating the cause of excessive, prolonged crying in 56 infants, aged 4 days to 245 months, who were brought to the emergency room of the Children's Hospital of Denver, a reason for the infant's distress was found for 46. The history provided a clue to the cause for 11 of the 56 infants, a careful physical examination resulted in a diagnosis for 23 patients, and a variety of laboratory tests revealed the cause for 11. The final diagnosis included a broad array of conditions, of which 61% were considered serious. The table below lists the diagnoses that explained the reason for excessive crying for these patients.

Diagnosis in 56 Infants with Unexplained, Excessive Crying

DIAGNOSIS	NO. WITH DIAGNOSIS	DIAGNOSIS	NO. WITH DIAGNOSIS
Idiopathic	10	Gastrointestinal tract	
Colic	6	Constipation	3
Infectious causes		Intussusception*	1
Otitis media*	10	Gastroesophageal reflux	1
Viral illness with anorexia, dehydration*	2	with esophagitis*	
		Central nervous system	
Urinary tract infection*	1	Subdural hematoma*	1
Mild prodrome of gastroenteritis	1	Encephalitis*	1
		Pseudotumor cerebri*	1
Herpangina*	1	Drug reaction/overdose	
Herpes stomatitis*	1	DTP† reaction*	1
Trauma		Inadvertent pseudoephe-	1
Corneal abrasion*	3	drine overdose*	
Foreign body in eye*	1	Behavior	
Foreign body in oropharynx*	1	Night terrors	1
		Overstimulation	1
Tibial fracture*	1	Cardiovascular	
Clavicular fracture*	1	Supraventricular tachycardia*	2
Brown recluse spider bite*	1	Metabolic	
Hair tourniquet syndrome (toe)*	1	Glutaric aciduria, type I*	1
		Total	56

* Indicates conditions considered serious.
† Diphtheria-tetanus-pertussis vaccine.

The components of the physical examination that were important in providing the diagnosis are listed below.

COMPONENT OF PHYSICAL EXAM	NO. OF PATIENTS WHOM COMPONENT PROVED USEFUL (n = 30)
Otoscopy	10
Rectal exam	4
Fluorescein staining of cornea	3
Inspection underneath clothing	2
Palpation of bones	2
Oral exam	2
Auscultation of heart (tachyarrhythmia)	2
Laryngoscopic exam of hypopharynx	1
Eversion of eyelid	1
Palpation of anterior fontanelle	1
Retinal exam	1
Neurologic exam	1

Laboratory studies that identified the diagnosis are listed in the following table.

DIAGNOSTIC STUDY	NO. OF PATIENTS (n = 11)
Skeletal roentgenography	2
Lumbar puncture/cerebrospinal fluid analysis	2*
Electrocardiography	2
Computed tomographic scan of the head	2*
Barium enema	1
Esophagram	1
Amino and organic acid studies	1
Urinalysis	1

*One patient, with pseudotumor cerebri, required lumbar puncture and computed tomographic scan of the head to make the diagnosis.

Reference: Poole SR: The infant with acute, unexplained, excessive crying. Pediatrics 88:450–455, 1991.

Colic, or Excessive Crying, in Young Infants

Colic, from the Latin *colicus*, strictly means related to or associated with the colon (and was originally an adjective). With respect to excessive crying in young infants, it has a poorly defined meaning that is connected to crying substantially more than the mean amount for age in an infant under 3 months. Usually this is thought to be a result of an intestinal (or "colic") disorder of paroxysmal pattern.

Normal Crying Time

In a 1962 study of 80 middle-class infants, Brazelton found the normal crying times, usually concentrated in the evening, to be as follows:

2 hr/day at 2 weeks of age
3 hr/day at 6 weeks of age
1 hr/day at 3 months of age

The clinical pattern of infant colic (also called paroxysmal fussing, infantile colic, evening colic, and 3-month colic) is well described:

1. Attacks occur suddenly, usually in the evening.
2. They are characterized by a loud, almost continuous cry.
3. They last several hours.
4. The face of the infant is flushed, with occasional circumoral pallor.
5. The abdomen is distended and tense.
6. Legs are drawn up on the abdomen and the feet often cold. Legs may extend periodically during forceful cries.
7. The fingers are clenched.
8. Relief is often noted from passage of flatus or feces.
9. The attack is not quelled for long by feeding, even though the infant may appear hungry and eats normally.
10. The attack usually terminates from apparent exhaustion.

No consistent etiology has been identified.

Reference: Brazelton TB: Crying in infants. Pediatrics 29:579, 1962.

Inconsolable Crying

Nothing is as troublesome both to parent and physician as an infant who cries inconsolably. Diagnoses to consider when confronted with an infant who cries continuously, particularly if it is shrill or high-pitched, include:

A corneal abrasion
An eyelash, or other foreign body, in the eye
Glaucoma
Colic and intussusception
Shaken baby syndrome
Meningitis
Fractures
A DPT reaction
An open diaper pin in the skin
Strand of hair wrapped around finger or penis

Reference: Harkness MJ: Corneal abrasion in infancy as a cause of inconsolable crying. Pediatric Emerg Care 5:242, 1989.

CYANOSIS

Common Causes

Acrocyanosis (especially cold stress)
Apnea of prematurity
Aspiration
    Direct (swallowing disorders,
      neuromuscular disease)
    Indirect (gastroesophageal
      reflux, emesis)
Atelectasis
Breath holding
Bronchiolitis
Congenital heart disease
    Decreased pulmonary blood flow
        (no pulmonary hypertension)
      Anomalous systemic venous
        return
      Ebstein's anomaly
      Hypoplastic right ventricle
      Pulmonary stenosis/atresia
      Tetralogy of Fallot
      Tricuspid stenosis/atresia/
        insufficiency
    Eisenmenger's syndrome
    Increased pulmonary blood flow
      Arteriovenous (AV) canal
      Coarctation (preductal)
      Hypoplastic left heart
      Total anomalous pulmonary
        venous return (TAPVR)

Congenital heart disease *(Cont.)*
    Increased pulmonary blood
      flow *(Cont.)*
    Transposition
    Truncus arteriosus
    Ventricular septal defect
      (VSD), large
    Pump failure
    Aortic stenosis (severe)
    Coarctation (postductal)
    Patent ductus arteriosus (PDA)
    VSD
Croup
Crying
Drugs—respiratory depressants
    (e.g., narcotics, benzodiazepines)
Hyaline membrane disease
Mucous plug
Nasal obstruction
Pneumonia
Pulmonary edema
Reactive airway disease
Seizures
Sepsis
Sleep apnea (tonsillar/adenoidal
    hypertrophy)

Uncommon Causes

Abdominal distention
Arterial thrombosis
Bronchopulmonary dysplasia
Chest wall abnormalities
    Congenital bone/cartilage
      abnormalities
    Pectus
    Flail chest
Cystic fibrosis
Epiglottitis
Foreign body
Hypovolemia
Mediastinal mass
Persistent fetal circulation
Pickwickian syndrome

Pleural effusion
Pneumothorax
Polycythemia
Pulmonary hemorrhage
Retropharyngeal/peritonsillar abscess
Scoliosis
Tracheal compression
    Abscess
    Adenopathy
    Hemorrhage
    Tumor
    Vascular ring
Tracheobronchomalacia/stenosis
Venous stasis

Rare Causes

Angioedema
Bronchogenic cyst
Central nervous system disease
  Edema
  Hemorrhage
  Infection
  Trauma
Chylothorax
Diaphragmatic hernia
Factitious (blue paint/dyes/makeup)
Glossoptosis
Hemoglobinopathy
  (M, low oxygen affinity)
Hypoplastic lungs
Laryngeal web
Lobar emphysema
Methemoglobinemia
  Methemoglobin reductase
    deficiency
  Oxidant stress
    Acetophenetidin
    Antimalarials
    Benzocaine
    Crayons
    Disinfectants
    EDTA
    Hydralazine
    Marking dyes
    Naphthalene
    Nitrites
      Amyl/butyl nitrate
      Nitrate-contaminated well water
      Nitrate food additive
      Nitroglycerin
      Plant nitrates (e.g., carrots grown in contaminated soil)

Methemoglobinemia *(Cont.)*
  Oxidant stress *(Cont.)*
    Nitroprusside
    Prilocaine
    Pyridium
    Sulfonamides
    Vitamin K analogs
Ondine's curse
Primary pulmonary hypertension
Pulmonary AV malformation/fistula
Pulmonary embolism/thrombosis
Pulmonary hemosiderosis
Pulmonary sequestration
Pulmonary tumor (primary
  or metastatic)
Respiratory muscle dysfunction
  Botulism
  Muscular dystrophy
  Myasthenia gravis
  Neuromuscular blockade
  Phrenic nerve damage
  Werdnig-Hoffmann disease
Superior vena cava (SVC) syndrome
Tracheoesophageal fistula
Tumor
Vocal cord paralysis

CYSTIC FIBROSIS

The Thirty Faces of Cystic Fibrosis

Cystic fibrosis is the great imitator. It may first present in utero with a picture of meconium peritonitis or its first manifestation may be sterility in the adult male. Listed below are 30 ways the disease may first manifest itself. Be suspicious and perform a sweat test when these problems are encountered without a plausible alternative explanation.

Meconium ileus and meconium
  peritonitis
Pancreatic insufficiency
  and growth failure
Recurrent pulmonary infections
Intestinal impaction and obstruction
Hypoproteinemia in infancy,
  with edema and anemia
Rectal prolapse
Cholestatic jaundice in neonates
Cirrhosis of the liver
Portal hypertension
Glucose intolerance
Diabetes
Acute or recurrent pancreatitis
Vitamin K deficiency and bleeding
Vitamin A deficiency
Vitamin E deficiency with
  neurologic abnormalities

Night cramps
Lactase deficiency
Duodenal ulcer
Cholelithiasis and cholecystitis
Chronic obstructive airway disease
Cor pulmonale
Recurrent episodes of asthma
Hypertrophic pulmonary
  osteoarthropathy
Nasal polyps
Optic neuritis
Salty taste of infant noted by
  the mother
Hyponatremic dehydration in warm
  weather
Hypochloremia metabolic alkalosis
Heat stroke
Infertility in males

CYSTITIS

Hemicystitis: Think Zoster!

There exists a fascinating clinical entity known as hemicystitis, which is an infection limited to one half of the bladder. It occurs with herpes zoster infection of the bladder in which vesicles are unilateral, conforming to the affected nerve supply.

Reference: Nelson JD, McCracken GH: Newsletter. Pediatr Infect Dis 16(8):16, 1990.

CYTOMEGALOVIRUS

Cytomegalovirus Infection in the Newborn

Cytomegalovirus (CMV) is the most common herpes infection that occurs during the neonatal period. Exposure to CMV can occur from a congenital source (e.g., either a primary infection in a seronegative mother or reactivation of latent virus in a seropositive mother), a natal source such as vaginal delivery in a mother shedding virus from the cervix, or postnatal sources (e.g., breast milk from a seropositive mother, blood transfusion from a seropositive donor, or close contact with individuals actively shedding CMV).

CMV is especially dangerous to the developing fetus when the pregnant woman is experiencing primary infection; in such cases there is a 30% mortality rate among those CMV-infected infants who were symptomatic at birth. Surviving infants who were symptomatic at birth encounter the following sequelae: microcephaly (70%), moderate-to-severe mental retardation (61%), hearing loss (30%), and chorioretinitis (22%). Symptomatic infants without neurologic signs at birth remain at risk for such sequelae as failure to thrive, microcephaly, spastic quadriplegia, and deafness during the first year of life. Asymptomatic infants of mothers experiencing a primary CMV infection are at risk for hearing defects and moderate-to-severe brain damage. Conversely, infants and fetuses who become infected with CMV as a result of recurrent viremia or perinatal exposure to a seropositive mother are generally protected from symptomatic infection of any kind. A minority of such infants, however, may be at risk for hearing defects and learning problems.

Clinical Manifestations of CMV Infection
(among infants born to previously seronegative mothers)

Prenatal Infection

Hepatomegaly
Hyperbilirubinemia
Petechiae/thrombocytopenia
Microcephaly
Hydrocephalus
Periventricular calcifications

Chorioretinitis
Optic atrophy
Strabismus
Microphthalmia
Cataracts
Deafness

Infection During Vaginal Delivery

Protracted pneumonitis

Postnatal Infection

Healthy infants and children who acquire CMV infection suffer no permanent sequelae and usually remain entirely asymptomatic. Symptomatic infection does occur rarely, however, and may include the following:

Fever
Hepatomegaly
Pneumonia

Reference: LaRussa P: Perinatal herpes virus infections. Ped Ann 13:659–670, 1984.

D

DAY CARE

What You Ought to Know About Your Day Care Center

With more and more parents relying on day care centers, clinicians need to be knowledgeable about what to look for in selecting such a center. One source of information both for parents and clinicians is the National Association for Child Care Resource and Referral Agency (NACCRRA), 2116 Campus Drive SE, Rochester, MN 55904 (507) 287-2220. This clearinghouse advises parents and others on how to select a safe and reliable day care center.

Clinicians should urge parents to visit their day care center frequently (and unannounced) in order to make sure their children are cared for in a loving and positive manner.

Parents also need to observe their children closely for behavioral changes such as depression, aggressiveness, fear of the day care center, and signs of physical abuse (e.g, bruises, abrasions) or neglect (e.g., diaper rash, bald spots on the back of the head indicating that the infant has been left supine all day, extreme hunger, etc.).

In the case of older toddlers who are left in day care, parents should ask the child what activities are offered during the day. Are constructive games and teaching employed or is the child merely parked in front of a television set?

Reference: Hoekelman RA: Day care, day care: Mayday! mayday! Pediatr Ann 20:403–404, 1991.

Pathogens Transmitted in Day Care Centers

Approximately 11 million children under the age of 6 years spend all or part of their day in a day care center. Some experts have predicted that by the year 2000, 80% of all American mothers will be a part of the nation's workforce. The result, of course, is an ever-increasing reliance upon day care. One of the most frequent questions that comes up regarding day care has to do with parents worrying about the risk of infections in the day care setting. The table below summarizes the most common pathogens you need to be aware of:

Pathogens Transmitted in Day Care Centers*

MODE OF TRANSMISSIONS	BACTERIA	VIRUSES	PARASITES
Direct	Group A streptococci *Staphylococcus aureus*	Herpes simplex Herpes zoster	Pediculosis Scabies

Table continued on next page.

Pathogens Transmitted in Day Care Centers* (Cont.)

MODE OF TRANSMISSIONS	BACTERIA	VIRUSES	PARASITES
Respiratory	*Haemophilus influenzae* *Neisseria meningitidis* *Bordetella pertussis* Mycobacterium tuberculosis	Adenovirus Coxsakie A16 (hand-foot-mouth disease) Epstein-Barr virus HHV6 (roseola) Influenza Measles Mumps Parainfluenza Parvovirus B19 (fifth disease) Respiratory syncytial virus Rhinovirus Rubella Varicella	
Fecal-oral	*Campylobacter* spp *Escherichia coli* *Salmonella* *Shigella* *Yersinia*	Enteroviruses Hepatitis A Rotavirus	*Cryptosporidium* *Entamoeba histolytica* *Giardia lamblia* *Hymenolepsis nana* (dwarf tapeworm) Pinworms
Contact with infected blood and secretions (urine, saliva)		Cytomegalovirus Hepatitis B Herpes simplex Human immunodeficiency virus[†]	

* Adapted from Hendley OJ: How germs are spread. In Donowitz LG (ed): Infection Control in the Child Care Center and Preschool. Baltimore, Williams & Wilkins, 1991.
[†] To date no reported cases of HIV infection are known to have resulted from transmission in day care centers.

Reference: Van R, Wun C-C, Morrow AL, Pickering LK: The effect of diaper type and overclothing on fecal contamination in day-care centers. JAMA 265:1840–1844, 1991.

DEHYDRATION

Predictable Fall of the Blood Urea Nitrogen (BUN) in a Dehydrated Child

Is the increased BUN in a child with diarrhea and vomiting always the result of simple dehydration or can it reflect the presence of associated renal disease? Brill and coworkers found that the rate of fall of BUN in a dehydrated child with normal renal function was predictable. They plotted BUN levels against time on semilogarithmic graph paper. BUN had fallen to one-half the admission level in 24 hours or less in all children with uncomplicated dehydration and diarrhea.

Line A in the accompanying figure represents the slope along which the BUN should fall in a child without renal disease or excess nitrogen load (e.g., gastrointestinal bleed). Lines B and C represent 2½ standard deviations on either side of that rate of fall.

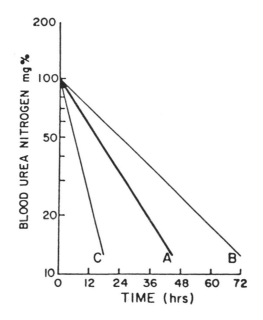

Complicating disease should be investigated in the dehydrated child whose BUN does not fall at a rate parallel to line A or within 2½ standard deviations from that rate.

Reference: Brill CB, Uretsky S, Gribetz D: J Pediatr 52:197, 1973. Adapted from McMillan JA, et al: The Whole Pediatrician Catalog. Philadelphia, W.B. Saunders, 1977, p 97.

DERMATOLOGY

Skin Lesions

Can you speak "dermatologese"? Or is it "dermaterminology"? In any event, understanding dermatology is impossible without a working knowledge of the sometimes exotic vocabulary of the specialty. The following list defines some (but by no means all) of the more commonly used terms for skin lesions and related structures and conditions.

Abscess—A localized accumulation of purulent material so deep in the dermis or subcutaneous tissue that pus is usually not visible on the surface of the skin.

Atrophy—An acquired loss of underlying tissue causing skin depression with intact epidermis.

Bulla—A relatively large vesicle (diameter 0.5 cm).

Carbuncle—Coalescence of several furuncles (see below).

Comedo (pl., comedones)—A greasy plug in a sebaceous follicle capped by a layer of melanin, hence its black appearance (blackhead).

Crust—Dried exudate of body fluids (serous and/or hemorrhagic).

Cyst—A sac that contains liquid or semisolid material.

Erosion—A superficial deficit of epithelium.

Erythema—Increased redness of skin from capillary dilatation.

Excoriations—Linear, angular erosions caused usually by scratching.

Furuncle—A deep necrotizing form of folliculitis with pus accumulation.

Figurate lesions—Lesions forming rings and arcs, usually erythematous.

Hyperpigmentation—Excessive pigmentation of any origin.

Hypopigmentation—Loss of pigmentation of any origin.

Keratosis—Benign horny lesion (also called *keratoma*).

Lichenification—A proliferation of keratinocytes and stratum corneum forming a plaque-like structure. The skin appears thickened, and the skin markings appear accentuated. The process results from repeated rubbing.

Macule—A circumscribed area of change (less than 2 cm in diameter) in normal skin color without elevation or depression of the surface in relation to the surrounding skin.

Milia—Small, firm, white papules filled with keratin.

Nodule—A palpable, solid, round, or ellipsoid lesion; it can be located in the epidermis or extend into the dermis or subcutaneous tissue.

Papule—A solid elevated lesion generally understood to be less than 1 cm in diameter.

Patch—A large, flat lesion (greater than 2 cm in diameter) with color different from surrounding skin. Differs from *macule* only in size.

Plaque—Elevation above the skin surface that occupies a relatively large surface area in comparison with its height above the skin.

Pustule—A circumscribed elevation of skin that contains a purulent exudate. (Follicular pustules are conical and usually contain a hair in the center.)

Rash—An inflammatory skin eruption.

Scale—A thin, platelike, external layer of horny epidermis.

Scar—Change in skin character—a mark—secondary to trauma or inflammation.

Sclerosis—Circumscribed or diffuse hardening or induration in the skin.

Tag—Small, sessile protuberance of skin.

Telangiectases—Permanent dilatations of blood capillaries that may or may not disappear with the pressure of a glass slide.

Tumor—A firm, solid, raised growth greater than 5 cm in diameter.

Ulcer—A deep, local deficit or excavation of skin and underlying tissue.

Vesicle—A small (less than 0.5 cm in diameter) fluid-filled lesion. A "dew-drop."

Wart—A benign keratotic tumor.

Wheal—A rounded or flat-topped elevation in the skin that is characteristically evanescent, disappearing within hours. Lesions are the result of edema in the upper layers of the dermis.

Dermatologic Manifestations of Viral and Bacterial Infections

There are a number of cutaneous manifestations associated with bacterial and viral infections common among children. The specific skin lesions that appear are usually the result of various pathways involved in inflammation and necrosis, such as the complement casacade, localized or generalized Schwartzman reactions, factors that yield hypotension and disseminated intravascular coagulation, and a host of yet undiscovered factors. The table lists the dermatologic manifestations of common pediatric bacterial and viral infections and should be useful in the bedside evaluation of the patient presenting with "fever and a rash."

References: Pediatric viral infections. In Roche Handbook of Differential Diagnosis 6(18):3–19, 1989. Yamanishi K, et al: Identification of human herpesvirus-6 as a causal agent for exanthem subitum. Lancet i:1065–1067, 1988.

Differential Diagnosis of Pediatric Infections with Dermatologic Manifestations

CLINICAL ENTITY	CAUSATIVE AGENT	AGE	CLINICAL SYNDROME	TYPE OF RASH	DISTRBUTION	SIMILAR ENTITIES
Roseola infantum (exanthem subitum)	Herpesvirus-6*	6 months–4 years	Fever, irritability; rapid lysis of fever with appearance of rash	Discrete macular or papular rash	Trunk with extension to neck, extremities, face	
Erythema infectiosum (fifth disease)	Parvovirus B-19	School-age children Infants, adults less common	Flu-like illness	Bilateral erythema of cheeks: "slapped cheeks" Lacy-reticular exanthem	Face, trunk, extremities; palms/soles spared	Scarlet fever Rubella
Measles	Measles virus	All ages	Fever, cough; coryza; conjunctivitis	Koplik spots Maculopapular eruption of upper trunk, face; spreads to lower trunk, extremities; becomes confluent	Starts on face, moves downward	Enteroviral infection Mycoplasma Drug eruption
Hand-foot-and-mouth disease	*Primary:* Coxsackie A viruses *Secondary:* Coxsackie B viruses; enterovirus 71	<10 years	Fever, anorexia; oral pain	Oral: discrete, ulcerative Skin: maculopapular, vesicular	Anterior mouth, hands, feet; occasionally trunk, face	Aphthous stomatitis Varicella Herpes simplex
Varicella	Varicella-zoster virus	90% of cases <15 years	Fever; pruritus; malaise	Maculopapular, then vesicles on erythematous base, which rupture Crusting as final stage	Diffuse, includes scalp, oral mucosa	Insect bites Herpes simplex
Periorbital buccal cellulitis	*Primary:* *H. influenzae* type B *Secondary:* *S. pneumoniae,* *S. aureus* β-hemolytic streptococci	3–36 months	Fever; bacteremia	Unilateral indurated cellulitis Indistinct borders Violaceous hue	Periorbital, cheek	Orbital cellulitis Parotitis
Staphylococcal scalded-skin syndrome	*S. aureus*	Infants	Fever, irritability; septicemia (rare); eye, nasal discharge	Tender, diffuse erythematous rash progressing to bullae Positive Nikolsky sign Exfoliation	Diffuse	Bullous impetigo *E. multiforme* Toxic epidermal necrolysis Pemphigus Epidermolysis bullosa Kawasaki disease

References: Pediatric viral infections. In Roche Handbook of Differential Diagnosis 6(18):3–19, 1989.
*Yamanishi K, et al: Identification of human herpesvirus-6 as a causal agent for exanthem subitum. Lancet i:1065–1067, 1988.

Seborrheic Dermatitis or Atopic Dermatitis?

Many clinicians have difficulty distinguishing these two common entities. Seborrhea is the excretion by the sebaceous glands of abnormally copius amounts of grease-like sebum. There is usually no underlying disorder. Atopy is a form of immediate hypersensitivity reaction to certain common allergens that produce the IgE antibody, reagin, and atopic dermatitis is the dermal manifestation of the allergic reaction. The following table should help you further to differentiate between the two conditions.

Seborrheic Dermatitis vs. Atopic Dermatitis

	SEBORRHEIC DERMATITIS	ATOPIC DERMATITIS
Family history of allergy	15–25%	40–60%
Character of individual lesions	Dry, scaly, "potato chip" lesion that may or may not appear greasy	Erythema, papules, vesicles, weeping, scales, lichenification, or a combination. May have superimposed pyoderma
Color of lesion	Only slightly erythematous, but more often of a salmon, yellow, or brown color	In acute phase, always red and often of an intense redness
Feature of lesion	More intense color at periphery—clearing at center. Appears sharply demarcated	More red at center. Gradually tapers out at periphery, fading into normal skin
Vesicles	Never present	Present in acute phase
Weeping and edema	Absent	Always present at some time in evolution of disease
Lichenification	Absent	Characteristic of late stage
Pruritus	Mild or moderate	Paroxysmal and severe

Reference: Perlman HH: Helpful diagnostic clues for differentiation of atopic dermatitis from seborrheic dermatitis. Ann Allergy 23:583, 1965.

DEVELOPMENT

Developmental Delay: Seeking the Etiology

As we learn from medical school on, the physician's best diagnostic tools are the history and physical exam. This dictum certainly holds true in the work-up of developmental delay.

Regardless of the age of the child at presentation, there are several strategies that the pediatrician can employ in the search for an etiology. The What, When, and How are invariably asked. The answers will often guide the parents in the decision to have another child and how to come to terms with their child's disability. The following guidelines and accompanying table should prove quite useful when confronted with a developmentally delayed patient.

1. Analyze the family's pedigree with attention paid to physical appearance, "birth defects," inheritance patterns of any disease, disabilities or dysmorphisms, consanguinity, and parental age. When possible, obtain photographs of the extended family.
2. Obtain a thorough prenatal history. Look for:
   a. First-trimester febrile illnesses; possible teratogenic exposures, including alcohol, cigarette, and drug use.
   b. First through second trimesters: viral illnesses, maternal diabetes mellitus, maternal medications, cardiorespiratory disease, and maternal metabolic abnormalities.
   c. First through third trimesters: see table.

Temporal Approach to the Etiology of Developmental Delay

CLASSIFICATION	ETIOLOGIC PERIOD	TYPICAL CAUSES
Genetic (Mendelian)	Preconceptional	Autosomal dominant Neurofibromatosis Tuberous sclerosis Autosomal recessive Phenylketonuria Galactosemia Tay-Sachs disease Sex-linked recessive Sex-linked nonspecific mental retardation Lesch-Nyhan syndrome Sex-linked dominant Albright's hereditary osteodystrophy
Chromosomal	Preconception or early mitotic phase	Polysomy Trisomy 21 (Down syndrome) Autosomal deletion Cri du chat syndrome (deletion of short arm 5) Sex chromosome aberrations Multiple-X syndromes Turner's syndrome
Multifactorial (genetic and environmental)	Preconception and first 12 weeks of gestation	Neural tube defects Meningomyelocele Encephalocele Hydrocephaly Cleft lip/cleft palate
Environmental	Prenatal First trimester (period of CNS morphogenesis and neuroblast proliferation)	Teratogenic agents (suspected) Phenytoin Maternal alcoholism Intrauterine infection
	Midpregnancy (period of neuroblast proliferation)	Intrauterine infection Maternal irradiation Teratogens

Table continued on next page.

Temporal Approach to the Etiology of Developmental Delay (Cont.)

CLASSIFICATION	ETIOLOGIC PERIOD	TYPICAL CAUSES	
Environmental *(Cont.)*	Prenatal *(Cont.)*		
	Midpregnancy to peri-natal period (rapid brain growth, glial cell prolifer-ation, myelinization, dendritic tree formation)	Intrauterine infection Preeclampsia Hemorrhage Hormonal disturbances Malnutrition Prematurity Teratogens	
	Perinatal	Intrapartum hemorrhage and anoxemia Trauma: Breech delivery Difficult delivery	
	Postnatal	Meningitis Malnutrition Head injury	Encephalitis Lead poisoning Near drowning

3. Obtain a birth history. Approximately 30% of the cases of developmental delay can be traced to difficulties in the prenatal period. It is wise, however, to avoid the temptation to overinterpret problems in labor and delivery. As often as possible, a hospital record of the birth and nursery stay should be procured.

4. Continue your detective work with a postnatal history. In addition to the causes listed in the table, inquire about any known metabolic diseases and their treatment, diarrheal illnesses with possible hypernatremia, failure to thrive, history of seizures, loss of milestones, and apparent receptive or expressive delays.

5. Examination of the patient: The physical exam should be undertaken with a fine-toothed comb.
   a. Height, weight, and head circumference are invaluable in the setting of developmental delay. [Refer to "Diagnosing Dysmorphism" (p. 95) or *Smith's Recognizable Patterns of Human Malformation: Genetic, Embryologic and Clinical Aspects* (Philadelphia, W.B. Saunders, 1988]. Microcephaly, macrocephaly, growth retardation, and growth acceleration may steer you toward a recognized syndrome and/or an etiology.
   b. Transilluminate the head if hydrocephaly, hydranencephaly, porencephaly, or cerebral cortical atrophy are in your differential. You may obviate the need for a CT scan with this simple test.
   c. Pay attention to the eye exam (see "Leukocoria: A Differential Diagnosis" [p. 204]). Look for a cherry red spot, chorioretinitis, retinitis pigmentosa, or rentrolental fibroplasia when examining the retina.
   d. Do not neglect to assess hearing. Unidentified hearing loss can lead to profound developmental delay.
   e. Proceed with the examination of the skin, facies, and body as if you were uncovering buried treasure. Remember that both major and minor abnormalities are more common in patients with developmental delay or frank mental retardation. Compile a list of your findings and consult the sources noted above, beginning with the least common abnormality.

6. Laboratory studies will often help secure a diagnosis, thus comforting the parents. They may also reveal chromosomal or metabolic abnormalities that will influence a couple's plans for other children. Consider pertinent laboratory studies, chromosomal analyses, viral cultures, computed tomography, and ultrasonography as you and the parents see the need.

References: Keele DK: The developmentally delayed child: Pursuing the etiologic work-up. Contemp Peds March:51–62, 1985.

Oski FA, et al: Principles and Practice of Pediatrics. Philadelphia, J.B. Lippincott, 1990.

The Draw-A-Person Test

Goodenough called her test the "Draw-a-man" test when she first introduced this superb simple screening test for intelligence. The name of the test has changed, but the test and its scoring have remained the same.

Basal age = 3 years. For each four criteria, add 1 year to arrive at mental age, between ages 3 and 10 years. Instruct child to draw *a complete person;* no further instructions.

$$\frac{\text{Maturation age}}{\text{Chronological age}} \times \frac{100}{1} = \text{IQ}$$

Twenty-eight criteria for scoring:
1. Head present
2. Legs present
3. Arms present
4. Trunk present
5. Length of trunk greater than breadth
6. Shoulder indicated
7. Both arms and legs attached to trunk
8. Legs attached to trunk and arms to trunk at correct point
9. Neck present
10. Outline of neck continuous with that of head or trunk, or both
11. Eyes present
12. Nose present
13. Mouth present
14. Both nose and mouth in two dimensions, two lips shown
15. Nostrils indicated
16. Hair shown
17. Hair on more than circumference of head, nontransparent, better than scribble
18. Clothing present
19. Two articles of clothing, nontransparent
20. Entire drawing, with sleeves and trousers shown, free from transparency
21. Four or more articles of clothing definitely indicated
22. Costume complete without incongruities
23. Fingers shown
24. Correct number of fingers shown
25. Fingers in two dimensions, length greater than breadth, angle subtended not greater than 180 degrees
26. Opposition of thumbs shown
27. Hand shown as distinct from fingers or arms
28. Arm joint shown; either elbow, shoulder, or both

Reference: Goodenough-Harris Drawing Test. New York, Harcourt Brace Jovanovich, 1963.

Watching for Developmental Lags

Parents often ask, "When should I expect my child to do _____?" When should you, as a clinician, begin to worry about the possibility of developmental delay? The following table includes many of the warning signs indicative of abnormal patterns of development. In many cases, the presence or absence of any one sign may mean nothing if the rest of development is normal, but certain signs, in and of themselves, are very important (e.g., no social smile at age 6 months).

Indications for Further Evaluation for Developmental Delay

At 3 mo.	Does not react to sudden noises. Does not appear to listen to a speaker's voice. Does not try to find the speaker's face with his or her eyes. Has not begun to vocalize sounds. Has been left to lie in a crib for hours without visual or auditory stimulation. Does not raise the head when lying on the stomach.
At 6 mo.	Does not turn to the speaking person. Does not respond to being played with. Is not visually alert. Never laughs or smiles. Is not babbling. Does not reach for or try to pick up a toy. Is not learning to sit up. Does not appear to be gaining weight. Does not arch the back when lying on the stomach and raising the head.
At 1 yr.	Has not been responding to "Pat-a-Cake," "Peek-A-Boo," or other baby games. Is not imitating a variety of speech sounds. Is not saying two or three words such as "bye-bye, mama, dada." Is not pulling up to a standing position.
At 18 mo.	Is not yet beginning to feed itself with a spoon. Does not imitate speech or vocalize in jargon. Is not moving about to explore. Does not give eye contact. Has not or does not spontaneously squat when picking up objects.
At 2 yrs.	Is not naming a few familiar objects and using a few two- or three-word phrases. Is not noticing animals, cars, trucks, trains. Is not beginning to play symbolically with housekeeping toys, little cars. Is not moving about vigorously, running, climbing, exploring. Avoids eye contact. Does not seem to focus eyes on a large picture. Engages in rocking or head banging for extensive periods of time. Is not walking up stairs.
At 3 yrs.	Does not seem aware of other children, of adults, of the weather, traffic, and so forth Uses little or no speech. Does not engage in imitative play symbolic of adult activities. Avoids looking at pictures or pointing to pictures of familiar objects Does not follow simple directions.

Table continued on next page.

Indications for Further Evaluation for Developmental Delay (Cont.)

At 3 yrs. *(Cont.)*	Engages for long periods of time in repetitive behaviors like flipping pages of a magazine, or spinning a wheel on a little truck, head banging, and so forth. Cannot ride a tricycle if given plenty of opportunity to do so.
At 4 yrs.	Does not have at least partially understandable speech with sentences. Uses echolalic speech or frequent, bizarre, meaningless sounds. Does not focus visually on pictures. Does not seem interested in listening to a simple story about his or her experiences. Repeatedly tests all limits. Is so quiet and conforming that he or she never tests or tries anything new. Has pronounced fears and phobias. Frequently engages in flapping of the arms or flipping of the hands to express excitement. Runs about from one thing to another every minute or so without getting fully involved in an activity. Is still untrained in toileting (occasional slips do occur at this age). Does not draw some sort of representation of human beings (at least a head and a few features), if crayons or pencils have been available to the child. Stays on the periphery of the playroom, paying no attention to other children for some weeks, after most children have overcome shyness and begun to play with or near other children. Avoids eye contact. Engages in head banging or rocking. Cannot tolerate change or frustration without frequent 2-year-old tantrums.

Reference: Accardo, PJ, Capute AJ: The Pediatrician and the Developmentally Delayed Child: A Clinical Textbook on Mental Retardation. Baltimore, University Park Press, 1979.

DIABETES

Classification and Etiology of Diabetes Mellitus

Classification of Diabetes Mellitus

IDIOPATHIC	SECONDARY
Insulin-dependent (type I)	Pancreatic trauma, disease, or resection
Non-insulin dependent (type II)	Hormone-induced
Maturity onset diabetes of youth (MODY)	Drugs and chemical agents
	Genetic syndromes
	Insulin receptor abnormalities
	Other types

From Lebovitz HE: Etiology and pathogenesis of diabetes mellitus. Pediatr Clin North Am 31:524, 1984, with permission.

Although the majority of cases of pediatric diabetes mellitus will be of the type I classification, the remaining idiopathic and secondary etiologies cannot be overlooked. Some clues in establishing a diagnosis between type I and type II are provided in the following table:

Insulin-Dependent vs. Non-Insulin-Dependent Diabetes

	INSULIN-DEPENDENT	NON-INSULIN-DEPENDENT
1. Association with HLA B8/D3 or HLA B15/D4	2.5 × expected frequency	Same frequency as normal population
2. Pancreatic insulin content	0	>50% of normal
3. Anti-islet antibodies	85%	<5%
4. Primary insulin resistance	Minimal	Marked
5. Concordance rate of identical twins for diabetes mellitus	25 to 50%	~100%

From Lebovitz HE: Etiology and pathogenesis of diabetes mellitus. Pediatr Clin North Am 31:525, 1984, with permission.

The secondary causes of diabetes mellitus are too numerous to cover adequately in this text. There are, however, a number of hormonal and chemical causes that deserve mention, principally because treatment of the primary disorder in hormonal abnormalities and removal of the offending agent in chemically induced diabetes mellitus frequently reverse the disease process.

Hormonally Induced Diabetes Mellitus

ABNORMALITY	PREVALENCE (WHERE KNOWN)
Acromegaly	20%
Cushing's syndrome	20%
Primary aldosteronism	—
Pheochromocytomas	—
Glucagonoma	—

Diabetogenic Drugs

Diuretics and Antihypertensives	Psychoactive Agents	Analgesic, Antipyretic and Anti-inflammatory Agents
Chlorthalidone	Chlorprothixene	Indomethacin
Clonidine	Haloperidol	
Diazoxide	Lithium carbonate	**Antineoplastic Agents**
Furosemide	Phenothiazines	Alloxan
Metalazone	Tricyclic antidepressants	L-Asparaginase
Thiazides	**Catecholamine and Other Neurologically Active Agents**	Streptozotocin
Hormonally Active Agents	Diphenylhydantoin	**Miscellaneous**
ACTH	Epinephrine	Isoniazid
Glucagon	Isoproterenol	Nicotinic acid
Glucocorticoids	Levodopa	
Oral contraceptives	Norepinephrine	
Growth hormones		
Thyroid hormones (thyrotoxic doses)		

From Lebovitz HE: Etiology and pathogenesis of diabetes mellitus. Pediatr Clin North Am 31:527, 1984, with permission.

Diagnosis of Diabetes Mellitus

In the presence of symptoms, the diagnosis of diabetes mellitus is an uncomplicated task: a child presenting with polydipsia, polyuria, polyphagia, and weight loss with an accompanying elevation of blood glucose and/or ketonemia leads the pediatrician to a rapid answer. In the absence of symptoms or the presence of mild symptoms, however, the diagnosis of diabetes mellitus is much more difficult.

In children, the diagnostic criteria for diabetes mellitus are as follows:

1. Presence of symptoms of diabetes, such as polydipsia, polyuria, ketonuria, and weight loss, together with a random plasma glucose of 200 mg/dl

or

2. In asymptomatic children, both an elevated fasting glucose concentration and a sustained elevated glucose concentration during an oral glucose tolerance test (1.75 g/kg up to maximum of 75 g) on two or more occasions.

Fasting value:

Venous plasma $\geq$ 140 mg/dl
Venous blood $\geq$ 120 mg/dl
Capillary blood $\geq$ 120 mg/dl

2-hour OGTT value and an intervening value:

Venous plasma $\geq$ 200 mg/dl
Venous blood $\geq$ 180 mg/dl
Capillary blood $\geq$ 200 mg/dl

Reference: Adapted from Lebovitz HE: Etiology and pathogenesis of diabetes mellitus. Pediatr Clin North Am 31:521–523, 1984.

Diabetic Ketoacidosis

Despite continued advances in control of the diabetic child, diabetic ketoacidosis remains an acute medical emergency. In the known and presenting diabetic child, ketoacidosis is defined as "hyperglycemia with a blood glucose exceeding 300 mg/dl, ketonemia with total ketones (β hydroxybutyrate and acetoacetate) in serum exceeding 3 mmol/L or positive at a 1:2 dilution in serum or undiluted urine with the sodium nitroprusside reaction (Acetest; Ketostix; Chemstrips UGK), and acidosis with pH reduced to less than 7.30 or reduced serum bicarbonate to less than 15 mEq/L." The maintenance requirements for fluid and electrolyte therapy for diabetic ketoacidosis are outlined below. The clinician should keep in mind that these values represent averages and that the extent of dehydration and electrolyte imbalances vary with the duration of symptoms, the possible presence of vomiting, and prior insulin administration.

Fluid and Electrolyte Maintenance in Diabetic Ketoacidosis

	MAINTENANCE REQUIREMENTS*	LOSSES[†]
Water	1500 ml/m²	100 ml/kg (range 60–100 ml/kg)
Sodium	45 mEq/m²	6 mEq/kg (range 5–13 mEq/kg)
Potassium	35 mEq/m²	5 mEq/kg (range 4–6 mEq/kg)
Chloride	30 mEq/m²	4 mEq/kg (range 3–9 mEq/kg)
Phosphate	~10 mEq/m²	3 mEq/kg (range 2–5 mEq/kg)

* Maintenance is expressed in surface area to permit uniformity because fluid requirements change as weight increases.
[†] Losses are expressed per unit of body weight, since the losses remain relatively constant as a function of total body weight.

Reference: Sperling M: Diabetic ketoacidosis. Pediatr Clin North Am 31:591–610, 1984, with permission.

Glycosylated Hemoglobin Assay

The glycosylated hemoglobin assay provides the clinician with a profile of glycemia during the previous 60 to 120 days. This is helpful in ascertaining inter-visit glycemia control and to determine the relationship between complications and compliance. The issue of compliance is particularly important in early adolescence, when responsibility for glycemic control shifts from the parents to the teenager.

Estimate of Blood Glucose Control Using Glycosylated Hemoglobin Assay

GLYCOSYLATED HEMOGLOBIN (%)	PROBABLE BLOOD GLUCOSE RANGE (mg/dl)	ESTIMATE OF "CONTROL"
5.4–7.4	60–120	Normal range
8– 9	120–150	Excellent
9–10	150–180	Good
10–11	180–220	Fair
11–12	220–260	Fair
12–13	260–300	Fair to poor
> 13	> 300	Very poor

Reference: Spack NP: Diabetes mellitus in adolescence. Adolescent Medicine State of the Art Reviews 2:529, 1991, with permission.

The Diabetic Patient with Concomitant Systemic Disease

The following guidelines are intended to assist the clinician or other caregiver in managing the diabetic patient with additional illness:

Guidelines to Sick Day Management

1. Never skip insulin administration.

2. Check blood glucose and urinary ketones every 4–6 hours

3. Give supplemental short-acting insulin every 4 hours for elevated blood sugar and additional dose amounts for hyperglycemia with ketonuria.

4. Evaluate and treat the underlying illness.

5. If blood glucose levels are low (less than 120 mg/dl), reduce short-acting insulin and give glucose-containing fluids.

6. If adequate fluid intake cannot be maintained or vomiting persists for more than 2 hours, intravenous hydration is necessary.

7. Notify a clinician if blood glucose is more than 400 mg/dl with moderate to large acetone or change in patient's level of alertness or signs of dehydration (weighing every 6 hours may be a useful guide.

Reference: Spack NP: Diabetes mellitus in adolescents. Adolescent Medicine State of the Art Reviews 2:511, 1991, with permission.

DIARRHEA—CHRONIC

Common Causes

Antibiotic-induced
Carbohydrate malabsorption, hereditary
   Lactose
Chemotherapy-induced
Cystic fibrosis
Dietary
   Allergy (milk, soy, other)
   Overfeeding

Infection
   Bacterial
   Human immunodeficiency
     virus (HIV)
   Parasitic
Postinfectious
   Carbohydrate malabsorption

Uncommon Causes

Anatomic lesions
   Hirschsprung's disease
   Malrotation
Celiac disease
Irritable bowel syndrome
Malnutrition, starvation

Necrotizing enterocolitis
Parenteral infections
   Otitis media
   Urinary tract infections
Regional enteritis
Ulcerative colitis

Rare Causes

Abeta- and hypobetalipoproteinemia
Adrenal insufficiency
Biliary atresia
Blind loop syndrome
Carbohydrate malabsorption
   Sucrose, isomaltose, glucose, galactose
Chronic hepatitis
Enterokinase deficiency
Familial chloride diarrhea
Ganglioneuroma
Hyperthyroidism
Immune deficiency
   Combined immune deficiency
   Hypogammaglobulinemia
   IgA deficiency

Intestinal ischemia
Intestinal lymphangiectasia
Intestinal pseudo-obstruction
Mesenteric artery insufficiency
Neuroblastoma
Pancreatic insufficiency and
   neutropenia (Schwachman-
     Diamond-Oski syndrome)
Pancreatic tumors
Radiation-induced
Short gut syndrome
Small bowel tumors;
   lymphosarcoma
Wolman's disease

The Common Bacterial Causes of Bloody Diarrhea

The association of diarrhea and the passage of small amounts of blood in the stool (hematochezia) can be due simply to hemorrhoids or mucosal tears caused by spasm, hypermotility, or irritation at the mucocutaneous junction. The persistent case of hematochezia associated with diarrhea, however, is most likely indicative of an infectious or inflammatory etiology. In the pediatric patient, bloody diarrhea is usually a result of an infectious enteric pathogen.

The following table summarizes the types and manifestations of bloody diarrhea caused by bacterial pathogens.

Bloody Diarrhea of Bacterial Origin

INFECTIOUS AGENT	AGE CHILD MOST AFFECTED	USUAL INCUBATION PERIOD	USUAL SOURCE OF ACQUISITION	SEASON	PRESENTING SIGNS & SYMPTOMS	MAIN PATHO-PHYSIOLOGICAL MECHANISM
Shigella	6 mo–3 yr	36–72°	Fecal-oral; contaminated food or water	Warm months	Fever, abdominal pain watery diarrhea becoming bloody	Enteroinvasive; cytopathic
Salmonella	Infants <2 yr sometimes older	24–48°	Oral via contaminated food or water	Warm months	Vomiting, abdominal pain, diarrhea—dysentery-like	Enteroinvasive
Campylobacter	Infants and children <6 yr	2–7 d	Oral via contaminated food or water; infected pets	Warm months	Severe abdominal pain, bloody diarrhea	Cytolytic exotoxin
Yersinia	Toddlers to teenagers	3–4 d	Oral via contaminated food or water; person-to-person	Cooler months	Fever, abdominal pain, vomiting, diarrhea	Enteroinvasive; enterotoxigenic
C. difficile	All ages after neonatal period	1–6 wk	Almost always requires prior exposure to antibiotics, especially ampicillin, clindamycin, cephalosporins	All year	Abdominal pain, diarrhea, distention, blood in stool	Cytotoxin
Escherichia coli a. Enteroinvasive	All ages	24–72°	Fecal-oral; contaminated food or water	Warm months	Fever, chills, abdominal pain, watery diarrhea becoming dysentery-like	Enteroinvasive; cytopathic
b. Entero-pathogenic	All ages	1–3 d	Fecal-oral; contaminated food or water	Warm months	Fever, nausea, cramps watery or bloody diarrhea in some serotypes	Cytotoxin; enteroinvasive
N. gonorrheae	Teenagers	2–7 d	Anal intercourse	All year	Dysentery, odynochezia	Enteroinvasive; cytotoxic
C. trachomatis	Teenagers	2–3 wk	Anal intercourse	All year	Dysentery, odynochezia	Enteroinvasive; cytotoxic

Bloody Diarrhea of Bacterial Origin (Cont.)

INFECTIOUS AGENT	STOOL FINDINGS	LABORATORY	ENDOSCOPY	HISTOLOGY	BARIUM ENEMA	Rx
Shigella	Blood, WBCs	Band forms > segmented forms	Mild-to-severe colitis	Acute inflammation	Normal to colitis-like, mucosal ulcers	Trimethoprim-sulfamethoxazole
Salmonella	Blood, WBCs	Normal to ↑WBC L shift	Mild colitis	Acute focal inflammation	Normal to colitis-like	None except in sick infant <1 yr: chloramphenicol, ampicillin, trimethoprim-sulfamethoxazole
Campylobacter	Blood, WBCs	Normal to ↑WBC	Colitis-like	Focal or diffuse acute inflammation	Colitis-like	Erythromycin stearate
Yersinia	Rare PMNs, blood	↑WBC and sed rate	Crohn's-like aphthous lesions	Focal inflammation; monos > PMNs	Spasm cecum, abnormal terminal ileum	Seldom needed: tetracycline, ampicillin, chloramphenicol, trimethoprim-sulfamethoxazole
C. difficile	Blood, few WBCs	Normal to slight ↑WBC	Hyperemia; plaques, focal or diffuse	Pseudomembranes, distended glands, acute inflammation locally	"Dirty"-colon, mucosal irregularities, nodular	Vancomycin, Bacitracin, metronidazole, cholestyramine
Escherichia coli						
a. Enteroinvasive	Blood, few WBCs	Normal or ↑WBC	Lesion in R colon; hyperemic exudate, sm ulcers	Mild inflammatory erosions	—	Ampicillin, gentamicin, trimethoprim-sulfamethoxazole
b. Entero-pathogenic	Blood, few WBCs	↑WBC L shift	Hyperemia, hemorrhage, superficial ulceration	Nonspecific colitis	"Thumb printing" R colon	None needed
N. gonorrheae	Mucopus, blood	↑WBC L shift	Severe proctitis to 10–15 cm	Acute diffuse inflammation	Normal or proctitis	Penicillin, tetracycline
C. trachomatis	Blood, WBCs	Slight ↑WBC	Proctitis to 15 cm	Acute inflammation giant cells	Proctitis, stricture rectum	Tetracycline, trimethoprim-sulfamethoxazole

The stool culture, of course, yields the most definitive information in the consideration of a patient with bloody diarrhea of an infectious source. Other useful tests that can be performed immediately include a microscopic examination of the stool for the presence of mucus, red blood cells, and white blood cells, using either methylene blue or Wright's stain, a Gram stain, and visual examination for ova and parasites. Immunoassays for the diagnosis of possible viral etiologies of diarrhea (e.g., rotavirus, adenovirus, Norwalk virus, etc.) can also be helpful.

Reference: Silverman A: Common bacterial causes of bloody diarrhea. Pediatr Ann 14:39–50, 1985, with permission.

Management Plan for an Infant Less Than 1 Year of Age with Diarrhea Who Does Not Require Hospitalization at the Initial Evaluation

1. First evaluation

   a. Colitis (fecal leukocytes)   0–12 mo   Stool culture; blood culture if <3 mo

   b. No colitis; diarrhea <5 days   0–12 mo   No stool culture

   c. History of exposure to *Salmonella*   0–3 mo   Stool culture

2. Follow-up evaluation

   a. Diarrhea >5 days   0–12 mo   Stool culture

   b. Stool culture positive Blood culture positive   0–12 mo   Admit; look for focal infection in meninges bone, urinary tract

   c. Stool culture positive; blood culture negative   0–12 mo   Admit, as above

      i. Toxic or immuno-compromised   Admit; do blood culture and give antibiotics

      ii. Febrile   <3 mo   Admit; do blood culture and give antibiotics

      iii. Febrile   >3 mo   Admit; do blood culture; withhold antibiotics pending culture results

      iv. Afebrile, improving   0–12 mo   Reexamine, observe at home

   d. Stool culture positive; blood culture not obtained at first visit.   See 2-c.

Antibiotics of choice: cefotaxime or ceftriaxone.

Reference: St. Geme JW III, et al: Consensus: Management of *Salmonella* infection in the first year of life. Pediatr Infect Dis 7:615–621, 1988.

DYSMENORRHEA

Primary and Secondary Dysmenorrhea

Dysmenorrhea is a cramping pain in the lower abdomen and lower back that is temporally associated with menstrual blood flow. It may also be accompanied by headache, nausea, or diarrhea. Epidemiologic studies reveal, with great consistency, the high prevalence rate of dysmenorrhea among adolescent girls. During adolescence, dysmenorrhea becomes more common as age increases. This is probably because primary dysmenorrhea—the more common of the two types—is associated with ovulatory menstrual cycles, and most girls are anovulatory 18 to 24 months after menarche.

Primary dysmenorrhea is associated with no clinically detectable pelvic disease or other disorder. It usually begins 18 months after menarche (with the onset of ovulation). The pain starts on the same day as blood flow, lasting a few hours to 3 days, and is frequently accompanied by diarrhea in moderate or severe cases. The etiology of primary dysmenorrhea remains unclear, although it is known that women who suffer from this disorder produce increased amounts of prostaglandins E_2 and $F_{2\alpha}$ in their menstrual fluids. These prostaglandins cause the myometrium to increase its resting muscle tone, which yields excessive uterine contractions. The result is uterine ischemia and painful cramping.

Secondary dysmenorrhea, which presents far less frequently among the adolescent age group, is usually associated with some pathologic process in the pelvis. The pain is unusually severe and it (1) begins at menarche (obstructive form of secondary dysmenorrhea); (2) begins more than 3 years after menarche (e.g., endometriosis); or (3) is acute and related to one particular menstrual period (e.g., a complication of sexual activity such as a sexually transmitted infection or pregnancy).

Conditions Associated with Secondary Dysmenorrhea

1. Genital tract infections, specifically sexually transmitted endometritis or salpingitis	4. Congenital malformations of the genital tract (with or without a component of blood flow obstruction)
2. Complications of pregnancy, e.g., threatened or ectopic pregnancy	5. Genital tract cysts and neoplasms
3. Endometriosis	6. Intrauterine devices

Reference: Coupey SM, Ahlstrom P: Common menstrual disorders. Pediatr Clin North Am 36:551–571, 1989.

DYSMORPHISM

Diagnosing Dysmorphism

The dysmorphic infant or child presents the pediatrician and the parent with several unsettling requirements: a correct diagnosis and, where possible, an etiology; a comprehensive management guide; and, a careful assessment of recurrence risks and rates.

The pediatrician's best tools in the diagnosis of the dysmorphic child are his or her eyes, the child's parents and other family members, and several guiding principles. The task involves the determination of the pathogenesis and close attention to the appearance of marked or subtle patterns (Table 1).

Table 1. Pathogenic Mechanisms of Dysmorphism

TYPE OF DYSMORPHISM	DEFINITION	ASSOCIATED FACTORS	EXAMPLES
Malformation	A rudimentary abnormality involving differentiation or organization of an organ part, an organ, or body part representing an embryologic field. Occurs during embryogenesis.	Genetic or chromosomal abnormality; teratogenic effect	Cleft lip/palate Spina bifida Congenital heart defects Down syndrome
Deformation	Represents a response of normal tissue to abnormal external forces. Tends to occur late in pregnancy.	**Fetal:** Large fetus Multiple fetuses Malformed fetus Oligohydramnios Unusual placental site **Maternal:** Primigravida Small mother Small uterus Malformed uterus Uterine fibroids	Craniostenosis Plagiocephaly-torticollis sequence Micrognathia Ear deformities Pectus carinatum Scoliosis Dorsiflexion of foot Clubfoot Facial nerve palsies Erb's palsy
Disruption	Abnormality involving a destructive process in a normally formed organ.	**Disruptive agent** Radiation Infection Early amnion rupture Ischemia Vascular mechanism, hemorrhage Occlusion	**Anomaly** Microcephaly TORCHES syndrome Anencephaly, unusual facial clefting, eye defects, clefts, limb/digit abnormalities or amputations Porencephalic cysts, ileal atresia Hemifacial microsomia/Goldenhar's syndrome Streeter's bands Limb/digit amputations Gastroschisis
Dysplasia	Abnormality in the development (organization or differentiation) of cells and tissues as opposed to whole organs.	Genetic or unknown	Tuberous sclerosus Ectodermal dysplasia Neurofibromatosis Presacral teratoma Neuroblastoma Retinoblastoma Beckwith-Wiedemann syndrome—as example of dysplasia-malformation combination

Looking for patterns:

The anomalies described in the above table can be characterized as "major" (those with functional, surgical, or cosmetic consequences) or "minor" (those without consequences). Bear in mind that normal variants may constitute minor anomalies in the context of a syndrome.

A pattern of anomalies will often reveal the diagnosis and can present as syndromes, sequences, or associations.

Sequence:

A sequence refers to an isolated developmental abnormality and its subsequent structural consequences. An example is the initial mandibular hypoplasia of the Pierre Robin sequence that results in small chin, cleft palate, obstructive airway, and anoxia. The cause of a sequence is not necessarily defined.

Syndrome:

A syndrome consists of a pattern of malformations that are recognized to result from a specified cause, such as trisomies.

Association:

Associations are recognized as nonrandom and significant groupings of malformations without known etiologies. Two of the common associations are VACTERL and CHARGE. VACTERL, previously known as VATER, describes vertebral anomalies, anal atresia, cardiac defects, tracheoesophageal fistula with atresia, radial and renal defects, and limb defects. CHARGE consists of coloboma of the eye, heart defects, atresia of the choanae, growth and mental retardation, genital anomalies in the male, and ear anomalies.

In addition to the examination directed at recognition of patterns, there are several measurements that can be made to facilitate a diagnosis. The size of the hands and feet as well as the ratio of upper body length (crown to pubis symphysis) to lower body length (symphysis to soles) can signal dwarfing syndromes. The measurement of inner canthal distance, interpupillary distance, corneal diameter, internipple distance, and penile length may lead to diagnostic clues.

Be aware of the risk factors for structural anomalies (Tables 2 and 3).

Table 2. Children at Risk for Structural Anomalies

1. The child with a family history of structural anomalies	4. The infant of a mother with diabetes mellitus, phenylketonuria, epilepsy, or alcoholism
2. The child with one known structural anomaly	5. The mentally retarded child
3. The small-for-dates infant	6. The "strange-looking" child

Table 3. Anomalies and Associated Conditions

LOCATION	ANOMALY	CONDITION*
Back	Scoliosis	Stickler syndrome, neurofibromatosis
Chest	Pectus excavatum	Marfan's syndrome
Digits	Curved fifth fingers (clinodactyly)	Russell-Silver syndrome
	Finger-like thumbs	Holt-Oram syndrome, Aase syndrome

*These are illustrative conditions; often other conditions will also have the anomaly.

Table continued on next page.

Table 3. Anomalies and Associated Conditions (Cont.)

LOCATION	ANOMALY	CONDITION*
Digits (Cont.)	Polydactyly	Carpenter's syndrome, trisomy 13 syndrome
	Broad thumbs/great toes	Rubinstein-Taybi syndrome
	Syndactyly	Apert's syndrome
	Nail hypoplasia	Fetal hydantoin syndrome, Coffin-Siris syndrome
	Second finger overlaps third finger, fifth finger overlaps fourth finger	Trisomy 18, trisomy 13
Ears	Low-set	Trisomy 18, Treacher Collins' syndrome
	Crumpled	Beal syndrome
	Small	Down syndrome
	Large	Sotos' syndrome
	Preauricular tags	Goldenhar's syndrome
	Preauricular pits	BOR syndrome
Eyes	Microphthalmos	Oculodentodigital dysplasia
	Coloboma of iris	CHARGE association
	Stellate pattern of iris	Williams syndrome
	Absent iris	Aniridia-Wilms' tumor
	Cataracts	Hallermann-Streiff syndrome
Face	Unique facial gestalt	Down syndrome, Williams syndrome, Prader-Willi syndrome, Cornelia de Lange syndrome, whistling face syndrome
Genitalia	Hypospadias	Smith-Lemli-Opitz syndrome
	Micropenis	Robinow's syndrome
	Scrotal shawl	Aarskog's syndrome
	Hypoplasia of labia majora	Escobar syndrome
Hair	Widow's peak	Frontonasal dysplasia
	White forelock	Waardenburg syndrome
	Low posterior hairline	Turner's syndrome, Noonan's syndrome
	Scalp defect	Trisomy 13
	Sparse to absent	Hypohidrotic ectodermal dysplasia
	Kinky	Menkes' syndrome
Hands/feet	Short	Prader-Willi syndrome
	Long	Marfan's syndrome
	Abnormal palm/sole creases	Sotos' syndrome, Down syndrome
Head	Macrocephaly	Hydrocephalus, Sotos' syndrome
	Microcephaly	Many syndromes
Joints	Dislocations	Larsen's syndrome
	Elbow abnormalities	Turner's syndrome, XXXXY syndrome
	Absent patella	Trisomy 8
	Contractures	Beal syndrome, arthrogrypotic conditions
Limbs	Long	Beal syndrome, Stickler syndrome, XYY syndrome
	Short	Many short-limbed dwarfing syndromes
	Radial hypoplasia	VATER association
Mandible	Hypoplasia	Pierre Robin sequence
Maxilla	Hypoplasia	Nager syndrome
Mouth	Large	Goldenhar's syndrome
	Multiple frenula	Orofaciodigital syndrome
	Large tongue	Beckwith-Wiedemann syndrome

Table continued on next page.

Table 3. Anomalies and Associated Conditions (Cont.)

LOCATION	ANOMALY	CONDITION*
Neck	Webbed	Noonan's syndrome
	Short	Klippel-Feil syndrome
Nose	Small	Fetal warfarin effect
	Large	Seckel's syndrome
	Choanal atresia	CHARGE association
Ocular region	Hypertelorism	Opitz syndrome, Aarskog's syndrome
	Hypotelorism	Holoprosencephaly
	Short palpebral fissures	Fetal alcohol syndrome, blepharophimosis
	Epicanthic fold	Fetal trimethadione syndrome
	Upward slant of palpebral fissures	Down syndrome
	Downward slant of palpebral fissures	Treacher Collins' syndrome
	Synophrys (fusion of eyebrows in midline	Cornelia de Lange syndrome
Philtrum	Prominent	Trichorhinophalangeal syndrome
	Long	Williams syndrome
	Short	Cohen syndrome
	Smooth	Fetal alcohol syndrome
Skin	Café au lait spots	Neurofibromatosis, Russell-Silver syndrome, Bloom's syndrome
	Pigmented nevi	Turner's syndrome
	Multiple lentigines	Leopard syndrome
	Telangiectases	Ataxis-telangiectasia syndrome, Bloom's syndrome, Rothmund-Thomson syndrome
	Hemangiomata	Sturge-Weber syndrome
Teeth	Hypodontia	Hypohidrotic ectodermal dysplasia
	Caries	Dentinogenesis imperfecta
	Neonatal	Ellis-van Creveld syndrome
Thorax	Small	Jeune's syndrome

Lastly, the pediatrician must be armed with the knowledge of recurrence risks and be able to appropriately counsel the concerned parent(s) (Table 4).

Table 4. Recurrence Risk in Families of Dysmorphic Children

RISK IN SIBLINGS	PERCENTAGE	CONDITION
Low	1–2	Trisomy 21 syndrome, trisomy 13, trisomy 18
	3–7	Spina bifida, cleft palate/lip, hypospadias
Moderate	25	Autosomal recessive disease: Smith-Lemli-Opitz syndrome
		X-linked recessive disease: X-linked hydrocephalus
High	50	Autosomal dominant disease: neurofibromatosis, tuberous sclerosis
Total	100	Chromosomal disorder: 21/21 translocation
		Down's syndrome with carrier parent

Reference: Keele DK: A diagnostic approach to the dysmorphic child. Contemp Ped Nov:63–84, 1985. Tables 2 to 4 from this reference, with permission.
Oski FA, et al: Principles and Practice of Pediatrics. Philadelphia, J.B. Lippincott, 1990.

DYSPHAGIA

Common Causes

Chemical mucositis
   Caustic ingestion
   Gastroesophageal reflux
     with esophagitis
   Radiation/chemotherapy
Immature sucking/swallowing
   mechanism

Oropharyngeal infections
   Cervical adenitis
   Epiglottitis
   Gingivitis
   Herpetic stomatitis
   Peritonsillar abscess
   Pharyngitis
   Retropharyngeal abscess
   Tooth abscess
Physiologic expulsion reflux

Uncommon Causes

Cerebral palsy
Cleft palate
Esophageal spasm
Esophageal stricture
External compression of the esophagus
   Esophageal diverticuli
   Esophageal duplication
   Mediastinal masses/tumors
   Vascular anomalies

Foreign body
Infectious esophagitis
   Candida, herpes
Macroglossia (any cause)
Micrognathia
Pharyngeal diverticuli
Physiologic (globus hystericus)
Submucosal cleft
Tracheoesophageal fistula

Rare Causes

Choanal atresia
Collagen vascular disease
   Dermatomyositis
   Scleroderma
Diphtheria
Esophageal atresia, web, cyst
Laryngeal cyst, cleft
Muscular hypertrophy of the esophagus
Neuromuscular causes
   Botulism
   Bulbar and suprabulbar palsy
     Mobius syndrome
   Chalasia/achalasia of the esophagus
   Congenital laryngeal stridor
   Cranial nerve palsy

Neuromuscular causes (*Cont.*)
   Demyelinating disease
   Guillain-Barré syndrome
   Hypotonias
   Muscular dystrophy
   Myasthenia gravis
   Myotonic dystrophy
   Pharyngeal or cricopharyngeal
     incoordination
   Tetanus
Pharyngeal cyst, cleft
Rumination
Temporomandibular ankylosis/
   hypoplasia
Tumors (oropharynx, esophagus)

DYSRHYTHMIA

Common Causes

Acidemia
Congenital heart disease
Drugs
    Antiarrhythmics
    Beta blockers
    Caffeine
    Cocaine

Drugs *(Cont.)*
    Psychotropics
    Sympathomimetics
Hypoxemia
Idiopathic
Postoperative (cardiac procedures)

Uncommon Causes

Cardiomyopathy (dilated, hypertrophic,
    infiltrative)
Electrolyte disturbances (especially
    K, Ca, Mg)
Myocarditis

Sickle-cell disease
Sick-sinus syndrome
Wolff-Parkinson-White syndrome
    (and/or other necessary bypass
    tracts)

Rare Causes

Anomalous coronary artery
Central nervous system
    Hemorrhage
    Infection
    Trauma
Collagen vascular disease
Complete congenital heart block
Endocrine (thyrotoxicosis, secondary
    electrolyte disturbance)

Kawasaki disease
Myocardial ischemia
Myocardial trauma
Myocardial tumors
Neonatal lupus
Prolonged QT syndrome
Rheumatic fever

DYSURIA

Common Causes

Candidal dermatitis/vaginitis
Chemical urethritis (bubble bath)
Contact dermatitis/vulvitis

Urethritis
Urinary tract infection
Viral cystitis

Uncommon Causes

Foreign body
Herpes simplex
Meatitis

Pinworms
Urethral trauma

Rare Causes

Appendicitis
Bladder diverticulum
Bladder outlet obstruction
   Posterior urethral valves
Bladder stones
Constipation
Drugs
   Amitriptyline
   Cytoxan
Hematospermia
Interstitial cystitis

Meatal stenosis
Posthitis
Prostatitis
Reiter's syndrome
Schistosomiasis
Stevens-Johnson syndrome
Tuberculosis
Urethral prolapse
Urethral stricture
Varicella

I'm sorry you are wiser,
   I'm sorry you are taller;
I liked you better foolish,
   And I liked you better smaller.

Aline (Mrs. Joyce) Kilmer
*For the Birthday of a Middle-
Aged Child, Stanza 1*

E

EARS

Low-set Ears

Because of their association with various syndromes, low-set ears can be a finding of extreme importance. There is still a controversy over what constitutes low-set ears. We prefer a method of evaluation suggested by Dr. Murray Feingold. In the figure, the face has a sheet of x-ray film held over it. On the margins of the film are measurement scales, and the center of the film is bisected by a horizontal line that is aligned with the medial canthi of the eyes. The amount of the ear lying above the line is measured as well as the overall length of the ear. If the ear is below the center line, the ear is low set. If 10% or less of the overall length of the ear is above the line, the ears are said to be low set. If low-set ears are found, look carefully for other physical abnormalities.

If $\frac{a}{b} \times 100 \leq 10$, the ears are low set.

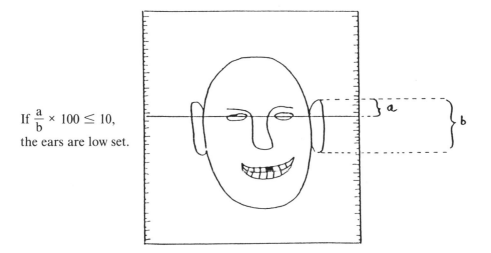

Some Syndromes Associated with Low-set Ears

Apert's syndrome	Down's syndrome	Seckel's syndrome
Camptomelic syndrome	Fetal hydantoin syndrome	Trisomy 13 syndrome
Carpenter's syndrome	Hallermann-Streiff	Trisomy 18 syndrome
Cri-du-chat syndrome	syndrome	Treacher-Collins
Deletion of the short arm	Noonan's syndrome	syndrome
of chromosome 13	Saethre-Chotzen syndrome	Turner's syndrome

Reference: Feingold M: Commentary, Yearbook of Pediatrics, p 152, 1977.

ENCOPRESIS

Common Causes

Chronic constipation
Diarrheal disorders
Emotional disturbance

Uncommon Causes

Hirschsprung's disease

Rare Causes

Diastematomyelia
Epidural abscess
Poliomyelitis
Postanorectal
  surgery
Osteomyelitis of the
  vertebral body

Sacral agenesis
Spinal cord tumor
Syringomyelia
Transverse myelitis

ENDOTRACHEAL INTUBATION

Complications of Endotracheal Intubation

Endotracheal intubation in the setting of an intensive care unit, emergency room, or delivery suite is rarely as controlled a procedure as the same performed in an operating room. Unrecognized esophageal placement of an endotracheal tube is the most common complication of emergency intubations and can lead rapidly to brain damage or death. Below are the phases of progressive hypoxemia, their clinical pictures, and recommended resuscitative maneuvers.

Precritical Phase: Arterial oxygen content decreases from normal 19 vol% to 12 vol% ($\pm$ 70% saturation).
    Sympathetic tone increases: HR increases by approximately 10 bpm.
        Systolic BP increases 10–15 mmHg.
        Diastolic BP unchanged.
        Pulse pressure widens.

Critical Phase: Arterial oxygen content ranges from 12 vol% to 9 vol% (50% saturation).
    Vagal tone increases: systolic BP decreases, HR decreases.
    Cyanosis evident in nonanemic patients.

Terminal Phase: Arterial oxygen content falls below 9 vol% (<50% saturation).
    HR slow to 40 or fewer bpm.
    BP readings cannot be obtained.
    ECG readings may show marked sinus bradycardia in the absence of a
      palpable pulse.

Resuscitation

In the absence of a known and immediately remediable problem, the tube should be removed quickly and an oral or nasal airway should be placed. The patient should be administered 100% oxygen with a bag and mask until an unhurried reintubation can be performed. The use of atropine or vasopressors will not correct the hypoxia.

Recognition and correction of the hypoxemia during the precritical and critical phases will generally avert any catastrophic event. Terminal phase may require initiation of BLS and ALS.*

---

*BLS = basic life support; ALS = advanced life support.

Other Complications

Foreign bodies: Due to excessive lymphoid tissue in childhood, semirigid naso-tracheal tubes may cause dislodging of adenoid tissue and subsequent obstruction.

Bronchial intubation: The right bronchus is more susceptible to catheterization due to the obtuse angle at its junction with the trachea. Partial catheterization of the right bronchus may result in occlusion and collapse of the right upper lobe.

Tube distortion: Tubes constructed from soft rubber or metal reinforced plastic are less likely to kink, compress, or twist, but even they may distort, leading to occlusion and hypoxemia.

Effect of tube size: Due to the diameter of the pediatric airway, increased airway resistance is a significant problem with thick-walled tubes. Refer to the chart below for selection of the appropriate thin-walled endotracheal tube.

Selection of Endotracheal Tube

INFANT WEIGHT (g)	ENDOTRACHEAL TUBE INTERNAL DIAMETER	SUCTION CATHETER SIZE (FRENCH GAUGE)
<1250	2.5	5 Fr
1250–3000	3.0	6 Fr
>3000	3.5	8 Fr
BY AGE		
Full term–9 mo	3.5	
12–20 mo	4.0	
2 yr	4.5	
>2 yr	$4.5 + \dfrac{age\ (yr)}{4}$	

References: Adriani J, et al: Complications of endotracheal intubations. South Med J 81:739–744, 1988.
Firestone LL, et al (eds): Clinical Anesthesia Procedures of the Massachusetts General Hospital. Boston, Little, Brown, 1988.

Verification Techniques for Proper Placement

Although no verification technique for the placement of endotracheal tubes is completely infallible, there are several methods that are quite reliable and ought to be routinely performed after intubation.

1. The most reliable method of verification, **detection of end-expired CO_2**, requires instruments that may not be available in all emergency situations. As carbon dioxide analyzers become less cumbersome and more available, this will be the method of choice.

2. **Auscultation of breath sounds** is historically accepted as a reliable method for verification of tracheal intubation. Recent studies have found that it may be dependable only two-thirds of the time. Confounding factors in the pediatric age group include short necks and obesity. An important point: auscultation is most useful when performed both before and after intubation. Nonidentical sounds or unequal chest expansion should alert the pediatrician to a possible problem.

3. **Pulse oximetry**, now widely available, is a good adjunct to auscultation but in general should not be the sole method of verification. Oximetry is an excellent monitoring device for the intubated child at risk for mucous plugging or compression. Regardless of the patient's risk status, pulse oximetry is useful because pediatric patients tend to desaturate more quickly than their adult counterparts.

4. **Mouth-to-tube-insufflation** remains a reliable, simple, and universally available technique for verifying tube placement. A quick, but not too forceful, breath is expired into the tube connector by the physician. A properly placed tube will allow gradual insufflation of the lungs. Expiration, against minimal resistance, should be felt against the physician's turned cheek. If esophageal placement has occurred, the expired air will not equal the insufflated amount, the expulsion will be rapid, and the air will not be felt on the cheek.

Reference: Adriani J, et al: Complications of endotracheal intubation. South Med J 81:739–744, 1988.

Firestone LL, et al (eds): Clinical Anesthesia Procedures of the Massachusetts General Hospital. Boston, Little, Brown, 1988.

ENURESIS

Common Causes

Developmental delay of bladder function and capacity
Psychological

Uncommon Causes

Diabetes	Obstructive abnormalities of the urinary tract
Food allergy	Urinary tract infections

Rare Causes

Compulsive water drinking	Lumbosacral anomalies
Diabetes insipidus,	Sickle-cell anemia
central or nephrogenic	Spinal cord tumors

Natural History of Nocturnal Enuresis

Most children stop wetting their beds between 2 and 4 years of age. Does that mean that persistent bedwetting after 4 indicates an abnormality? Almost certainly not. An organic disorder is rarely found in enuretic children, that is, children who are bedwetting after the age of 5.

Bedwetting after age 5 years is more common in boys, in children from large families, and in children from lower socioeconomic groups, and it occurs more commonly in families where one of the parents may have been a bedwetter. Nocturnal enuresis occurs once a month or more in 8% of school-age children.

When bedwetting recurs after a period of dryness (termed regressive or secondary enuresis), an explanation should be sought. The polyuria of diabetes mellitus may frequently present in this way. Also rule out urinary tract disease and diabetes insipidus.

Age by Which Bedwetting Stopped

	BOYS		GIRLS	
AGE	White (%)	Black (%)	White (%)	Black (%)
<2	28	37	37	35
2–3	70	73	80	77
4–5	85	83	89	90
6–7	91	89	92	92

What becomes of the children, about 10 to 15%, who continue to wet after 4 to 5 years of age?

There is a relative constancy to the percentage of children who spontaneously remit from their enuresis each year. The figure to remember is that any one child during the course of 1 year has about a 15% chance of this problem going away by itself. Thus, a child who wets his bed at age 5 will have about a 3% chance of bedwetting by age 20. These figures apply only to the natural history of bedwetting and not to those children whose bedwetting is related to an environmental factor.

Percentage Spontaneously Ceasing Bedwetting per Year

AGES	5 TO 9	10 TO 14	15 TO 19
Percentage	14	16	16

Diurnal or daytime enuresis occurs much less frequently than nocturnal, with an incidence of less than 1% in a 7- to 12-year-old group.

References: Dodge WF, West EF, Bridgforth EB, et al: Am J Dis Child 120:32, 1970.
Forsythe WI, Redmond A: Arch Dis Child 49:259, 1974.
Adapted from McMillan JA, et al: The Whole Pediatrician Catalog, Vol. 1 and Vol. 2. Philadelphia, W.B. Saunders, 1977, pp 299–300; 1979, p 84.

EOSINOPHILS

Cerebrospinal Fluid Eosinophilia

Many laboratories now perform cytocentrifugation and differential cytologic staining of the WBCs found in cerebrospinal fluid. The finding of CSF eosinophilia using this technique has led to the development of a list of the various agents—infectious and otherwise—that can cause eosinophilic pleocytosis in the central nervous system. The following list includes the reported causes of "eosinophilic meningitis." For most of the causes listed, a careful history and physical examination will provide the diagnosis.

Fungal infection
Coccidiomycosis meningitis
Viral infection
Coxsackie virus meningitis
Chronic lymphocytic
choriomeningitis virus
Subacute sclerosing panencephalitis
Bacterial infection
Tuberculous meningitis
Neurosyphilis
CSF inflammation
Radiologic dye used in myelography
Rubber CSF shunt tubing
CNS malignancy
Multiple sclerosis
CNS hemorrhage

Parasitic infection
Neurocysticercosis (caused by the
tapeworm *Taenia solium* and
found in Asia and Africa)
Toxocara canis and *T. cati*
Trichinella
Nematode meningoencephalitis,
including that due to *Angio-
strongylus cantonensis* and
Gnathostoma spinigerum, found
in Taiwan, Thailand, and the
Pacific islands
Amebic meningitis caused by the
free-living amebae *Naegleria
fowleri* and *Acanthamoeba*
found in warm fresh or brackish
water all over the world.

EPIDIDYMITIS

Epididymitis in Children and Adolescents

Epididymitis, though considered rare in prepubertal males, is also a common cause of acute scrotum in childhood. Like torsion of the spermatic cord, the common clinical presentation includes pain, swelling, and erythema. Unlike torsion, the onset tends to be less acute.

Although definitive differentiation between epididymitis and testicular torsion requires radionuclide scanning or surgery, the history and physical exam should point the pediatrician in the correct direction. Once established, the diagnosis of epididymitis often suggests further urologic investigation.

Epididymitis Compared with Testicular Torsion

FEATURE	EPIDIDYMITIS	TESTICULAR TORSION
Onset:	Insidious onset often accompanied by signs and symptoms of urethritis or systemic bacterial and/or viral infection. History may be significant for recent trauma.	Acute onset of pain
Physical signs:	Elevation of testis *decreases* pain.	Elevation of testis *increases* pain.
	Gastrointestinal symptoms rare.	Abdominal pain and gastrointestinal symptoms common.
	Cremasteric reflex present.	Cremasteric reflex present.
Causes:	Bacterial: Coliform organisms, gonorrhea, *Staphylococcus, M. Tuberculosis, C. trachomatis;* viral; traumatic; chemical (i.e., reflux); systemic diseases such as sarcoid, Kawasaki's, Henoch-Schönlein purpura; idiopathic	Anatomical defect

In the infant with suspected epididymitis, a thorough work-up for sepsis is indicated, because epididymitis in infancy is often a signpost of systemic illness. In the child less than 2 years of age and in older patients with recurrent episodes, a urologic work-up with an IVP and VCUG is recommended to rule out any associated genitourinary abnormality.

Reference: Likitnukul S, et al: Epididymitis in children and adolescents. Am J Dis Child 141:41–44, 1987.

EPISTAXIS

Common Causes

Allergic rhinitis
Repeated sneezing
Secondary to dryness and crusting
   over anterior portion of nasal septum

Trauma
  External
   Self-inflicted (nose picking)
Upper respiratory infection

Uncommon Causes

Factor XI deficiency
Hypertension
Platelet dysfunction syndrome

Sickle cell anemia
Thrombocytopenia from any cause
von Willebrand's disease

Rare Causes

Angiofibroma
Ataxia-telangiectasia
Congenital syphilis
Ehlers-Danlos syndrome
Foreign body
Malaria
Measles
Nasal angiomas
Nasal diphtheria
Nasal polyp
Oral contraceptives

Osler-Weber-Rendu disease
  (hereditary hemorrhagic
  telangiectasia)
Pertussis
Rheumatic fever
Scarlet fever
Scurvy
Typhoid fever
Varicella
Wegener's granulomatosis

EPSTEIN-BARR VIRUS

Epstein-Barr Viral Antibody Titers

Although the heterophile antibody test is sometimes positive in young children with infection caused by the Epstein-Barr virus, heterophile positivity is certainly not as reliable in pediatric patients as it is in adults. But don't despair. More specific antibody assays are available. They allow you to determine on a single serum sample whether a patient is currently infected or has had the infection at some time in the past. The most helpful tests are the following:

Interpretation of EBV Serum Antibody Patterns

INTERPRETATION	IgM CAPSID ANTIGEN	IgG CAPSID ANTIGEN	IgG EARLY ANTIGEN		ANTINUCLEAR ANTIGEN
			D	R	
Susceptible	−	−	−	−	−
Acute primary infection (IM presentation)	+	+	+	−*	−†
Acute primary infection (non-IM presentation or asymptomatic)	+	+	−	+	−†
Old, quiescent infection	−	+	−	−‡	+§
Reactivated infection	±	+	+ or +		+//

* A few (<10%) adults and an even greater number (10% to 20%) of children with acute IM develop an antibody response directed to R instead of D component.
† A low antibody titer (≤1:5 in our laboratory) may also be detected in acute infection.
‡ Occasionally a weak, probably nonspecific, antibody response to R component is present.
§ Moderate, stable titers of antibody should be present.
// Stable levels of antibody, although in low or absent levels in immunosuppressed and immunodeficient patients, are present.
From Sumaya CV, Epstein-Barr virus serologic testing: Diagnostic indication and interpretations. Pediatr Infect Dis 5:337, 1986. Reproduced by permission of Williams & Wilkins Co.

The timing of these antibody rises is depicted in the accompanying figure.

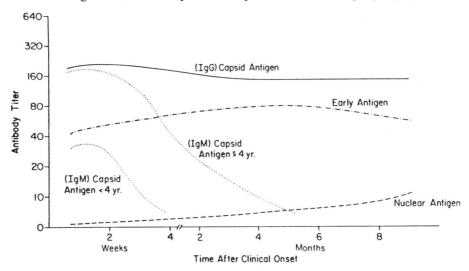

Duration of serum IgM and IgG antibody responses to EBV early antigen and nuclear antigen. The antibody response to EBV early antigen components may persist for years after an episode of EBV infectious mononucleosis. Antibodies to EBV nuclear antigen may be absent during acute infection but, once present, remain for life. (From Sumaya CV, Ench Y. Pediatrics 75:1011, 1985. Reproduced by permission of the American Academy of Pediatrics.)

Heterophile antibodies are nonspecific and not directed against the virus. They cause agglutination of sheep, horse, beef, and goat red blood cells. Since other antibodies may cause such agglutination, care should be taken to avoid false-positive reporting. Testing sera with horse RBCs is the most sensitive method, whereas the beef cell hemolysin test gives the most specific results. The most reliable method for single slide tests is to absorb the sera with guinea pig kidney cells before adding horse RBCs. When the antibody is due to EBV infection, the test should remain positive after such absorption. Many of the rapid test kits include guinea pig kidney cells for this purpose. Rapid test kits may be accurate and helpful, but experienced personnel and fresh testing material are essential for best results.

The list below provides a summary of the contents of some of the commercially available kits.

TRADE NAME	RED BLOOD CELL USED	USE OF GUINEA PIG KIDNEY ABSORPTION	MANUFACTURER
Mono-test	Horse	No	Wampole Labs.
Mono-Diff	Horse	Yes	Wampole Labs.
Monospot	Horse	Yes	Ortho Diagnostics
Diagluto	Horse	Yes	Beckman Instruments, Inc.
Monosticon	Sheep	Yes	Organon Diagnostic Products
Mono-Stat	Native and papain-treated sheep	Not needed	Colab Labs., Inc.
Confirmikit	Native and enzyme-treated horse	Not needed	BBL-BioQuest, Div. of Becton, Dickinson & Co.
Heterol	Native and enzyme-treated horse	Not needed	Difco

Reference: Andiman WA: J Pediatr 95:171, 1980. Figure—courtesy of Dr. John Sullivan, X-Linked Lymphoproliferative Syndrome Registry. Department of Pathology, University of Massachusetts Medical Center, Worcester, MA.

Adapted from McMillan JA, et al: The Whole Pediatrician Catalog, Vol. 3. Philadelphia, W.B. Saunders, 1982, with permission.

ERYTHROCYTE SEDIMENTATION RATE

The Slow Sedimentation Rate

All of the factors responsible for determining the rate at which erythrocytes sediment have not been identified. Factors that are known to influence the sedimentation rate include the quantity of fibrinogen, alpha$_1$-globulin, the gamma-M globulin, and the serum cholesterol, with the quantity of fibrinogen perhaps playing the most important role. In addition, alterations in the morphologic characteristics of the red cell or in cell surface charge that hinder rouleau formation will affect the erythrocyte sedimentation rate.

Everyone is familiar with the long and nondescript list of diseases that produce an increase in the erythrocyte sedimentation rate. It is generally not appreciated that certain disorders or drugs characteristically produce a slow sedimentation rate or a rate that is slower than would be anticipated. Disorders that produce a slow sedimentation rate include:

Anorexia nervosa
Hypofibrinogenemia, congenital
  or acquired
Abetalipoproteinemia (acanthocytosis)
Sickle cell anemia (if many sickled
  forms are present)
Pyruvate kinase deficiency (usually
  postsplenectomy if associated with marked
  morphologic alterations of the erythrocytes)

Hereditary spherocytosis
Congestive heart failure
Nephrotic syndrome
Steroid therapy
Aspirin administration
Serum sickness
Hepatitis B

In patients with the nephrotic syndrome in whom an infection is suspected, the measurement of the C-reactive protein provides a useful alternate screening test.

From McMillan JA: The Whole Pediatrician Catalog, Vol. 1. Philadelphia, W.B. Saunders, 1977, pp 226–227, with permission.

EYE

Causes of Severe Eye Injuries in Children

Approximately 160,000 school age children in the U.S. suffer from traumatic eye injuries of varying severity each year. Indeed, the only more common pediatric ophthalmologic entity requiring hospital admission is strabismus. Although trauma is the usual descriptive word for these eye injuries among children, a variety of offending etiologies is responsible, including balls, sticks, fists, fingers, falls, glass, animal bites, and metallic foreign bodies. Listed below are the most frequent diagnoses made among children with eye trauma severe enough to warrant hospital admission, subdivided into age groups.

Primary Diagnoses of Eye Trauma

DIAGNOSIS	TOTAL (%)	AGE GROUP, NO. OF CASES			
		0–5 YR	6–10 YR	11–15 YR	16–20 YR
Hyphema	81 (31.4)	11	23	30	17
Globe lacerations	48 (18.6)	15	7	12	14
Traumatic cataract	31 (12)	5	10	5	11
Eyelid laceration	28 (10.9)	12	10	3	3
Retinal detachment	19 (7.4)	0	2	9	8
Foreign body in eye	18 (7)	2	3	7	6
Orbital fractures	10 (3.9)	0	0	7	3
Injury to orbital tissue	7 (2.7)	2	0	4	1
Burns	4 (1.6)	2	0	1	1
Vitreous hemorrhage	4 (1.6)	1	0	1	2
Traumatic glaucoma	3 (1.2)	1	1	1	0
Corneal abrasion	2 (<1)	0	2	0	0
Lens subluxation	2 (<1)	0	1	0	1
Conjunctival laceration	1 (<1)	0	0	0	1
Total (%)	258 (100)	51 (19.8)	59 (22.8)	80 (31.0)	68 (26.4)

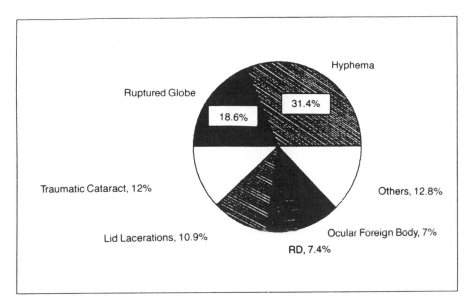

Primary admitting diagnoses of pediatric patients with ocular trauma (ages 0 to 20 years). Others include those less-frequent diagnoses listed in the table. RD indicates retinal detachments.

Reference: DeRespinis PA, Caputo AR, Fiore PM, Wagner RS: A survey of severe eye injuries in children. Am J Dis Child 143:711–716, 1989, with permission.

The Eyelash Syndrome

Adults can appreciate the fact that a foreign body in the eye is both annoying and painful. Indoors the most common foreign body to produce such discomfort is the eyelash. We frequently forget that eyelashes may get into the eyes of infants as well. The next time you are confronted with the problem of an irritable, crying baby for which you cannot find a suitable explanation, be sure to check the eyes for a foreign body. If you find it, you can produce an instant cure.

If an older child complains of the sensation of a foreign body, there usually is one, particularly indoors. Oblique illumination with a flashlight can aid detection. If nothing is seen, check the upper tarsal conjunctiva by eversion of the lid. This may call for instillation of a local anesthetic.

Most foreign bodies on or in the cornea or conjunctiva can be removed by irrigation or gentle wiping with a wet cotton applicator (also see next entry). In the event of an abrasion, instill an antibacterial ointment and follow up within 24 hours to check on healing and for the presence of infection.

Removal of a Foreign Body

You may be called upon to remove a simple nonpenetrating foreign body from the eye—objects such as eyelashes, dust, or dirt. All you need is a clean Band-Aid. Simply touch the foreign body with the adhesive portion of the Band-Aid. You can even do this to yourself with the aid of a mirror when necessary.

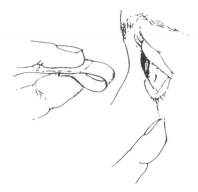

Reference: Pryatel W: Another use for a Band-Aid. Resident & Staff Physician, January, 1977, p 99.

Remember that as a teenager you are at the last stage in your life when you will be happy to hear that the phone is for you.

Fran Lebowitz

F

FAILURE TO THRIVE

Common Causes

Neglect
  Inadequate ingestion/metabolism
    of calories
    Depression with anorexia
    Manipulative behavior
    Rumination as self-
      stimulation
    Secondary malabsorption
      Self-induced (vomiting,
        laxative abuse)
      Specific deficiency
        (e.g., zinc, biotin)
      Starvation
    Secondary neuroendocrine
      abnormalities
      Abnormal cycling of
        growth hormone
      Cortisol deficiency
  Physical neglect/abuse
  Psychosocial deprivation
  Withholding of food as
    neglect/abuse
    Intentional withholding
      of food
    "Unintentional" withholding
      of food
    "Overwhelmed" caretaker
    Lack of support systems
      (financial/social)
    Primary personal needs
      (e.g., drug/alcohol abuse)
    Time constraints (e.g.,
      unsupervised eating,
      bottle propping)
    Psychotic or depressed
      caretaker

Nonorganic failure to thrive
  Inadequate volume of feeds
    Two feeds per day
    Too little per feed
      Colic
      "Difficult" feeder
      Financial factors
      Ignorance
      Inexperienced/impatient
        ± compounding child
        factors
  Inappropriate foods for age
    Cultural factors
    Fad diets
    Financial factors
    Ignorance
  Incorrect preparation of formula
    Chronic dilution
      Financial factors
      Ignorance
      Prolonged use after gastro-
        enteritis
    Inappropriate additives
Normal variants
  Delayed growth spurt
  Early onset growth retardation
  Genetic "slightness"
Organic failure to thrive
  CNS etiologies
    Mental retardation/cerebral
      palsy
    Neurodevelopmental retardation
  Gastrointestinal etiologies
    Chronic gastroenteritis
    Gastroesophageal reflux
    Pyloric stenosis
Prematurity
Small for gestational age

Uncommon Causes

Defective utilization of calories
  Chronic hypoxemia
  Diabetes mellitus
Defects in absorption
  Cystic fibrosis
  Enzymatic deficiencies
  Food sensitivity/intolerance
  Hepatitis
  Inflammatory bowel disease
  Milk allergy
  Starvation
Inadequacy of food intake
  Cleft lip/palate
  Dyspnea of any cause
    Congenital heart disease
    Respiratory disease/insufficiency

Inadequacy of food intake *(Cont.)*
  Immature suck/swallow
  Pharyngeal incoordination
Increased metabolism
  Chronic anemias
  Chronic/recurrent infections
    Otitis, sinusitis, pneumonia
    Parasites
    Tuberculosis
    Urinary tract infection
  Chronic respiratory insufficiency
  Congentital heart disease
  Malignancies

Rare Causes

Defective utilization of calories
  Adrenal insufficiency
  Chromosomal syndromes
  Diabetes insipidus
  Diencephalic syndrome
  Drugs/toxins
  Dysmorphogenic syndromes
  Fetal exposure syndromes
  Hypopituitarism
  Hypothyroidism
  Metabolic disorders
    Aminoacidopathies
    Galactosemia
    Organic acidurias
    Storage diseases
  Parathyroid disorders
  Renal tubular acidosis
Defects in absorption
  Acrodermatitis enteropathica
  Biliary atresia/cirrhosis
  Celiac disease
  Hirschsprung's disease
  Immunologic deficiency
Necrotizing entercolitis
  Pancreatic insufficiency
  Short gut syndrome

Inadequacy of food intake
  Choanal atresia
  CNS disorders
    Cerebral insults
    Degenerative diseases
    Drugs/toxins
    Subdural hematoma
  Diaphragmatic hernia/hiatal hernia
  Esophageal atresia
  Generalized muscle weakness
    Congenital hypotonia
    Myasthenia gravis
    Werdnig-Hoffmann disease
  Micrognathia/glossoptosis
  Tracheoesophageal fistual
Increased metabolism
  Acquired heart disease
  Adrenocortical excess
  Chronic inflammation
    (e.g., JRA, SLE)
  Chronic seizure disorder
  Drugs/toxins
  Hyperaldosteronism
  Hyperthyroidism

FATIGUE

Common Causes

Acute recovery from surgery,
 trauma, most illnesses
Anemia
Chronic atopy
Eating disorders
 Excessive dieting ($\pm$ anorexia
  nervosa, bulimia)
Excessive physical exertion
Mononucleosis (and most
 viral infections)
Obesity

Pregnancy
Psychosocial
 Chronic boredom
 Chronic depression/anxiety
 Grief
 Stress (prolonged and severe)
Sedentary lifestyle
Sleep disorders
 Insomnia
 Sleep pattern disruption
  (lack of REM sleep)

Uncommon Causes

Acute bacterial infections
 Bacteremia
 Meningitis
Chronic hypoxemia
 Asthma
 Cardiomyopathy
 Chronic pulmonary disease
 Congenital heart disease
 Congestive heart failure
 Cystic fibrosis
 Heart disease
 Pericarditis
 Pulmonary hypertension
Chronic infections
 Brucellosis
 Cytomegalic inclusion disease

Chronic infections *(Cont.)*
 Histoplasmosis
 Osteomyelitis
 Parasitic infestations
 Pyelonephritis
 Sinusitis
 Subacute bacterial endocarditis
 Toxoplasmosis
 Tuberculosis
 Urinary tract infection
Dehydration
Hepatitis
Upper airway obstruction
 (sleep apnea)
 Pickwickian syndrome
 Tonsillar-adenoidal hypertrophy

Rare Causes

Acquired immunodeficiency
 syndrome (AIDS)
Allergic tension fatigue syndrome
Connective tissue diseases
 Dermatomyositis
 Juvenile rheumatoid arthritis
 Mixed connective tissue disease
 Scleroderma
 Systemic lupus erythematosus
Endocrine disorders
 Diabetes insipidus
 Diabetes mellitus

Endocrine disorders *(Cont.)*
 Hyper/hypoadrenalism
 Hyper/hypopituitarism
 Hyper/hypothyroidism
 Hyperparathyroidism
Hepatic insufficiency
Hypoglycemia
Inborn errors of metabolism
Inflammatory bowel disease
Intussusception
Malignancy
 Leukemia

Malignancy *(Cont.)*
  Lymphoma
  Solid tumors
Metabolic disturbances
  Hypermagnesemia
  Hypokalemia
  Hypomagnesemia
  Hyponatremia
Neurologic
  Intracranial hematomas
  Myasthenia gravis
  Narcolepsy
Renal tubular acidosis
Toxins and drugs
  Alcohol
  Analgesics and salicylates
  Anticonvulsants

Toxins and drugs *(Cont.)*
  Antihistamines
  Barbiturates
  Carbon monoxide
  Corticosteroids
  Digitalis
  Heavy metals
  Insulin
  Nicotine
  Pesticides
  Progesterones
  Sedatives
  Tetracycline
  Vitamin A
  Vitamin D
Uremia

FEVER

Fever of Unknown Origin

Fever is defined here as a temperature, higher than 38.5°C for more than 2 weeks.

Common Causes

Collagen vascular disease
  Juvenile rheumatoid arthritis
  Lupus erythematosus
  Periarteritis nodosa
Factitious
Infections
  Atypical mycobacterial infections
  Epstein-Barr virus infections
  Osteomyelitis
  Sinusitis, mastoiditis
  Urinary tract infections
  "Viral syndromes"

Inflammatory bowel diseases
  Regional enteritis
  Ulcerative colitis
Malignancy
  Acute lymphoblastic leukemia
  Neuroblastoma
  Hodgkin's disease
  Non-Hodgkin's lymphoma

Uncommon Causes

Drug-induced
Infections
  Cat-scratch disease
  Cytomegalic inclusion disease
  Lung abscess
  Hepatitis

Infections *(Cont.)*
  Histoplasmosis
  Pelvic inflammatory disease
  Salmonellosis
Kawasaki disease
Lyme disease

Rare Causes

Infection
  Behcet's syndrome
  Diabetes insipidus
    Central
    Nephrogenic
  Diencephalic syndrome
  Ectodermal dysplasia
  Familial dysautonomia
  Hepatoma
  Infection
    Blastomycosis
    Brucellosis
    Human immunodeficiency
      virus infection
    Leptospirosis
    Liver abscess
    Lymphogranuloma venereum
    Malaria
    Perinephric abscess

Infection *(Cont.)*
  Psittacosis
  Q fever
  Rocky Mountain spotted fever
  Streptococcosis
  Subdiaphragmatic abscess
  Toxoplasmosis
  Tuberculosis
  Tularemia
  Viral encephalitis
  Visceral larva migrains
Myelogenous leukemia
Pancreatitis
Periodic disease (familial fever)
Reticulum-cell sarcoma
Sarcoidosis
Serum sickness
Thyrotoxicosis

Fever of Unknown Origin—Continued

Prolonged episodes of fever without an apparent explanation are an uncommon diagnostic problem in pediatrics. Because of their rarity, they represent an exacting challenge and provide the clinician with an unequaled opportunity to demonstrate his skills in both careful history taking and physical examination. At least 50% of "fevers of unknown origin" can be diagnosed by thoughtful attention to details and very simple laboratory studies. Unfortunately, the designation "fever of unknown origin" often prompts a myriad of tests and radiographic procedures in a nonsystematic fashion.

What are the usual causes of obscure, prolonged fevers in children and how do they differ in etiology from those observed in adults? The accompanying table summarizes the findings in two studies involving infants and children and contrasts them with a representative study of adult patients. Fever was defined as the presence of a rectal temperature of 38.5°C (99.8°F) on at least four occasions over a minimum period of 2 weeks.

Causes of Fever of Unknown Origin

INFANTS AND CHILDREN				ADULTS	
Pizzo and Associates		McClung		Jacoby and Swartz	
Infections	*(52%)*	*Infections*	*(29%)*	*Infections*	*(40%)*
Viral syndromes		Respiratory		Tuberculosis	
Respiratory		Central nervous system		Endocarditis	
Central nervous system		Salmonellosis		Localized to peritoneum,	
Urinary tract		Endocarditis		urinary tract, or liver	
Osteomyelitis		Histoplasmosis			

Table continued on next page.

Causes of Fever of Unknown Origin (Cont.)

INFANTS AND CHILDREN		ADULTS
Pizzo and Associates	McClung	Jacoby and Swartz
Infections (Cont.) (52%)	*Infections (Cont.)* (29%)	*Infections (Cont.)* (40%)
Endocarditis Tuberculosis Herpes simplex, generalized Sinusitis Salmonellosis	Brucellosis Epstein-Barr infection	
Collagen-Vascular (20%)	*Collagen-Vascular* (11%)	*Collagen-Vascular* (15%)
Rheumatoid arthritis Vasculitis Anaphylactoid purpura Lupus erythematosus	Rheumatoid arthritis Lupus Unclassified	Rheumatoid arthritis Rheumatic fever Lupus Polyarteritis Temporal arteritis Wegener's granulo- matosis
Neoplastic (6%)	*Neoplastic* (8%)	*Neoplastic* (20%)

Leukemia
Lymphoma
	Leukemia
	Lymphoma
	Neuroblastoma
	Reticulum cell sarcoma
		Leukemia
		Lymphoma
		Multiple myeloma
		Colonic, pancreatic, and
		  renal tumors
		Metastatic disease to
		  bone and liver

Miscellaneous (10%)	*Miscellaneous* (10%)	*Miscellaneous* (20%)

Agranulocytosis
Lamellar ichthyosis
Milk allergy
Agammaglobulinemia
Behçet's syndrome
Anicteric hepatitis
Ruptured appendix
Central nervous system
  fever
Aspiration pneumonia
	Regional enteritis
	Thyroiditis
	Salicylate toxicity
	Diencephalic syndrome
	Dehydration fever
	Immunodeficiency
		Granulomatous disease
		  Sarcoid
		  Hepatitis
		Regional enteritis
		Ulcerative colitis
		Thrombophlebitis
		Factitious fever
		Mediterranean fever
		Cirrhosis
		Whipple's disease

	Physically well children (9%)	
Undiagnosed (12%)	*Undiagnosed* (32%)	*Undiagnosed* (5%)

The Diagnostic Evaluation

1. *Initial studies* should be determined by clues provided by the history and physical examination. One must particularly search for a history of recent immunizations, transfusions, travel, risk factors for HIV infection, and exposure to animals or other sick individuals.

2. *Initial diagnostic procedures* should include a complete blood count, urinalysis, erythrocyte sedimentation rate, chest film, and serum protein electrophoresis in addition to more specific studies indicated from the history and physical examination.

3. If sedimentation rate is elevated, if serum electrophoresis reveals a reversed albumin-globulin ratio or increase in the alpha globulin fraction, or if leukocytosis exists, these should all be considered evidence of an active disease process.

4. If initial studies fail to provide a diagnosis, other useful studies might include:

   Blood cultures, urine cultures, stool cultures
   Liver function tests
   Bone marrow biopsy and culture
   Antinuclear antibodies
   Latex fixation text
   Lupus erythematosus preparations
   Upper gastrointestinal films
   Barium enema
   Intravenous pyelogram
   Bone scan
   Sinus films

5. Ultimately, the diagnosis may require a biopsy of skin, muscle, and/or liver.

6. It is useful to establish an orderly timetable for the pursuit of the diagnosis. All too often the investigation proceeds in an aimless fashion without a logical schedule.

References: Pizzo PA, Lovejoy FH Jr, Smith DH: Pediatrics 55:468, 1975. McClung J: Am J Dis Child 124:544, 1972. Jacoby GA, Swartz MN: N Engl J Med 289:1407, 1972.
From McMillan JA, et al: The Whole Pediatrician Catalog. Philadelphia, W.B. Saunders, 1977, with permission.

The Symptomatic Treatment of Fever

Would you throw cold water on the walls of an overheated room or would you turn down the thermostat? The answer seems obvious, yet the same logic is often not present when it comes to the management of fever in children. The rational treatment of fever requires an understanding of its pathophysiologic basis. Most febrile states in infants and children result from an abnormal elevation in the hypothalamic setpoint triggered by the release of interleukins. When this occurs, heat production is increased and heat loss is minimized. Much less commonly, fever is a result of excessive heat production alone, or when heat production is normal but heat loss is faulty.

The accompanying table examines the pathophysiologic basis for fever and describes the corresponding appropriate treatment.

Reference: Lorin M: The Febrile Child. New York, John Wiley, 1982.

Pathophysiologic Basis for Symptomatic Treatment of Fever

DISEASE PROCESS CAUSING FEVER	PATHOPHYSIOLOGY OF FEVER	CLINICAL FINDINGS	APPROPRIATE NONSPECIFIC TREATMENT	INAPPROPRIATE NONSPECIFIC TREATMENT
Infection, malignancy, allergy, steroid fever, collagen disease	Endogenous pyrogen causes rise in hypothalamic setpoint	Patient complains of feeling cold; piloerection; cold extremities; absent of minimal sweating; body positioned to minimize surface area, shivering	Drug-induced lowering of hypothalamic setpoint (e.g., with aspirin, acetaminophen); supply sufficient clothing and covers for maximal comfort; avoid shivering	Physical removal of heat, e.g., sponging, ice blanket, ice water enemas; without change in setpoint, these measures will cause discomfort, increase metabolic rate and will only lower body temperature for brief period
CNS lesion, DDT poisoning, scorpion venom, radiation, epinephrine and norepinephrine overdose	Agent or illness acts directly on hypothalamus to raise setpoint	Same as above	Drug-induced lowering of hypothalamic setpoint theoretically indicated as above; it is not clearly established, however, as possible with presently available drugs	Same as above
Malignant hyperthermia, hyperthyroidism, hypernatremia, primary defect in energy metabolism, aspirin overdose	Heat production exceeds heat loss mechanisms	Patient complains of feeling hot; no piloerection; hot extremities; active sweating; body positioned to maximize surface area	Undress patient; physical removal of heat, e.g., ice blanket, sponging	Attempt to lower setpoint (which is already set normally) with drugs, e.g., aspirin—possible toxicity of drug without potential benefit
Overuse of sauna, exposure to industrial heat, over dressing	Environmental heat load exceeds normal heat loss mechanisms	Same as above	Eliminate heat source; undress patient; physical removal of heat is effective but is not usually necessary	Same as above
Ectodermal dysplasia, burns, phenothiazine, anticholinergic overdose, heat stroke	Defective heat loss mechanisms cannot cope with normal heat load	Patient complains of feeling hot; sweating decreased (secondary to disease process); hot extremities; body positioned to maximize surface area	Provide cool environment; undress patient; physical removal of heat may be necessary	Same as above

Reference: Lorin M: The Febrile Child. New York, John Wiley, 1982.

Decline in Fever Following Acetaminophen—What Does It Mean?

Many physicians assume that a febrile child who exhibits a reduction in fever along with an improvement in general appearance following acetaminophen administration is not likely to have a bacterial infection. In fact, the degree of fever reduction does not distinguish between viral and bacterial infection, nor does it help in selecting those children who are bacteremic. Comparison of the degree of fever reduction in children with their eventual etiologic diagnosis has yielded the following conclusions:

1. The improvement in clinical appearance following fever reduction makes the identification of patients with potentially life-threatening infection more difficult.
2. Patients with occult bacteremia and bacterial deep tissue infections experience at least as great a reduction in fever 1 and 2 hours following acetaminophen administration as do patients with self-limited viral infections.
3. Even patients with bacterial meningitis experience a mean temperature reduction of 1.1°C following acetominophen administration.

These studies demonstrate that neither the observation of clinical improvement nor the history of defervescence following antipyretic administration should comfort the physician when the patient's condition prior to antipyretic therapy gave cause for concern.

References: Baker MD, Fosarelli PD, Carpenter RO: Pediatrics 80:315, 1987. Weisse ME, Miller G, Brien JH: Pediatr Infect Dis J 6:1091, 1987. Baker RC, Tiller T, Bauscher JC, et al: Pediatrics 83:1016, 1989.

Hospitalization of Febrile Infants—What Is the Risk?

When we hospitalize young infants and treat them with intravenous antibiotics for presumed sepsis, we believe we are decreasing their risk of serious disease and complications. In fact, hospitalization of young febrile infants is not only costly, it is risky. Of 190 febrile infants under 2 months of age evaluated in the outpatient clinics of The Johns Hopkins University Hospital and hospitalized for observation and treatment, 37 patients (19.5%) had 48 separate complications. Twenty-four (50%) of the complications resulted from intravenous administration of fluids and/or antibiotics.

Complications During In-hospital Treatment of Febrile Infants

TYPE OF COMPLICATION	NO. OF COMPLICATIONS
Preventable	
IV infiltrates requiring compresses	13
Sloughing of skin with IV therapy	10
Fluid overload	1
Gentamicin overdose	1
Fever secondary to high isolette temperature	1
Untreated urinary tract infection	1
Distraught mother secondary to multiple lumbar punctures	1
Stolen Infant	1
Total	**29**

Table continued on next page.

Complications During In-hospital Treatment of Febrile Infants (Cont.)

TYPE OF COMPLICATION	NO. OF COMPLICATIONS
Other	
Diarrhea with onset > 72 hr after admission	12
Thrush/candidiasis	6
Chloramphenicol sodium succinate-induced bone marrow suppression	1
Total	**19**

In addition to the complications listed above, diagnostic misadventures during hospitalization can lead to unnecessary costs and patient trauma. The table below lists the diagnostic misadventures encountered during the hospitalization of the same 190 infants mentioned above.

Misadventures During In-hospital Treatment of Febrile Infants

TYPE OF MISADVENTURE	NO.
Contaminated CSF cultures	12
Contaminated blood cultures	4
Abnormal urinalysis findings with no follow-up	4
3 normal chest roentgenograms in 1 patient	1
Suprapubic examination done to check contaminated, improperly labeled urine culture	1
2 repeated lumbar punctures, both negative after positive counterimmunoelectrophoresis	1
Traumatized infant 2° to multiple lumbar punctures	2
Kept 48 hr for neurologic consultation that was not done	1
Total	**26**

The next time you consider hospitalizing an infant "just for observation," remember these potential complications and try to assure more good than harm comes from your decision.

References: DeAngelis C, Joffe A, Wilson M, Willis E: Iatrogenic risks and financial costs of hospitalizing febrile infants. Am J Dis Child 137:1146, 1983, with permission.

Baskin MN, O'Rourke EJ, Fleisher GR: Outpatient treatment of febrile infants 28 to 89 days of age with intramuscular administration of ceftriaxone. J Pediatr 120:22–27, 1992.

FONTANELS

How Many Fontanels Are Present at Birth in the Infant's Skull?

There are actually six fontanels, but only two, the anterior and posterior, are normally palpable.

The anterior fontanel is at the meeting place of the coronal, sagittal, and frontal sutures. It is a diamond-shaped, fibrous tissue membrane covering a transient defect in ossification. It is the largest fontanel and measures about 4 cm in the A-P direction, and 2.5 cm transversely. The membrane pulses with the infant's pulse and can be observed to be slightly depressed when the baby is upright and quiet. Molding of the skull from pressures during labor and delivery can cause temporary overriding of the sutures and the impression of a smaller fontanel. Other less benign conditions causing smaller fontanel size are discussed in the following section.

The posterior fontanel is at the meeting place of the saggital and lambdoid sutures. It is triangular and usually less than 1 cm at the widest point.

Two pairs of fontanels, the sphenoidal and mastoid, appear on each side of the skull, are small and irregular, and are difficult to palpate.

Abnormal Fontanel Size

An abnormality in size of the anterior fontanel may be a tip-off to abnormality in the infant. The figure displays the fontanel size,

defined as $\dfrac{\text{length} + \text{width}}{2}$, as measured with a steel tape in 201 normal infants.

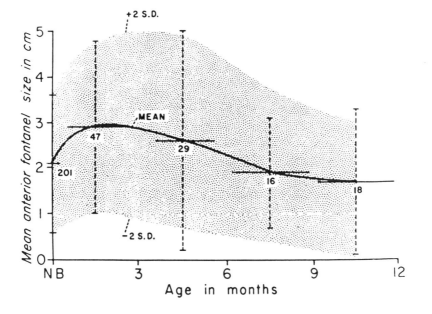

The following tables list conditions associated with an unusually small (or prematurely closed) fontanel or with an unusually large fontanel.

Disorders in Which Premature Closure
or Small Fontanel for Age May Be a Feature

Microcephaly
High Ca++/vitamin D ratio in pregnancy
Craniosynostosis
Hyperthyroidism
Normal variant

Disorders in Which Large Fontanel for Age May Be a Feature

SKELETAL DISORDERS	CHROMOSOMAL ABNORMALITIES	OTHER CONDITIONS
Achondroplasia	Down's syndrome	Athyrotic hypothyroidism
Aminopterin-induced syndrome	13 Trisomy syndrome	Hallermann-Streiff syndrome
Apert's syndrome	18 Trisomy syndrome	Malnutrition
Cleidocranial dysostosis		Progeria
Hypophosphatasia		Rubella syndrome
Kenny's syndrome		Russell-Silver syndrome
Osteogenesis imperfecta		
Pyknodysostosis		
Vitamin D deficiency rickets		

References: Popich GA, Smith DW: J Pediatr 80:749, 1972. Barness LA: Manual of Pediatric Physical Diagnosis, 6th ed. Chicago, Mosby-Year Book, 1990.

The Bulging Fontanel

A bulging fontanel in an infant is generally regarded as a sign of serious CNS disease, such as:

Meningitis	Cerebral hemorrhage	Lead poisoning
Encephalitis	Intracranial abscess	Sinus thrombosis
Hydrocephalus	Subdural hematoma	Tumor

The history, however, may suggest a benign cause. A congenital subgaleal cyst over the anterior fontanel may simulate a bulging fontanel. *Benign intracranial hypertension*, a syndrome of increased intracranial pressure, normal ventricular system and CSF composition, and absence of focal neurologic signs can also produce a bulging fontanel.

The causes of benign intracranial hypertension in infancy:

Impaired CSF absorption
  Obstructed inferior vena cava
    secondary to intrathoracic mass
    or obstructive lung disease
  Obstruction of sagittal sinus secondary
    to skull fracture or other cause
Endocrine/Metabolic
  Galactosemia
  Addison's disease
  Hypophosphatasia
  Hypoparathyroidism
  Hypothyroidism
Drugs
  Hypervitaminosis A
  Tetracyclines

Drugs *(Cont.)*
  Nalidixic acid
Infections
  Roseola infantum (herpes virus 6)
  Guillain-Barré syndrome
Nutritional
  Hypovitaminosis A
  Rapid brain growth following
    starvation
Miscellaneous
  Polycythemia vera
  Heart disease
  Allergic diseases
  Anemia (severe)
  Wiskott-Aldrich syndrome

References: Hagberg B, Silinpää M: Acta Paediatr Scand 59:328–339, 1970.
Barnett HL: Pediatrics. New York, Appleton-Century-Crofts, 1972.
From McMillan JA, et al: The Whole Pediatrician Catalog. Philadelphia, W.B. Saunders, 1977, with permission.

FOREIGN BODY

Where Is the Coin—in the Esophagus or Trachea?

The list of foreign bodies encountered in various openings of children's bodies is almost endless. A frequent problem is the swallowing or aspiration of objects. Coins are favored for this purpose (but note that hot dogs are one of the most common causes of fatal aspiration). Opaque objects such as coins are accurately localized with radiography. However, a frequent question that comes up in removing a coin is whether it is in the esophagus or trachea.

In the esophagus, foreign bodies are usually found at one of three areas of physiologic narrowing: (1) below the cricopharyngeal muscle; (2) at the level of the aortic arch; or (3) just above the diaphragm. Foreign bodies lie in the plane of least resistance, and if a coin enters the esophagus, it will lie in a frontal plane and thus appear head-on in the anterior-posterior film of the chest and on-edge in a lateral film. In contrast, a coin in the trachea will come to rest in the sagittal plane and will appear on-edge in the A-P view and head-on in the lateral view.

Of course foreign bodies can lodge in the larynx and in bronchi, as well as in the trachea. Objects in the upper airway can cause dysphagia from swelling, and objects in the esophagus can cause airway problems from compression or overflow of food or other secretions.

Other common locations for foreign bodies in children are the eye (see entry under "EYE"), ear, nose, stomach and intestine.

Reference: Hollinger PH, Johnson KC: Foreign bodies in the air and food passages. Pediatr Clin North Am 1:827, 1954.

Foreign Bodies in the Air and Food Passages

A wise pediatrician once said, "When deliberating over a difficult diagnosis in a child, even if it's as clear-cut a case as otitis media, *always* consider the ingestion of a foreign body!" The following should facilitate that thought process.

1. **Underlying factors leading to foreign bodies of the esophagus**
   Neuromuscular disorders (uncoordinated swallowing)
   Vascular compression (double aortic arch, etc.)
   Stricture or stenosis secondary to:
      Congenital deformity
      Repaired tracheoesophageal fistula
      Reflux esophagitis
      Caustic injestion
   Altered mental status (e.g., poor judgment secondary to age, underlying
      medical condition)
   Alteration of sensation

2. **Signs and symptoms of esophageal foreign bodies**

Refusal to take oral feedings	Gagging
Increased salivation	"Foreign body" sensation
Vomiting	Pain radiating to the sternal
Pain or discomfort with swallowing	or back area
Drooling	

3. **Signs and symptoms of foreign bodies of the airway**

Foreign Bodies of the Airway

SIGNS/SYMPTOMS	LOCATION OF FOREIGN BODY		
	LARYNX	TRACHEA	BRONCHI
Hoarseness	+		
Aphonia	+		
Odynophagia	+		
Drooling	+		
Audible slap		+	
Cough	+	+	+
Hemoptysis	+	+	+
Stridor	+	+	+
Wheeze	+	+	+
Dyspnea	+	+	+
Airway obstruction	+	+	+
Sudden death	+	+	+

4. **Progression of radiographs: Imaging that may be required for diagnosis**
   Chest x-ray (anteroposterior and lateral)
   Lateral neck (if indicated)
   Inspiratory/expiratory films (if patient is cooperative)
   Chest fluoroscopy
   Ultrasound; overpenetrated films of unresolved areas of density
   Possible computed tomography; possible contrast studies

5. **An ounce of prevention**
   Certain foods are more easily aspirated than others (e.g., peanuts—the most commonly aspirated food, chunks of carrots and apples, hot dogs, etc.). These foods should be withheld from children 0–4 years until they can chew them properly (i.e., after their molars have erupted). Small objects, such as tiny plastic toys, etc., should always be avoided in this age group.

Reference: Kenna MA, Bluestone CD: Foreign bodies in the air and food passages. Pediatrics in Review 10(1):25–31, 1988.

FRAGILE X SYNDROME

Recognition of the Fragile X Syndrome in Young Children

Fragile X syndrome is the most commonly inherited form of mental retardation. Although it is thought to be an X-linked recessive trait with variable expression and incomplete penetrance, 30% of all carrier women are also affected. The syndrome is named "fragile X" because there exists a fragile site or gap at the end of the long arm of the X-chromosome in lymphocytes of affected patients when grown in a folate-deficient medium. Carrier females typically have a 30 to 40% chance of giving birth to a retarded male and a 15 to 20% chance of having a retarded female. Further, there frequently exists a maternal family history for a relative with mental retardation or developmental and learning disabilities. Most studies have dealt with recognition of this syndrome in older children and young adults, but many of the physical features, behavioral characteristics, and family history features are apparent far earlier.

Prominent parental concerns that might bring such a child to a pediatrician's attention include:

Developmental delay
Speech delay
Short attention span or hyperactivity
Mouthing of objects persisting at an age beyond when it would be expected
Difficulty in disciplining the child
Frequent temper tantrums
Autistic-like behaviors such as rocking, talking to oneself, spinning, unusual hand movements, difficulty with transitions, preference for being alone, echolalia, and poor eye contact
Poor gross motor coordination
History of vomiting, spitting up, or colic during infancy
History of frequent otitis media
Self-abusive behaviors
Hand flapping
Drooling persisting at an age beyond when it would be expected
Hypotonia
Fighting with others
Pica
Hand/thumb sucking

While older children (8 to 12 years of age) are more likely to display the classic physical features of fragile X syndrome (long face with a prominent jaw, large prominent ears, and post-pubertal macroorchidism), patients as young as 2 or 3 years have been noted to exhibit the following physical findings:

Long and/or wide and/or protruding ears
Prominent jaw or long face
High arched palate
Flattened nasal bridge
Microcephaly or relative macrocephaly
Apparent hypertelorism
Epicanthic folds
Simian creases of palms; vertical creases of soles
Long philtrum
Hemangioma
Hyperextensible joints
Antimongoloid slant to eyes
Clinical impression of macroorchidism
Prominent forehead

It is not feasible or sound to recommend chromosomal studies on all children with developmental, learning, and behavioral disabilities. But these problems (particularly speech delay, unusual behaviors, and developmental delay) taken in context with a maternal family history of mental retardation or developmental disabilities and the physical findings of long, wide, or protruding ears, a long face, flat nasal bridge, and a high arched palate probably warrant a search for the fragile X chromosome. A new method of identifying carriers of these mutations by direct DNA analysis has recently been described.

References: Simkoi A, Hornstein L, Soukup S, Bagamery N: Fragile X syndrome: Recognition in young children. Pediatrics 83:547–552, 1989.
Rousseau F, Hertz D, Biancalana V, et al: Direct diagnosis by DNA analysis of the fragile X syndrome of mental retardation. N Engl J Med 325:1673–1681, 1991.

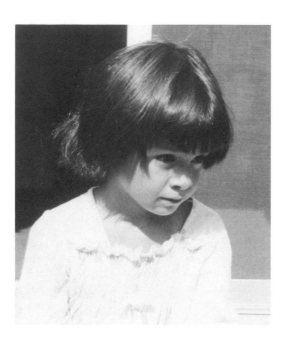

To make a prairie it takes a clover
    and one bee,—
One clover, and a bee,
And revery.
The revery alone will do
If bees are few.

                    Emily Dickinson

GASTROENTERITIS

Rotavirus Versus Astrovirus

Over the past 20 years, pediatricians and virologists have gained great insights into the causes and nature of gastroenteritis. The enteric adenoviruses, such as rotavirus, have been of particular focus as a cause of diarrhea in infants and young children. Recently, reports of astrovirus-caused gastroenteritis has come to the attention of clinicians, although their medical importance remains poorly defined. Offered below is a comparison of the clinical findings associated with astrovirus and rotavirus gastroenteritis:

Clinical Findings Associated with Astrovirus and Rotavirus Gastroenteritis*

FINDINGS	ASTROVIRUS INFECTION (N = 44) (percent)	ROTAVIRUS INFECTION (N = 175) (percent)
Watery stools	61	67
Loose stools	41	35
Mucoid stools	55	51
Bloody stools	7	6
Nausea[†]	71	88
Abdominal pain[†]	58	63
Vomiting	61	67
Fever	80	83
Dehydration ≥5%	5	15

* Only stool samples in which no bacterial, parasitic, or other viral pathogens were detected are included.
† Includes data from Study 1 only (33 children with astroviruses and 116 with rotaviruses).

Reference: Herrmann JE, Taylor DN, Echeverria P, Blacklow NR: Astroviruses as a cause of gastroenteritis in children. N Engl J Med 324:1757–1760, 1991, with permission.

Chitterlings: Another *Yersinia* Food Group

Yersinia enterocolitica was first recognized as a cause of human infection in 1933. In young children, infection generally causes acute gastroenteritis. In older children a picture of mesenteric adenitis that can easily be confused with appendicitis predominates. A 1988–89 outbreak of *Yersinia enterocolitica* in Atlanta has added chitterlings (also *chitlins*), the small intestines of pigs, to the list of agents of transmission. Although the epidemiology remains poorly understood, previously cited agents include contaminated milk products, contact with sick pets, transfusion of contaminated blood products, and ingestion of raw pork.

The Atlanta outbreak was traced to households where chitterlings were prepared for holiday meals. Preparation of chitterlings involves boiling the raw small intestines of pigs after fat and fecal matter have been removed. In nearly all of the Atlanta cases, the affected infants and children had contact with the chitterlings' preparers, although not the raw intestines themselves.

The take-home message is that when an infant or child presents with a picture of acute gastroenteritis, a thorough investigation into intrahousehold contacts as well as ingestion of possible contaminants is called for.

Clinical Manifestations of Yersiniosis

Diarrhea	Fever
Mucoid stools	Vomiting
Bloody diarrhea or pus (10–20%)	Abdominal pain—colicky, diffuse or localized to RLQ

Differential Diagnosis

Shigella
Enteroinvasive *E. coli*
Salmonella
Campylobacter

Yersinia pseudotuberculosis can cause identical picture to the mesenteric adenitis of older children.

References: Lee LA, et al: Yersinia enterocolitica 0:3 infections in infants and children, associated with the household preparation of chitterlings. N Engl J Med 322: 984–987, 1990.
Oski FA, et al: Principles and Practice of Pediatrics. Philadelphia, J.B. Lippincott, 1990.

GASTROINTESTINAL BLEEDING

In the Neonate

Common Causes

Esophagitis
Gastritis
Ingested maternal blood
Necrotizing entercolitis
Stress ulcer (gastric)

Uncommon Causes

Acquired coagulopathy
Gastroenteritis (*Campylobacter* infections)
Hemophilia
Rectal trauma or gastrointestinal trauma
Thrombocytopenia
Vitamin K deficiency
Volvulus

Rare Causes

Acute ulcerative colitis
Gastric polyp
Gastrointestinal duplication cyst
Intussusception
Leiomyoma
Milk allergy
Nasal or pharyngeal bleeding
Severe cyanotic congenital heart disease
Vascular malformation of the gut (hemangioma, telangiectasia, arteriovenous malformation)

In Infancy

Common Causes

Anal fissures
Esophagitis
Gastritis (possibly due to
    drug ingestion)
Gastroenteritis
Polyps

Uncommon Causes

Acquired coagulation disturbance
Hemophilia
Henoch-Schönlein purpura
Inflammatory bowel disease
Meckel's diverticulum
Parasitism
Peptic ulcer
Thrombocytopenia

Rare Causes

Chronic granulomatous disease
Diverticulitis
Esophageal varices
Hemangiomas and telangiectasia
Hemolytic-uremic syndrome
Hemorrhoids
Intestinal foreign body
Lymphosarcoma
Peutz-Jegher syndrome
Pseudoxanthoma elasticum
Scurvy

Using the BUN/Creatinine Ratio in Localizing the Source of Gastrointestinal Bleeding in Children

Although most children with gastrointestinal bleeding make the diagnostician's job somewhat easier by presenting with a chief complaint of either hematemesis or bright red blood per rectum, there exists a gray zone in localizing the source of bleeding when a child presents with melena or altered blood in the stool. Frequently, this child undergoes a wide variety of costly and invasive diagnostic procedures in order to determine the site of blood loss. A useful and inexpensive means of identifying upper gastrointestinal bleeding, however, lies in an evaluation of the blood urea nitrogen to creatinine ratio (BUN/Cr).

In a retrospective study of 40 children hospitalized for evaluation and treatment of gastrointestinal bleeding at the Children's Hospital of Los Angeles, a BUN/Cr ratio >30 indicated an upper gastrointestinal bleeding source with a specificity of 100%. Documentation of the source of bleeding was confirmed by endoscopy, surgery, or presence of hematemesis or bright red blood per rectum. The rise in BUN after an upper gastrointestinal hemorrhage is probably a result of increased hepatic catabolism of the absorbed amino acid load from the intraluminal blood. The bleeding, therefore, must occur proximal to the small intestine's absorptive surface (e.g., proximal to the ligament of Treitz) in order to cause a significant rise in the BUN/Cr ratio. The sensitivity of the BUN/Cr ratio for upper gastrointestinal bleeding, however, was 39%, because there existed a wide range of BUN/Cr ratios among the upper GI bleeders (range = 10–140; mean = 34 ± 29 SD) in comparison to the lower GI bleeders (range = 3.3–30; mean = 16 ± 8.5 SD). A BUN/Cr ratio less than or equal to 30, therefore, can be consistent with either an upper or a lower gastrointestinal bleeding site. The wide range of BUN/Cr ratios seen in children with upper gastrointestinal bleeding may have been due to smaller volumes of blood loss, vomiting, or more rapid gastro-intestinal transit times in children when compared to adults.

Reference: Felber S, Rosenthal P, Henton D: The BUN/Creatinine ratio in localizing gastrointestinal bleeding in pediatric patients. J Pediatr Gastroenterol Nutr 7:685–687, 1988.

Kool-Aid Colitis

A mother brings her child to your Emergency Room frightened by the new onset of bright red stools in the child's diaper. The child appears hemodynamically stable and is without abdominal tenderness. What do you do?

If the stool guaiac is negative, ask the mother whether her child has had any cherry- or strawberry-containing beverages. Don't stop there. Ask about beets, tomato-containing products, and cherry or strawberry candies. Any and all of these substances can be the culprit when an alarmingly scarlet, nonclotting effluent accompanies a stool.

Reference: Sack J: "Kool-Aid colitis" (letter). N Engl J Med 322:1012, 1990.

GENETICS

What is a Human Being's "Unique Genetic Make-up"?

The uniqueness of each individual stems from the fact that over one-fifth of his or her genes (i.e., proteins) are in a form that differs from that present in the majority of the population. All human diseases are a result of the interaction of the person's unique genetic make-up and the environment, and therefore genetics can be considered the basis of all medicine.

Reference: Goldstein JL, Brown MS: Genetics. In Wilson JD, et al (eds): Harrison's Principles of Internal Medicine, 12th ed. New York, McGraw-Hill, 1991, p 21.

Ethnicity As a Risk Factor

Disorders transmitted by the inheritance of a single mutant gene, termed mendelian or "simply inherited disorders," occur with increased frequency in specific ethnic groups. Some examples of these relationships are listed in the table below.

Examples of Simply Inherited Disorders that Occur with Increased Frequency in Specific Ethnic Groups

ETHNIC GROUP	SIMPLY INHERITED DISORDER
African blacks	Hemoglobinopathies, especially Hb S, Hb C, persistent Hb F, α and β thalassemias Glucose-6-phosphate dehydrogenase deficiency
Armenians	Familial Mediterranean fever

Table continued on next page.

Examples of Simply Inherited Disorders that Occur with Increased Frequency in Specific Ethnic Groups (Cont.)

ETHNIC GROUP	SIMPLY INHERITED DISORDER
Ashkenazi Jews	Abetalipoproteinemia
	Bloom's syndrome
	Dystonia musculorum deformans (recessive form)
	Factor XI (PTA) deficiency
	Familial dysautonomia (Riley-Day syndrome)
	Gaucher's disease (adult form)
	Neimann-Pick disease
	Pentosuria
	Tay-Sachs disease
Chinese	α-Thalassemia
	Glucose-6-phosphate dehydrogenase deficiency
	Adult lactase deficiency
Eskimos	Pseudocholinesterase deficiency
	Adrenogenital syndrome
Finns	Congenital nephrosis
	Mulibrey nanism
French Canadians	Tyrosinemia
Japanese	Acatalasemia
Lebanese	Homozygous familial hypercholesterolemia
Mediterranean peoples (Italians, Greeks, Sephardic Jews)	β-Thalassemia
	Glucose-6-phosphate dehydrogenase deficiency
	Familial Mediterranean fever
	Glycogen storage disease, type III
Northern Europeans	Cystic fibrosis
Scandinavians	Alpha$_1$-antitrypsin deficiency
	LCAT (lecithin:cholesterol acyltransferase) deficiency
South African whites	Porphyria variegata
	Homozygous familial hypercholesterolemia

From Wilson JD, et al (eds): Harrison's Principles of Internal Medicine, 12th ed. New York, McGraw-Hill, 1991, with permission.

GROWTH

Predicted Weight and Height from Age

If you know the age of a child and want a rough estimate of the weight and height:

For 3–12 mo:	Weight (lb) = age (mo) + 11
For 1–6 yr:	Weight (lb) = age (yr) × 5 + 17
For 7–12 yr:	Weight (lb) = age (yr) × 7 + 5
For 2–14 yr:	Height (in) = (2½ × age) + 30

Reference: Graef JW, Cone TE: In Manual of Pediatric Therapeutics, 6th ed. Boston, Little, Brown, 1991.

More on Predicted Heights

The formula of Tanner et al. demonstrates that height at age 3 years correlates better with height at maturity than it does at any other age:

Adult height (cm) = 1.27 × height (at 3 yr) + 54.9 cm (males)

Adult height (cm) = 1.29 × height (at 3 yr) + 42.3 cm (females)

If you cannot remember these formulas or your programmable calculator has been stolen, the commonly accepted statement that the child at age 2 has achieved one half his or her final height is quite satisfactory. For girls, however, 10 to 12 cm (2.54 to 4.00 in) must be subtracted from this predicted height. If the height at 3 years is known, an alternative to the Tanner equation to predict final adult height is to multiply the age 3 height by 1.87 for boys and 1.73 for girls.

Reference: Tanner et al: Arch Dis Child 31:372, 1956.
Adapted from McMillan JA, et al: The Whole Pediatrician Catalog, Vol. 3. Philadelphia, W.B. Saunders, 1982, p 74.

Growth During Infancy: Weight

When assessing the growth of infants in a well-child care setting, a handy rule of thumb is offered: the newborn infant typically loses between 5 and 10% of his or her birth weight during the first few days of life (due to water loss). After that, the infant should gain 1 ounce or 30 grams, on average, per day. This weight gain, approximately 1 to 2 pounds per month, results in a doubling of the birth weight by six months of age. By the age of 2 years, weight gain should slow down to about one-half pound per month. Please note that although this tip is quite useful in the growing infant, it is not sensitive in the older child.

Growth During Infancy: Length

The greatest rise in linear growth occurs during infancy (the first 2 years of life). The average length of a newborn American infant is 50.4 cm (2.0 SD) or 19.8 inches (0.8 SD) in males and 49.7 cm (1.9 SD) or 19.6 inches (0.75 SD) in females. The growth increment during this period should be 25 to 30 cm (10 to 12 in) during the first year of life and 12 cm (5 in) during the second year of life. Male infants are typically heavier (by about 0.5 kg) and longer (by about 0.5 cm) than their female counterparts.

Growth During Infancy: Cranial and Brain Growth

The human brain begins its peak growth rate at birth and during the postnatal period. It should be noted that at birth, the infant's brain is only one-sixth of its final weight. Consequently, the growth of the cranial vault parallels this rapid development in order to accommodate the increasing brain size. In fact, careful evaluation of the skull size (head circumference) and shape gives the pediatrician a great deal of insight into the infant's neurologic development.

Mean head circumference at birth is approximately 35.3 cm (1.2 SD) or 13.9 inches (0.5 SD). There should be a 5 cm increase in head circumference during the first 3 months of life and an additional 6 cm increase by the end of the first year of life. Whereas the head circumference of a newborn infant is greater than his or her chest, this ratio should approximate 1:1 by age 1 year.

(N.B.: Closure of the fontanel is covered under "Fontanels.")

GYNECOMASTIA

The Differential Diagnosis of Gynecomastia

Gynecomastia is defined as the visible or palpable development of breast tissue in boys or men. It has been divided into four types:

Type I gynecomastia (pubertal gynecomastia or benign adolescent breast hypertrophy) refers to the common entity seen in pubertal males. In fact, many cite an incidence of 60 to 70% in this population. It is typically a firm, tender subareolar mass anywhere from 1 to 5 cm in diameter. The pubertal adolescent frequently complains of pain in the breasts, particularly when wearing binding clothing. It usually spontaneously resolves within 2 years.

Type II gynecomastia (physiologic gynecomastia without evidence of underlying disease, or with evidence of organic disease including the effects of specific drugs) refers to a generalized, nonpainful breast enlargement. It is essential to differentiate between physiologic gynecomastia and breast enlargement due either to a pathologic process or to the use of a specific drug. The physician should, therefore, obtain a careful history regarding the time of onset, family history, duration of the enlargement, history of systemic illness, weight change, and drug or medication use. Physical examiantion should include height, weight, blood pressure, breast size, and Tanner staging of both breasts and genitals, in addition to a neurologic assessment. The most frequent causes of Type II gynecomastia are listed in tabular form below.

Type III gynecomastia is general obesity simulating gynecomastia, and **Type IV gynecomastia** is pectoral muscle hypertrophy.

Common Causes of Type II Gynecomastia

I. Idiopathic
II. Familial causes
    a. Associated with anosmia and testicular atrophy
    b. Reifenstein's syndrome (a type of familial male pseudohermaphroditism secondary to partial androgen insensitivity)
    c. Associated with hypogonadism and small penis
    d. Others
III. Specific illnesses or syndromes
    a. Kleinfelter's syndrome
    b. Male pseudohermaphroditism
    c. Testicular feminization syndrome
    d. Tumors (e.g., seminoma, Leydig cell tumor, teratoma, feminizing adrenal tumor, hepatoma, bronchogenic carcinoma)
    e. Leukemia
    f. Hemophilia
    g. Leprosy
    h. Thyroid dysfunction (hyper- and hypothyroidism)
    i. Cirrhosis of the liver
    j. Traumatic paraplegia
    k. Chronic glomerulonephritis
    l. Starvation (on refeeding)

IV. Miscellaneous Drugs
   a. Amphetamines
   b. Anabolic steroids
   c. Birth control pills
   d. Busulfan (and other chemotherapeutic agents)
   e. Cimetidine
   f. Clomiphene
   g. Diazepam
   h. Corticosteroids
   i. Digitalis
   j. Estrogens
   k. Human chorionic gonadotropin
   l. Insulin
   m. Isoniazid (and other antituberculosis drugs)
   n. Ketoconazole
   o. Marijuana
   p. Methadone (and other narcotics)
   q. Methyldopa
   r. Reserpine
   s. Spironolactone
   t. Testosterone
   u. Tricyclic antidepressants

Adapted from: Greydanus DE, Parks DS, Farrell EG: Breast disorders in children and adolescents. Pediatr Clin North Am 36:601–638, 1989.

H

HEAD

Head Circumference in Term Infants

When you are stuck without your growth grid, there is still a simple means of determining if a head is growing normally. The little table below lists the expected rate of increases in head circumference for term infants during the first year of life.

Rate of Increases in Head Circumference

PERIOD	HEAD CIRCUMFERENCE INCREMENTS
First 3 months	2 cm/month = 6 cm
4–6 months	1 cm/month = 3 cm
6–12 months	0.5 cm/month = 3 cm
First year	12 cm

HEADACHE

Common Causes

Extracranial infection
    Otitis/mastoiditis
    Pharyngitis
    Sinusitis
    Tooth abscess

Febrile illness
Migraine
Tension
    Anxiety
    Environmental stress

Uncommon Causes

Depression
Eye strain
Meningitis/encephalitis
Temporomandibular joint disease

Trauma
    Concussion
    Occipital neuralgia

Rare Causes

Allergy
Arnold-Chiari malformation
Cervical osteoarthritis
Chronic renal disease

Congenital erythropoietic porphyria
Cranial bone disease
Decreased intracranial pressure
    Post-lumbar puncture

Drugs
  Amphetamines
  Carbon monoxide
  Heavy metals
  Indomethacin
  Malidixic acid
  Nitrates/nitrites
  Oral contraceptives
  Steroids
  Sulfa
  Tetracycline
  Vitamin A
Epilepsy
Hyperventilation
Increased intracranial pressure
  Hydrocephalus
  Mass/tumor/abscess
  Pseudotumor cerebri
Leukemia infiltration
Metabolic
  Hyperammonemia
  Hypercarbia
  Hypoglycemia
  Hyponatremia
  Hypoxia
  Metabolic acidosis
Myositis

Psychogenic
  Conversion reaction
  Mimicry
  Secondary gain
Orbit
  Glaucoma
  Orbital tumor
Vascular
  Anemia
  Aneurysm
  Arteritis
    Giant cell
    Periarteritis nodosa
    Subacute bacterial endocarditis
    Systemic lupus erythematosis (SLE)
  AV malformation
  Cerebral infarct
    Embolism
    Thrombosis
  Cluster headache
  Hemorrhage
    Epidural
    Parenchymal
    Subdural
  Hypertension
  Phlebitis
  Venous sinus thrombosis

HEARING

Which Infant Is at Risk for Hearing Loss?

Long before a delay in language development secondary to a hearing loss is noted by a parent or physician, the astute pediatrician can single out infants at risk. Screening for hearing loss is relatively inexpensive and easy to perform, and the benefits of early detection are immeasurable. Be aware of the risk factors and look for the absence of the normal newborn's response to sound: startling, blinking, crying, quieting, or other forms of alertness are the normal newborn's reactions to sound.

Factors that Mandate Screening for Hearing Loss

A blood relative with childhood hearing impairment.
Anatomic malformations involving the head and neck.
Bacterial meningitis—especially *H. influenzae*.
Birthweight less than 1,500 g.
Severe asphyxia as evidenced by low Apgar scores, arterial pH $\leq$ 7.25, coma, seizures, or the need for continuous assisted ventilation.
Unconjugated bilirubin $>$ 17 mg/100 ml of serum.
Viral or other nonbacterial intrauterine fetal infections.

Any neonate with known congenital defect: Recessive syndromes constitute 4% to 40% of childhood deafness; dominant syndromes constitute about 15%; x-linked syndromes about 2%; and rubella, 9 to 20% of cases of childhood deafness.

Screening Tests

These screening tests allow evaluation of the infant at risk as early as 2 weeks of age:

1. Crib-o-gram: Crib movement is recorded in response to sound stimulus application.
2. Brainstem auditory evoked response (BAER): More sensitive than a crib-o-gram, BAERs record electrical potential at the skin overlying the nuclei and tracts of the auditory pathway.
3. Behavior assessment: See "Speech and Language Milestones."

References: Rowe LD: Hearing loss: The profound benefits of early diagnosis. Contemp Peds October:77–85, 1985.

Oski FA, et al: Principles and Practice of Pediatrics. Philadelphia, J.B. Lippincott, 1990.

Exogenous Causes of Hearing Loss

In addition to heredity, gestational age, dysmorphisms, and asphyxia, there are several exogenous causes of hearing loss to consider in the evaluation of communicative delay in infants and children.

Preconception and Prenatal

Cytomegalovirus
Hypoxia
Maternal drug abuse and alcoholism
Ototoxic drugs (quinine)
Irradiation of parent

Rubella
Syphilis
Toxemia, diabetes, or other severe
    maternal systemic disease
Toxoplasmosis

Perinatal

Hypoxia
Maternal infection
Ototoxic drugs (aminoglycosides)

Prematurity
Traumatic delivery

Neonatal and Postnatal

Erythroblastosis fetalis
Hypoxia
Infantile measles or mumps

Meningitis, encephalitis
Ototoxic drugs (aminoglycosides)

Reference: Rowe LD: Hearing loss: The profound benefits of early diagnosis. Contemp Pediatr October: 77–85, 1985.

HEMATOLOGY

Laboratory Test Results in Disorders Producing Hypochromia and Microcytosis

DISORDER	SERUM IRON	IRON-BINDING CAPACITY	FERRITIN	FEP*	HEMOGLOBIN ELECTRO-PHORESIS	MARROW IRON STORES
Iron deficiency	Decreased	Increased	Decreased	Increased	Normal	Decreased
Chronic disease anemia	Decreased	Decreased	Increased	Increased	Normal	Increased
Sideroblastic anemia	Increased	Normal	Increased	Decreased	Normal	Ring sideroblasts
β-thalassemia trait	Normal	Normal	Normal	Normal	Hemoglobin A_2 increased	Normal
α-thalassemia trait	Normal	Normal	Normal	Normal	Normal	Normal

*FEP indicates free erythrocyte protoporphyrin.
Adapted from Steinberg MH, Dreiling BJ: Microcytosis. JAMA 249:85, 1983, with permission.

HEMATURIA

Common Causes

Benign causes
    Benign recurrent hematuria
    Familial hematuria
    Idiopathic recurrent gross hematuria
    Postural hematuria
Contamination
    Menstrual
    Munchausen's syndrome
    Munchausen's syndrome by proxy
    Pregnancy-related bleeding
Hemoglobinopathies
    Hgb C
    Hgb SC
    Sickle-cell disease/trait (Hgb SS/SA)
    Sickle-thalassemia trait
Hypercalciuria
    Distal renal tubular acidosis
    Diuretic therapy
    Endocrine disorders
        Diabetes mellitus

Hypercalciuria *(Cont.)*
    Endocrine disorders *(Cont.)*
        Hyperadrenocorticism
        Hyperparathyroidism
        Hypothyroidism
    Hypercalcemia
    Hyperphosphatemia
    Hypertension
    Immobilization
    Juvenile rheumatoid arthritis
    Medullary sponge kidney
    Metabolic acidosis
    Neoplasm
    Renal tubular dysfunction
    Sarcoidosis
    Vitamin D excess
Hypoxia, asphyxia, and circulatory compromise
    Acute tubular necrosis
    Cortical and medullary necrosis

Infections
  Cystitis (viral, bacterial)
  Pyelonephritis
  Urethritis
Meatal stenosis
Noninfectious cystitis
  Cytoxan
  Radiation
Perineal irritation
Phimosis

Post-infectious glomerulonephritis
Trauma
  Fractured pelvis
  Postcatheterization
  Postcircumcision
  Postsurgery
  Renal contusion
  Renal fracture
  Urethral trauma
  Urethral ulceration

Uncommon Causes

Bladder diverticuli/polyps
Coagulopathies
Drug-induced
  Analgesic nephropathy
  Cephalosporins
  Cytoxan
  Penicillin
  Sulfonamides
Exercise
Glomerular disorders
  Mesangioproliferative
  Minimal change disease
Hydronephrosis

Infections
  Epididymitis
  Prostatitis
Masturbation
Periureteritis (appendicitis, ileitis)
Polycystic disease
Reflux nephropathy
Renal calculi
Renal vein thrombosis
Thrombocytopenia
Ureteropelvic junction obstruction
Urethral foreign body
Wilms' tumor

Rare Causes

Allergy
"Apparent"
  "Beeturia"
  Betadine
  Biliuria
  Desferoxamine
  Dyes
    Analine
    Congo red
  Hemoglobinuria
  Myoglobinuria
  Phenothiazines
  Porphyria
Diabetic nephropathy
Glomerular disorders
  Amyloidosis
  Crescentic glomerulonephritis (GN)
  Familial nephiritis (Alport's)
  Focal segmented proliferative GN
  Focal segmental sclerosis

  Goodpasture's syndrome
  IgA nephropathy
  Membranous GN
  Mesangiocapillary GN
  Subacute bacterial endocarditis
  Systemic lupus erythematosus
    (SLE)
  Wegener's granulomatosis
Hemangioma
Hematospermia
Immunologic
  Hemolytic-uremic syndrome
  Henoch-Schönlein purpura
  Polyarteritis nodosa
  SLE
Infections
  Leptospirosis
  Malaria
  Schistosomiasis
  Toxoplasmosis

Infections *(Cont.)*
  Tuberculosis
  Varicella
Malignant hypertension
Medullary sponge kidney
Neoplasms
  Bladder cancer

Neoplasms *(Cont.)*
  Prostatic concer
  Renal infarction
  Retroperitoneal fibrosis
  Vitamin deficiency
    Scurvy
    Vitamin K deficiency

Evaluation of Hematuria in Children and Adolescents

After urinary tract infections, hematuria is the most frequently occurring abnormality in the genitourinary tract. One must carefully assess the complaint of hematuria in order to rule out or diagnose from a large list of potentially serious disorders. It is important, first, to assess whether or not actual blood or simply a red substance is being excreted into the urine. A reagent strip (impregnated with orthotolodine-peroxide and enhanced with 6-methoxyquinolone) makes this quite simple. False-negative results with the dipstick method are rare but can result from the presence of high urinary concentrations of ascorbic acid. False-positive results, which are also rare, can occur in the presence of a raging urinary tract infection where bacterial peroxidase is released in high quantities. Following a positive dipstick microscopic evaluation is required; if no red blood cells (RBCs) are noted in a fresh urine sample, one should entertain the diagnosis of hemoglobinuria or myoglobinuria.

Although gross hematuria is easily recognized upon visual inspection, the urine should always be examined with dipstick and microscopic analysis to rule out other causes of red urine. Microscopic hematuria is usually defined as (a) three or more consecutive urine samples with positive reagent strip test results and either two or more RBCs per cubic millimeter in a fresh, uncentrifuged urine sample or (b) six or more RBCs per high-power field in a fresh urine sediment specimen.

Common Causes of Red Urine

1. **Negative Dipstick Test** (e.g., dyes, drugs, pigments)
   a. Pink, red, Coca-Cola, burgundy-colored urine (drug and food ingestion): Aminopyrine, anthocyanin, azo dyes, beets,* blackberries, chloroquine, desferoxamine, mesylate, ibuprofen, methyldopa, nitrofurantoin, phenazopyridine, phenolphthalein, rifampin, rhodamine B, sulfasalazine, urates.
   b. Dark brown, black:
      i. Disease-associated: alkaptonuria, homogentisic aciduria, melanin, methemoglobinemia, tyrosinosis
      ii. Drug and food ingestion: alanine, resorcinol, thymol.

2. **Positive Dipstick Test but No RBCs on Microscopic Examination**
   a. Hemoglobinuria
      i. Drugs and chemicals: aspidium, betanaphthyl, carbolic acid, carbon monoxide, chloroform, fava beans, mushrooms, naphthalene, pamaquine, phenylhydrazine, quinine, snake venom, sulfonamides.

---

*The excretion of red-purple or beet-colored urine (beeturia) after ingesting beets should prompt the clinician to work up the patient for iron-deficiency anemia.

ii. Disease-associated and other causes: all types of hemolytic anemias, hemolytic-uremic syndrome, septicemia, paroxysmal nocturnal hemoglobinuria, freshwater drowning, mismatched blood transfusions, cardiopulmonary bypass.

3. **Positive Dipstick Tests with RBCs on Microscopic Examination**
   a. No RBC casts present: tumors, cysts, stones, obstruction
   b. RBC casts present:
      i. Without proteinuria: IgA nephropathy, familial nephritis, benign or familial hematuria (in association with hypercalciuria)
      ii. With proteinuria: Acute glomerulonephritis, Henoch-Schönlein purpura, systemic lupus erythematosus, chronic glomerulonephritis
      iii. Heavy proteinuria: Nephrotic syndrome

The basic work-up and evaluation for the patient with hematuria should proceed as follows:

1. History (associated symptoms, precipitating events, pattern of hematuria, familial occurrence).

2. Physical examination (presence of edema, elevated blood pressure, skin lesions, joint involvement).

3. Laboratory tests

   a. Urinalysis (with confirmation of microscopic hematuria on two or more occasions).
   b. Urine culture (gross hematuria occurs in 5% to 10% of children with symptomatic urinary tract infection; the frequency of those children with symptomatic urinary tract infection and microscopic hematuria is not known).
   c. Complete blood count with examination of peripheral smear
   d. Serum creatinine
   e. ASO titer, streptozyme, C3 complement, anti-DNA antibody (e.g., poststreptococcal glomerulonephritis, SLE, proliferative GN)
   f. Quantitative urine protein, calcium, creatinine excretion
   g. Imaging studies (e.g., ultrasonography of the urine tract, intravenous pyelography, voiding cystourethrography).

References: Adapted from Boineau FG, Lewy JE: Evaluation of hematuria in children and adolescents. Pediatr Rev 11:101–107, 1989.
Norman ME: An office approach to hematuria and proteinuria. Pediatr Clin North Am 34:545–560, 1987.

Hematuria After Blunt Trauma

Hematuria is a common finding in the aftermath of blunt trauma to the abdomen. Traditional thinking suggests that hematuria is a significant consequence of genitourinary (GU) injury, and its presence typically elicits consideration of radiologic imaging of the GU tract. Which patient, in fact, requires a study and which study should you choose?

Asymptomatic hematuria is not an indication for computed tomography (CT) of the abdomen. In a study of 378 consecutive children evaluated by CT of the abdomen, those who were asymptomatic had no evidence of organ injury. A child with no signs or symptoms of abdominal injury (e.g., tenderness, ecchymoses, distention) despite the presence of hematuria does not warrant a CT exam. Children with asymptomatic hematuria may be evaluated on a nonemergent basis with Doppler ultrasonography, excretory urography, or a radioactive renal scan. In contrast, hematuria with abdominal symptoms is a significant marker of injury to both urinary and nonurinary organs in the setting of blunt abdominal trauma.

References: Taylor GA, et al: Hematuria: A marker of abdominal injury in children after blunt trauma. Ann Surg 208:688–693, 1988.

Jaffe D, Wesson D: Emergency management of blunt trauma in children. N Engl J Med 324:1477–1482, 1991.

Drug-induced Causes of Hematuria

THE DRUG	THE DISORDER
Penicillin and cephalosporin analogues, phenytoin	Allergic interstitial nephritis
Phenacetin, nonsteroidal anti-inflammatory agents	Papillary necrosis
Cyclophosphamide, mitotane	Chemical cystitis
Cyclophosphamide, phenacetin	Malignant neoplasm of uroepithelium
Anticoagulants	Spontaneous bleeding or induction of bleeding from an occult lesion

Reference: Schoolwerth AC: Hematuria and proteinuria: Their causes and consequences. Hospital Practice 22 (Oct 30):45–62, 1987.

Neonatal Hematuria

Gross hematuria is a rare presentation during the first month of life. The findings in one series of 35 patients are demonstrated below.

Findings in Series of 35 Patients

CAUSE	NO. OF PATIENTS	AGE AT ONSET 1ST WEEK	2ND WEEK	3RD WEEK	4TH WEEK	DURATION (DAYS)	REMARKS
Unknown	11	8	2	1	—	1–3	1 died of hyaline membrane disease and pneumothorax; normal BUN level in 9, elevated in 2
Renal vein thrombosis	7	3	1	3	—	2–5	3 had diabetic mothers; Bun level > 40 mg/100 ml in all; 4 had thrombocytopenia

Table continued on next page.

Findings in Series of 35 Patients (Cont.)

CAUSE	NO. OF PATIENTS	1ST WEEK	2ND WEEK	3RD WEEK	4TH WEEK	DURATION (DAYS)	REMARKS
Polycystic disease of kidney	6	6	—	—	—	2–4	5 died in neonatal period, one at 4 months; all had increased BUN, 40 to 80 mg/100 ml
Obstructive uropathy							BUN level 25 to 30 mg/100 ml; 2 with hydronephrosis underwent difficult delivery; 3 had pyuria and bacteriuria; palpable mass present in 2
Hydronephrosis	3	1	—	2	—	1–5	
Ureteral valve	3	2	—	—	—	2–4	
Bladder neck	1	1	—	—	1	4	
Sponge kidney	3	—	—	2	1	1	Death within 4 to 6 months of age
Wilms' tumor	2	—	—	—	1	2	Survived, patient doing well 4 years later

Abdominal masses were palpated in all patients later found to have renal vein thrombosis or polycystic kidneys. Intravenous pyelograms were normal in all patients in whom no cause was found for the hematuria, in the patients with posterior urethral valves, and in the one with bladder neck obstruction. IVP was abnormal in all other patients. Voiding cystourethrogram demonstrated the abnormality in the patients with obstruction.

Conclusion: Abdominal palpation, IVP, and blood urea nitrogen levels are warranted in all newborns presenting with gross hematuria. If the diagnosis is still unavailable, voiding cystourethrogram is in order. A significant number of these patients, however, will have no evident cause for their hematuria, and will recover spontaneously.

Reference: Emanuel B, Aronson N: neonatal hematuria. Am J Dis Child 128:204, 1974.
Adapted from McMillan, et al (eds): The Whole Pediatrician Catalog. Philadelphia, W.B. Saunders, 1977, pp 314–315, with permission.

HEMOGLOBIN

Classification of Red Cell Hemolytic Disorders by Predominant Morphology

In the following lists, nonhemolytic disorders of similar morphology are enclosed in parentheses for reference.

Spherocytes
Hereditary spherocytosis
ABO incompatibility in neonates
Immunohemolytic anemias with IgG-
or C3-coated red cells
Acute oxidant injury (hexose monophos-
phate shunt defects during hemolytic
crisis, oxidant drugs and chemicals)
Hemolytic transfusion reactions
Clostridium welchii septicemia
Severe burns, other red cell thermal
injury
Spider, bee, and snake venoms
Severe hypophosphatemia
Hypersplenism*

Bizarre Poikilocytes
Red cell fragmentation syndromes
(micro- and macroangiopathic
hemolytic anemias)
Acute oxidant injury*
Hereditary elliptocytosis in neonates
Hereditary pyropoikilocytosis

Elliptocytes
Hereditary elliptocytosis
Thalassemias
(Other hypochromic-microcytic
anemias)
(Megaloblastic anemias)

Stomatocytes
Hereditary stomatocytosis
Rh_{null} blood group
Stomatocytosis with cold hemolysis
(Liver disease, especially acute
alcoholism)
(Mediterranean stomatocytosis)

Irreversibly Sickled Cells
Sickle cell anemia
Symptomatic sickle syndromes

Intraerythrocytic Parasites
Malaria
Babesiosis
Bartonellosis

Spiculated or Crenated Red Cells
Acute hepatic necrosis (spur cell
anemia)
Uremia
Red cell fragmentation syndromes*
Infantile pyknocytosis
Embden-Meyerhof pathway defects*
Vitamin E deficiency*
Abetalipoproteinemia
Heat stroke*
McLeod blood group
(Postsplenectomy)
(Transiently after massive
transfusion of stored blood)
(Anorexia nervosa)*

Target Cells
Hemoglobins S, C, D, and E
Hereditary xerocytosis
Thalassemias
(Other hypochromic-microcytic
anemias)
(Obstructive liver disease)
(Postsplenectomy)
(Lecithin:cholesterol acyltransferase
deficiency)

Prominent Basophilic Stippling
Thalassemias
Unstable hemoglobins
Lead poisoning*
Pyridine 5′-nucleotidase deficiency

Nonspecific or Normal Morphology
Embden-Meyerhof pathway defects
Hexose monophosphate shunt defects
Unstable hemoglobins
Paroxysmal nocturnal
hemoglobinuria
Dyserythropoietic anemias
Copper toxicity (Wilson's disease)
Cation permeability defects
Erythropoietic porphyria
Vitamin E deficiency
Hemolysis with infections*
Rh hemolytic disease in neonates
Paroxysmal cold hemoglobinuria*

---

* Disease sometimes associated with this morphology.
Reference: Oski FA: Differential diagnosis of anemia. In Nathan DC, Oski FA (eds):
Hematology of Infancy and Childhood, 3rd ed. Philadelphia, W.B. Saunders, 1987, p 270.

The Rise in Hemoglobin with Iron Therapy

How fast should the hemoglobin rise when you start treating your iron deficient patient with oral iron?

Two important factors must be considered when judging the adequacy of the hematologic response. They are (1) the initial hemoglobin value and (2) the duration of the period of observation. The lower the initial hemoglobin, the greater is the hemoglobin rise per day. The shorter the observation period, the greater is the calculated hemoglobin rise per day. As one gets closer to a normal hemoglobin value, the daily rise in hemoglobin is much less. In our own experience in treating patients with hemoglobin values of less than 8.0 g/100 ml, one may anticipate a hemoglobin rise of 0.2 to 0.3 g per day and during the first 7 to 10 days of therapy. During the period of 10 to 24 days, the hemoglobin rises at a rate of 0.15 g per day and slows after that point to a rate of 0.10 per day until a normal level is achieved. Normally, the reticulocyte count begins to increase in 48 to 72 hours and reaches a peak 7 to 10 days after the initiation of therapy.

Listed below is another guide to the expected response as a function of the initial hemoglobin level.

Hematologic Response to Oral Iron Therapy Based on Initial Hemoglobin Value

INITIAL HEMOGLOBIN (g/dl)	HEMOGLOBIN RISE IN ONE WEEK (g/dl)
2.0 – 5.0	1.61
5.1 – 6.0	1.53
6.1 – 7.0	1.17
7.1 – 8.0	1.11
8.1 – 9.0	0.98
9.1 – 10.0	0.57
10.1 – 11.0	0.72
11.1 – 12.0	0.40

Optimal responses to oral iron therapy are achieved by treating the patient with ferrous sulfate. A patient should receive 2 to 3 mg of elemental iron per kg three times per day. The iron should be given between meals and never administered with milk.

Reference: Mehta BC, Lotliker KS, Patel JC: Indian J Med Res 61:1818, 1973.

HEMOPTYSIS

The Child with Hemoptysis

Hemoptysis is defined as the spitting up of blood that originates from the lungs or bronchial tree. Although this is a rare sign in children, it can be potentially life-threatening. Rapid and thorough evaluation is vital in order to identify and control the source of bleeding.

In the work-up of the child with hemoptysis, it is necessary to begin by anatomically delineating where the bleeding is actually occurring. Most children who spit up blood have an identifiable source of bleeding outside of the lower respiratory tract, such as epistaxis or trauma to the oropharynx. Differentiating hemoptysis from hematemesis, on the other hand, can be difficult. Distinguishing features of these two signs are summarized below:

Hemoptysis

- Blood is usually bright red, frothy, and mixed with sputum (pus, organisms, and macrophages may be present).
- Anemia is not a common finding.
- Bleeding is often preceded by a gargling noise and is associated with coughing.
- pH of blood is alkaline.

Hematemesis

- Blood is usually dark red to brownish in color (e.g., coffee ground emesis).
- Often associated with anemia.
- Bleeding and emesis are often preceded or accompanied by nausea and retching.
- pH is acidic.

The different causes of hemoptysis are wide and varied, as detailed below:

1. Infectious Causes
   a. Bacterial
      i. Bronchiectasis (most commonly associated with cystic fibrosis, immunodeficiency disorders, dyskinetic cilia syndrome, and pertussis).
      ii. Necrotizing pneumonias (e.g., *Pseudomonas, Staphylococcus, Klebsiella*)
      iii. Pulmonary tuberculosis
      iv. Lung abscess
      v. Bronchitis
      vi. Tracheitis
      vii. Pertussis

   b. Fungal
      i. Aspergillosis
      ii. Coccidioidomycosis
      iii. Actinomycosis
      iv. Mucormycosis
      v. Candidiasis
   c. Parasitic
      i. Paragonimiasis
      ii. Echinococcosis
      iii. Strongylodiasis
      iv. Ancylostomiasis
   d. Viral
      i. Laryngitis
      ii. Laryngotracheobronchitis
      iii. Pneumonitis

2. Foreign Bodies

3. Intrathoracic Defects and Lesions (Congenital or Acquired)
   a. Pulmonary arteriovenous fistula
   b. Hemangiomatous malformation
   c. Neurenteric cyst
   d. Bronchogenic cyst
   e. Mitral stenosis
   f. Other cardiac anomalies
   g. Pulmonary embolism and infarction
   h. Aortic aneurysm
   i. Pulmonary sequestration
   j. Arteriovenous fistula
   k. Venous obstructive condition
   l. Anomalous vessel
   m. Congenital telangiectasia

4. Autoimmune Conditions
   a. Wegener's granulomatosis
   b. Pulmonary hemosiderosis
   c. Milk allergy
   d. Goodpasture's syndrome
   e. Collagen vascular disease

5. Trauma
   a. Compression, crush injury, or penetrating injury
   b. Iatrogenic (e.g., postsurgical, postdiagnostic lung puncture, posttrans-bronchial biopsy, barotrauma)

6. Neoplastic conditions
   a. Endobronchial metastasis (e.g., metastatic osteogenic sarcoma)
   b. Bronchial adenoma
   c. Mediastinal teratoma
   d. Choriocarcinoma
   e. Endometriosis
   f. Bronchiogenic carcinoma

7. Hemoglobinopathy with pulmonary infarct (e.g., the "chest syndrome" of sickle cell disease)

8. Factitious (as a manifestation of Munchausen syndrome)

References: Turcios NL, Vega M: The child with hemoptysis. Hospital Practice 22(Oct. 15):214–218, 1987.

Oski FA, et al: Principles and Practice of Pediatrics. Philadelphia, J.B. Lippincott, 1990.

HENOCH-SCHÖNLEIN PURPURA

Neurologic Manifestations of Henoch-Schönlein Purpura (HSP)

Although the classic triad of purpuric rash, arthritis, and crampy abdominal pain remains pathognomonic for Henoch-Schönlein purpura, nervous system involvement may be more common than we believe. Osler first described neurologic manifestations of HSP in 1914. It has not been until recently, however, that the protean neurologic symptoms have been recognized. Histopathology has demonstrated the characteristic fibrinoid necrosis in meningeal and cerebral parenchymal arterioles and small arteries that is found in the cutaneous lesions, GI blood vessel walls, and kidney mesangium (nephritis is also common in HSP).

The neurologic symptoms of HSP can be nonspecific or dramatic, transient or permanent, primary or late. Regardless of the case, the manifestations may be indicative of significant CNS disease requiring treatment and/or neurologic assessment and follow-up.

CNS Involvement in HSP

Headache
Mental status changes
  Behavior
  Depressed state of consciousness
Seizures
  Partial, partial complex, generalized
  Status epilepticus

Focal neurologic deficits
  Aphasia
  Hemiparesis
  Paraparesis
  Quadriplegia
  Cortical blindness
  Chorea
  Ataxia

Peripheral NS Involvement in HSP

Mononeuropathy
  Facial nerve
  Ulnar nerve
  Femoral nerve
  Sciatic nerve
  Peroneal nerve

Polyneuropathy
  Guillain-Barré
  Polyradiculoneuropathy
  Brachial plexopathy

References: Belman AL, et al: Neurologic manifestations of Schoenlein-Henoch purpura: Report of three cases and review of the literature. Pediatrics 75:687–691, 1985.
Oski FA, et al: Principles and Practice of Pediatrics. Philadelphia, J.B. Lippincott, 1990.
Markel H, McLean RH: Central nervous system involvement in hemolytic-uremic syndrome. J Pediatr 114:901–902, 1989.

HEPATOMEGALY

Common Causes

Benign cystic disease
Benign transient hepatomegaly
  (usually with GI viral illness)
Biliary tract obstruction
  Alagille's disease
  Ascending cholangitis
  Biliary atresia
  Choledochal cyst
Congestive heart failure
Cystic fibrosis
Diabetes mellitus
Hyperalimentation
Iron-deficiency anemia
Leukemia, lymphoma
Malnutrition
Maternal diabetes
Neonatal hepatitis

Pulmonary hyperinflation
  ("apparent" hepatomegaly)
Septicemia
Sickle-cell anemia
Toxin/drug reactions (hepatitis,
    cholestasis, fatty infiltration)
  Acetaminophen
  Birth-control pills
  Corticosteroids
  Hydantoins
  Phenobarbital
  Sulfonamides
  Tetracycline
Viral hepatitis
  CMV, EBV, coxsackievirus
  Hepatitis A, B, non-A, non-B

Uncommon Causes

Chronic active hepatitis
Chronic anemias
Erythroblastosis fetalis
Hamartoma
Hemangioma
Hemolytic anemias
Hepatic abscess (pyogenic)
Hepatoblastoma
Inflammatory bowel disease

Liver hemorrhage
Metastatic tumors
Pericarditis
Reye's syndrome
Rocky Mountain spotted fever
Systemic inflammatory disease
  (e.g., JRA, SLE)
Visceral larva migrans

Rare Causes

α_1-Antitrypsin deficiency
Amyloidosis
Beckwith-Wiedemann syndrome
Brucellosis
Budd-Chiari syndrome
Carnitine deficiency
Chediak-Higashi syndrome
Crigler-Najjar syndrome
Farber's disease
Galactosemia
Gangliosidosis M_1
Gaucher's disease
Glycogen storage disease
Granulomatous hepatitis
    Chronic granulomatous disease
    Sarcoidosis
    Tuberculosis
Hemochromatosis
Hemophagocytic syndrome
Hepatic porphyrias
Hepatocellular carcinoma
Hereditary fructose intolerance
Histiocytic syndromes
Histoplasmosis
Homocystinuria
Hyperlipoproteinemia 1
Hypervitaminosis A

Infantile pyknocytosis
Infantile sialidosis
Klippel-Trenaunary-Weber syndrome
Leptospirosis
Lipodystrophy
Malaria
Mannosidosis
Methylmalonic acidemia
Moore-Federmann syndrome
Mucolipidosis
Mucopolysacchardoses
Mulibrey nanism
Niemann-Pick disease
Parasitic infections
    Amebiasis
    Flukes
    Schistosomiasis
Rendu-Osler-Weber syndrome
Rickets
Tangier's disease
Tyrosinemia
Urea cycle defects
Veno-occlusive disease
Wilson's disease
Wolman disease
Zellweger syndrome

HERPES

Neonatal Herpes Simplex Virus Infections

Herpes simplex virus (HSV) infection of the newborn is a feared and potentially devastating illness. As herpes virus infections continue to rise among women in the child bearing years, so has the incidence of neonatal cases of HSV. To further complicate matters, at least 60% of neonates who develop HSV infections are born to women who have never recognized symptoms of genitourinary HSV infection. Common means of transmitting HSV to the neonate include: (1) vaginal delivery through an infected birth canal; (2) ascending infection after rupture of membranes in a woman shedding HSV from the cervix; (3) postnatal contact with individuals exhibiting active skin lesions; and (4) transplacental infections.

Serious neonatal HSV infection is less likely when the infant is born to a mother with recurrent lesions, apparently because maternal antibody provides some measure of protection. Eighty percent of neonatal HSV infections are caused by HSV-2 and 20% are due to HSV-1. Although serious neonatal disease due to HSV-1 has been described, neonates infected with HSV-1 are more likely to survive without serious morbidity than those infected with HSV-2. Listed below are the common clinical manifestations of neonates with HSV infections:

Disseminated HSV Disease (mean age of presentation = 7 days)

Fever	Shock
Lethargy	Bleeding
Convulsions or other CNS findings	Hepatosplenomegaly
Poor feeding	Jaundice
Respiratory distress	Skin lesions*
Pneumonitis	

Localized HSV Disease[†] (mean age of presentation = 11 days)

Skin and mucosal lesions (vesicular or ulcerated lesions on an erythematous base)
Keratoconjunctivitis
CNS findings

---

*Although 50% of all infants with disseminated HSV develop skin lesions, they may not be present with the onset of symptoms.
[†] Up to 60% of infants with local involvement of the skin, eyes, or mouth will progress to disseminated disease.
Reference: LaRussa P: Perinatal herpes virus infections. Ped Ann 13:659–670, 1984.

HIP

Congenital Dislocation of the Hip: A New Diagnostic Method

Congenital dislocation of the hip (CDH) is known to result from several etiologies (see below), including mechanical, hormonal, and hereditary factors. It occurs six times more frequently in otherwise normal females than in males. The Catch-22 of CDH is that it is difficult to diagnose in infants, but the success of treatment initiated after the child begins walking is poor.

In the past, pediatricians have relied on the Barlow and Ortolani tests to diagnose CDH in the neonate. These tests are only reliable in the newborn period but remain an effective screening test. Since approximately 60% of unstable hips in the newborn period resolve as laxity disappears, we need a reliable screening test for the infant from 2–4 months.

A recent study from Asahikawa, Japan, demonstrates the usefulness of abnormal or asymmetrical inguinal folds in the frog-leg position for diagnosing CDH in the 3–4 month old child. Although the number of false positives was high, the coincidence rates between radiographic diagnosis and abnormal inguinal folds for dislocation, subluxation, and acetabular dysplasia were 100%, 100%, and 47%, respectively. Comparative coincidence rates for the limited abduction test (Aliss' or Galeazzi's sign) were 0%, 60%, and 0%. Thus, abnormal inguinal folds are a more sensitive indicator of CDH than limited abduction and should reduce the number of radiologic exams performed on infants.

Factors Involved in CDH

Mechanical: Breech deliveries
First born child
Oligohydramnios
Hormonal: Generalized ligamentous laxity results from increased circulating estrogens and relaxin at the time of birth (6:1).
Hereditary: Positive family history in 20% of cases of CDH.

Physical Signs of CDH in 3-4 Month Old

Shortened leg
Limited passive abduction
Asymmetric folds of femoral skin
Abnormal inguinal folds

Tests for CDH

Barlow's and Ortolani's tests are performed with thumb and forefinger on the lesser and greater trochanters. Only one hip should be examined at a time.

Barlow: Adduction and posterior pressure may produce a "clunk" of subluxation or dislocation.
Ortolani: Abducting and "lifting" hip back into place relocates the dislocation caused by Barlow's test.

Abnormal inguinal folds: See figure.

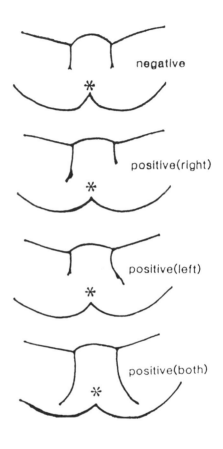

Findings of inguinal folds.

Ando M, Gotoh E: Significance of inguinal folds for diagnosis of congenital dislocation of the hip in infants aged three to four months. J Pediatr Orthop 10:331–334, 1990.
Oski FA, et al: Principles and Practice of Pediatrics. Philadelphia, J.B. Lippincott, 1990.

HIRSCHPRUNG'S DISEASE

Ruling Out Hirschprung's Disease

Hirschprung's disease, or congenital megacolon, is the most common cause of obstruction of the colon in the neonatal period (about 33% of all neonatal obstructions).

Clinically, it is difficult to distinguish which infants have Hirschprung's disease in the neonatal period. Meconium plug syndrome, cystic fibrosis, hypothyroidism, and many other abnormalities may present with constipation, obstruction, abdominal distention, or emesis. In contrast, infants who do not develop gastrointestinal signs or symptoms during the first 30 days of life do not have Hirschprung's disease and do not require biopsy to rule out the disease.

Reference: Landman GB: A five-year chart review of children biopsied to rule out Hirschprung's disease. Clin Pediatr 26:288–291, 1987.

HIRSUTISM

Common Causes

Familial or racial factors
Idiopathic hirsutism

Physiologic hirsutism
    Pregnancy
    Puberty

Uncommon Causes

Central nervous system injury
Drugs
    Anabolic steroids
    Birth-control pills
    Cyclosporine
    Diazoxide
    Dilantin

Drugs *(Cont.)*
    Minoxidil
    Progesterones
    Testosterone
Emotional stress (?)
Polycystic ovarian disease
Severe malnutrition

Rare Causes

Achard-Thiers syndrome
Acromegaly
Adrenal disorders
    Adrenal carcinoma
    Congenital adrenal hyperplasia
    Cushing's syndrome
    Virilizing adrenal adenoma
Congenital erythropoietic porphyria

Dysmorphogenic syndromes (many)
Hypothyroidism
Male pseudohermaphroditism
Ovarian disorders
    Pure gonadal dysgenesis
    Virilizing ovarian tumors
        Arrhenoblastoma
        Granulosa-theca cell tumors

HOARSENESS

Common Causes

Caustic ingestion
Excessive use of the voice
Foreign body
Infectious mononucleosis
Instrumentation (naso/orogastric
    tube)
Laryngitis

Laryngotracheitis
Laryngotracheobronchitis
Postintubation hoarseness
Postnasal drip
Vocal cord nodules
Vocal cord paralysis (postsurgical
    trauma)

Uncommon Causes

Congenital vocal cord paralysis
Epiglottitis
Hypocalcemia (e.g., hyper-
    parathyroidism)
Hypothyroidism
Laryngeal trauma

Laryngomalacia
Sicca syndrome
Toxins (chemotherapy, lead, mercury,
    irradiation, smoke)
Tracheitis (bacterial)
Vocal cord polyps

Rare Causes

Amyloidosis
Angioneurotic edema
Chromosomal abnormalities
    Achondroplasia
    Bloom's syndrome
    Cockayne's syndrome
    Cri du chat syndrome
    DeLange's syndrome
    Diastrophic dwarfism
    Dubowitz's syndrome
    Dysautonomia
    Williams' syndrome
Congenital abnormalities
    Arytenoid cartilage displacement
    Clefts
    Cysts
    Webs
Cricoarytenoid arthritis (JRA)
Diphtheria
Recurrent laryngeal nerve
        impingement
    Aberrant great vessels
    Cardiomegaly
    Hemorrhage
    Hilar adenopathy
    Neoplasm
Recurrent laryngeal nerve dysfunction
    Central nervous system disease
        Arnold-Chiari malformation
        Chediak-Higashi disease
        Encephalitis
        Hallervorden-Spatz disease
        Huntington's chorea
        Infection
        Ischemia
        Kernicterus
        Meningitis
        Metabolic disease
        Multiple sclerosis

Recurrent laryngeal nerve
        dysfunction *(Cont)*
    Central nervous system
            disease *(Cont.)*
        Polyneuritis
        Pseudobulbar palsy
        Ramsay Hunt syndrome
        Storage disease
        Syphilis
        Syringobulbia
        Toxin
        Trauma
        Tumor
        Wilson's disease
    Motor unit dysfunction
        Botulism
        Muscular dystrophy
        Myasthenia gravis
        Toxins
        Werdnig-Hoffmann disease
Sarcoidosis
Storage disease (e.g., lysosomal)
Tetany
Tuberculosis
Tumors of the larynx

Adenoma	Leukemia
Carcinoma	Lymphoma
Chondroma	Myoma
Ectopic thyroid	Myxoma
Fibroangioma	Neuroblastoma
Fibroma	Neurofibroma
Fibrosarcoma	Papilloma
Hamartoma	Rhabdomyo-
Hemangioma	sarcoma
Hygroma	Xanthoma

Vocal cord hemorrhage
    (nontraumatic)
Wegener's granulomatosis

HUMAN BITES

A Differential Diagnosis for Lesions That Mimic Human Bites

Human bites are a common occurrence, particularly in conjunction with fighting, abuse (both sexual and physical), patients who have been institutionalized, homicides, self-inflicted injuries, and in association with systemic illnesses (e.g., Lesch-Nyhan syndrome, bulimia). Although most human bites are superficial abrasions, deeper lesions can be quite difficult to treat because of polymicrobial infection and cellulitis. A thorough history and physical examination are important to differentiate human bite lesions from other dermatologic lesions that resemble them. Frequently, however, the history is inaccurate or absent in cases of human bites.

The lesion of a human bite is usually annular or ovoid in shape; teeth marks may be present but these usually become confluent with the passage of time. A key finding in distinguishing human bites from other dermatologic disorders is the presence or absence of scaly lesions; human bites are characteristically nonscaly. Listed below is a table of dermatologic disorders that can mimic human bites; identifying such lesions is of particular importance in suspected cases of child abuse.

Dermatologic Disorders That May Mimic Human Bites

DISEASE	DESCRIPTION OF LESION	HISTO-PATHOLOGY	PREDILECTION SITES	SPECIAL FEATURES
Fixed drug eruptions	One or several sharply demarcated erythematous lesions	Epidermis: hydropic degeneration of basal layer; dyskeratotic keratinocytes Dermis: pigment incontenence	Often involve face or genitalia	
Subacute cutaneous lupus erythema (LE)	Scaly erythematosus papules that enlarge, become confluent to form annular and polycyclic lesions	Epidermis: hyperkeratosis, follicular plugging, liquefaction degeneration of basal cells Dermis: patchy mononuclear infiltrate	Shoulders, extensor surfaces of arms, dorsum of hands, upper back, chest	Mild systemic illness; SS-A (Ro) and SS-B (La) antibodies
Pityriasis rosea	Herald patch: oval or round lesion with central salmon color and darker peripheral zone separated by collarette of scale Symmetric secondary eruption in "Christmas tree" distribution (smaller than herald patch)	Epidermis: hyperkeratosis, hypogranulosis, acanthosis, spongiosis Dermis: mixed superficial perivascular infiltrate with eosinophils	Usually on trunk	Variable prodromal symptoms

Table continued on next page.

Dermatologic Disorders That May Mimic Human Bites (Cont.)

DISEASE	DESCRIPTION OF LESION	HISTO-PATHOLOGY	PREDILECTION SITES	SPECIAL FEATURES
Dermatophy-tosis: tinea corporis	Most common shows annular lesion with active, erythematous border and central clearing; scales	Fungal organisms in stratum corneum	Glaborous skin	KOH positive
Granuloma annulare	Skin colored, erythem-atous, or violaceous papules that assume an annular configuration	Dermis: foci of collagen degeneration (necrobiosis)	Hands and feet; trunk	

Reference: Gold MH, Roenigk HH, Smith ES, Pierce LJ: Human bite marks. Differential diagnosis. Clin Pediatr 28:329–331, 1989, with permission.

HUMAN IMMUNODEFICIENCY VIRUS

Indicator Diseases for HIV Infection in Children

Acquired immunodeficiency syndrome (AIDS) is increasing among children as a result of perinatal transmission from infected mothers. By 1987 AIDS was the leading cause of death in the U.S. among children 1–4 years of age. Though many of these children are born to women known to be infected with the human immunodeficiency virus (HIV), mothers are often asymptomatic and undiagnosed at the time their children become ill. Recognizing the diseases with which AIDS in children is likely to present initially may allow for more rapid diagnosis among the children of undiagnosed mothers.

AIDS Indicator Diseases Among 1026 Patients with Perinatally Acquired HIV Infection

DISEASE	NO.	%*
Pneumocystis carinii pneumonia	345	34
Lymphoid interstitial pneumonitis	283	28
Recurrent bacterial infections	246	24
HIV wasting syndrome	165	16
Candida esophagitis	132	13
HIV encephalopathy	116	11
Cytomegalovirus disease	77	7
Pulmonary candidiasis	51	5
Cryptosporidiosis	31	3
Herpes simplex disease	30	3
Mycobacterium avium infection	29	3

*Some children had more than one reported disease.

References: Oxtoby MJ: Perinatally acquired human immunodeficiency virus infection. Pediatr Infect Dis J 9:606–619, 1990.

Hauger SB, Nicholas SW, Caspe WB: Guidelines for the care of children and adolescents with HIV infection. J Pediatr 119(1:2 suppl):S1–S66, 1991.

Recognition and Management of the Infant at Risk

As the incidence of pediatric AIDS continues to rise in the U.S., it becomes incumbent upon the pediatrician to be both facile and competent in its diagnosis and management. Listed below are some helpful hints:

Table 1. When to Suspect HIV Infection

Evidence of maternal HIV infection

Clinical evidence of HIV infection or immunodeficiency	From a geographic area where HIV infection is prevalent
Intravenous drug user and/or sexually promiscuous	Sexual partner of IV drug abuser or HIV-infected man

Evidence of infant HIV infection

Generalized lymphadenopathy	Unexplained wasting/failure to thrive
Hepatosplenomegaly	Chronic pneumonitis
Salivary gland enlargement	Immune thrombocytopenic purpura
Unexplained developmental delay or encephalopathy	Lymphoid malignancy
Recurrent or persistent infections	Unexplained hepatitis, nephropathy, or cardiomyopathy

Table 2. Initial Laboratory Evaluation for Neonatal HIV Infection

1. Perform an ELISA test for HIV antibody. If positive, repeat. If repeat ELISA is positive, perform Western blot. A positive Western blot confirms presence of HIV antibody. If possible, obtain a DNA PCR test, p24 antigen test, or HIV culture
2. If HIV ELISA test is negative and the patient is clinically well:
   Schedule regular (every other month) visits
   Consider repeat HIV ELISA test if child's condition changes
3. If HIV ELISA test is negative and patient is ill, obtain DNA PCR, p24 antigen test, or HIV culture

Table 3. Immunodeficiency Syndromes That May Present in Infancy

Fetal alcohol syndrome	Disorders of neutrophil function (chronic granulomatous disease)
DiGeorge syndrome	
Adenosine deaminase deficiency	Wiskott-Aldrich syndrome
Nucleoside phosphorylase deficiency	Severe combined immunodeficiency
Quantitative immunoglobulin disorders	Malignancy

Table 4. Assessment of Immune Function in Infants at Risk for HIV Infection

CBC with differential	Functional tests of cell-mediated immunity: skin testing for candida, trichophyton, mumps (if previously immunized for mumps)
Quantitative assay of IgG, IgA, and IgM	
Assay of IgG subclasses	Assay of isohemagglutinins or antibodies to previously administered vaccines
CD4/CD8 lymphocyte counts and ratio ("helper/suppressor" ratio)	Lymphocyte stimulation response to antigens and mitogens

Table 5. If the Infant Is HIV-positive but without Signs of Immune Deficiency

Mother should avoid breast-feeding	Recheck ELISA every 3 mo in healthy child
Physician should examine child every other month	Child should become HIV-negative (by ELISA) by 15 mo of age
Provide education for the mother/ household re: mechanisms of transfer of HIV, caring for baby, HIV transmission routes	Continue follow-up through at least 3 yr of age
	Recheck HIV ELISA later if change in clinical condition is suspicious

Table 6. Immunizing the Infant with HIV Infection

Do give:

DPT (regular schedule)	MMR (at 15 mo)
Hib (regular schedule)	Pneumococcal vaccine (at 2 yr)
Inactivated polio vaccine (same schedule as for OPV)*	Influenza vaccine (at 6 mo or later)

Do not give:

Live polio vaccine	BCG vaccine

* Inactivated polio vaccine should also be given to infants who are not infected but live in a household with an HIV-infected person.

Table 7. When to Start Prophylaxis for PCP*

AGE OF PATIENT	CD4 + COUNT (CELLS/μL)**	ACTION RECOMMENDED
1–11 mo	<1,500	Start PCP prophylaxis
	1,500–2,000	No prophylaxis; recheck CD4 + count in 1 mo
	>2,000	No prophylaxis; recheck CD4 + count every 3–4 mo
12–23 mo	<750	Start PCP prophylaxis
	750–1,000	No prophylaxis; recheck CD4 + count in 1 mo
	>1,000	No prophylaxis; recheck CD4 + count every 3–4 mo
24–72 mo	<500	Start PCP Prophylaxis
	500–750	No prophylaxis; recheck CD4 + count in 1 mo
	750–1,500	No prophylaxis; recheck CD4 + count every 3–4 mo
	>1,500	No prophylaxis; recheck CD4 + count every 6 mo
>72 mo	<200	Start PCP prophylaxis
	200–300	No prophylaxis; recheck CD4 + count in 1 mo
	>300–600	No prophylaxis; recheck CD4 + count every 3–4 mo
	>600	No prophylaxis; recheck CD4 + count every 6 mo

* Applies to children who are HIV-infected, HIV-seropositive, or less than 12 mo of age and born to an HIV-infected mother.
** Regardless of CD4 + count, start PCP prophylaxis if the CD4 + % is less than 20%. Prophylaxis is also indicated, regardless of age and CD4 + count, for any child who had an episode of PCP.
Adapted from Centers for Disease Control.

Reference: From Trowbridge GL, Marshall GS, Fahner JB, Barbour SD: HIV: Recognizing and managing the infant at risk. Contemp Pediatr 8:118–134, 1991, with permission.

HYDROPS

Nonimmune Hydrops Fetalis

The original definition of nonimmune hydrops fetalis is attributed to E.L. Potter who described the condition in 1943 as "universal edema of the fetus unassociated with erythroblastosis." Currently the term **hydrops** is used to describe the accumulation of fluid in specific interstitial tissues or body cavities, whereas **hydrops fetalis** refers to the generalized, pathologic accumulation of fluid in serous cavities in the fetus with edema of the soft tissue.

Ultrasound is the most common means of diagnosing this condition prenatally. The findings of such an examination typically reveal fetal skin edema, effusions in the body cavities (e.g., ascites), hydramnios, and placental edema. Upon delivery, the newborn infant displays gross edema and may be extremely difficult to resuscitate due to ascites, pleural effusions, and an associated lung hypoplasia.

Etiology

In general, hydrops fetalis is separated into two categories: immune and nonimmune. Immune hydrops is most commonly secondary to Rh isoimmunization. Since the advent of anti-D globulin in the early 1960s, the majority of cases of fetal hydrops are nonimmune in nature. The incidence of nonimmune hydrops fetalis is between 1/2500 to 1/3500 newborns.

The pathologic mechanisms leading to this condition can be categorized as follows:

1. Increased intracapillary hydrostatic pressure
2. Decreased intracapillary osmotic pressure
3. Damage to the peripheral capillary/vascular integrity.

Various combinations of these mechanisms in different conditions are seen (see accompanying table, "Causes of Nonimmune Hydrops").

The Investigation of Hydrops Fetalis

When hydrops fetalis is discovered, either by ultrasound during a pregnancy or at birth, the following approach is recommended in order to extract the maximum amount of information:

1. **Maternal work-up**
   Complete blood count and indices
   Hemoglobin electrophoresis
   Kleihauer-Betke stain of peripheral
     blood
   VDRL and TORCH titers
   Anti-Ro, systemic lupus erythematosis
     preparation, and sedimentation rate
   Oral glucose tolerance test

2. **Fetal assessment**
   Continued ultrasound-cardiac work-up
   Limb-length, fetal movement

3. **Amniocentesis**
   Karotype (α-fetoprotein)
   Virus cultures
   Establish culture for
     appropriate metabolic
     or DNA testing

4. **Fetal blood sampling**
   Kerotype
   Hemoglobin analysis
   IgM; specific cultures
   Albumin and total protein

5. **At delivery**

Karotyping (as appropriate)
Photography
X-ray films
Fluid from effusion, ascites
  (chyle, protein, culture)
Placental examination

Detailed autopsy
  (as appropriate)
Urinalysis
Complete blood count
Liver function studies
Viral titers

Causes of Nonimmune Hydrops

CATEGORY	CONDITIONS	APPROXIMATE % OF CASES
Hematologic	Homozygous α-thalassemia; chronic fetomaternal transfusion; twin-to-twin transfusion; acardius; atrioventricular shunts; hemorrhage or thrombosis; maternal drugs (chloramphenicol)	10
Cardiovascular	Severe congential heart disease (e.g, complex congenital heart defects, atrioventricular septal defects, premature closure of the foramen ovale, hypoplastic left and right heart); arrythmias or congential heart block; myocardial and endocardial disease; cardiac tumors (e.g., rhabdomyomas)	20
Respiratory	Cystic adenomatoid malformation of lung; diaphragmatic hernia; pulmonary lymphangiectasia; pulmonary sequestration; intrathoracic mass	5
Gastrointestinal	Bowel atresias; volvulus; duplications of the gut; peritonitis	5
Urinary/renal disorders	Urethral and ureteral atresia Bladder neck obstruction Posterior urethral valves Cloacal malformation Congenital nephrosis	5
Chromosomal	Turner syndrome; trisomies 13, 18, 21; triploidy; miscellaneous aneuploidy	16
Placenta	Umbilical vein thrombosis; torsion of cord; chorioangioma	
Intrauterine infection with or without hemolysis	Cytomegalovirus; toxoplasmosis; syphilis; parvovirus; parasitic diseases	8
Recognized syndromes	Dwarfing syndromes (e.g., thanatophoric, Jeune, hypophosphatasia, achondrogenesis); arthrogryposis; Neu-Laxova syndrome; Pena-Shokeir syndromes; Noonan syndrome; multiple pterygium syndromes; Meckel syndrome	11
Metabolic disorders	Lysosomal storage disorders (including mucopolysaccharidoses); Gaucher disease; gangliosidoses; sialidosis	5–10
Miscellaneous	Amniotic band syndrome; fetal tumors (e.g., teratoma, neuroblastomas, Wilms, angiomas)	

McGillivray BC, Hall JG: Nonimmune hydrops fetalis. Pediatrics in Review 9(6):197–202, 1987, with permission.

Reference: Potter EL: Universal edema of fetus unassociated with erythroblastosis. Am J Obstet Gynecol 46:130–134, 1943.

HYPERHIDROSIS

Common Causes

Emotional stimuli
Exercise
Fever, recovery from fever

Increased environmental temperature
Ingestion of spicy foods

Uncommon Causes

Atopic predisposition
Chronic illness
  Brucellosis
  Pulmonary tuberculosis
Cluster headaches

Congestive heart failure
Drug withdrawal
Hypoglycemia
Respiratory failure
Salicylate intoxication

Rare Causes

Acrodynia
Acromegaly
Auriculotemporal syndrome
Carbon monoxide poisoning
Carcinoid syndrome
Citrullinemia
Diencephalic syndrome
Familial dysautonomia
Familial periodic paralysis
Hyperthyroidism
Insulin overdose

Ipecac ingestion
Myocardial infarction
Organophosphate poisoning
Phenylketonuria
Pheochromocytoma
Pyridoxine deficiency
Spinal cord injury
Thrombocytopenia-absent radius
  syndrome (TAR)
Vasoactive intestinal peptide-
  secreting tumor

HYPERLEUKOCYTOSIS

Blood Gas Determinations with Extreme Leukocytosis

Patients with hyperleukocytosis—white cell counts in excess of 200,000 per mm^3, as seen with leukemia—may have respiratory distress and/or hypoxia secondary to leukocyte-thrombocyte aggregation in the lungs, to hyperviscosity, or to pneumonia. Because of these complications, arterial blood gas determinations are often essential to management of these patients. Because leukocytes consume oxygen, accurate determinations of arterial oxygen tension can only be made if blood samples are immersed immediately in crushed ice and injected into the gas analyzer within 1 minute. Blood gas measurements in patients with hyperleukocytosis should be considered unsuitable if there is a delay of more than 1 minute.

Reference: Shohat M, et al: Determination of blood gases in children with extreme leukocytosis. Crit Care Med 16:787–788, 1988.

HYPERLIPIDEMIA

Causes of Secondary Hyperlipidemia in Childhood

Drug use—steroids, thiazides,
 β-blockers, isotretinoin
 (Accutane), anticonvulsants,
 oral contraceptives, alcohol
Obesity
Diabetes mellitus
Hypothyroidism
Lipodystrophy
Pregnancy

Storage disease—Tay-Sachs, glycogen
 storage diseases, etc.
Renal failure
Nephrotic syndrome
Systemic lupus erythematosus
 and collagen diseases
Cholestasis
Anorexia nervosa
Idiopathic hypercalcemia

HYPERSENSITIVITY

Clinical Examples of Hypersensitivity Reactions

The immune system generally plays a protective role in maintaining a host's response to potentially dangerous immunologic and infectious stimuli, yet there are circumstances where the immune system's machinations, once set in motion, can produce tissue injury. These hypersensitivity reactions are divided into four types: (1) the immediate or anaphylactic type, (2) the cytotoxic type, (3) the immune complex or Arthus type, and (4) the delayed hypersensitivity reaction. Listed below are clinical examples of each reaction.

1. **Type 1 hypersensitivity (allergic reactions mediated by IgE)**
   a. Urticaria
   b. Hay fever
   c. Allergic rhinitis
   d. Allergic conjunctivitis
   e. Allergic asthma
   f. Systemic anaphylaxis (e.g., reactions to antibiotics, vaccines, foreign sera, hormones, medications, contrast agents, hymenoptera stings, snake venom, blood products, and foods)

2. **Type 2 hypersensitivity (antibody = dependent cytotoxicity)**
   a. Erythroblastosis fetalis
   b. Acquired hemolytic anemia
   c. Thrombocytopenia
   d. Pemphigus
   e. Goodpasture's syndrome (glomerulonephritis associated with hemoptysis)
   f. Graft rejection
   g. Neutropenia
   h. Chronic keratitis

3. **Type 3 hypersensitivity (immune complex or Arthus type)**
   a. Microbial infection
      i. Bacterial (e.g., streptococcal, glomerulonephritis, and lepromatous leprosy)
      ii. Viral (e.g., cytomegaloviral choriomeningitis)
      iii. Parasitic (e.g., toxoplasma retinochoroiditis)
   b. Malignancy (e.g., solid tumor metastases, lymphoma, and leukemia)
   c. Autoimmune disorders (e.g., systemic lupus erythematosus, sympathetic ophthalmia, rheumatoid arthritis, Sjogren's syndrome, lens-induced uveitis)

d. Vasculitis
  i. Secondary to immune complexes involving any infection or tissue antigens
  ii. Erythema multiforme (Stevens-Johnson)
  iii. Serum sickness

4. **Type 4 hypersensitivity (delayed cell-mediated immunity)**
  a. Mantoux tuberculin test (which only becomes positive after 48 hours)
  b. Reactions to poison ivy, poison sumac, and poison oak contact
  c. Hashimoto's thyroiditis
  d. Transplantation reaction and graft rejection

References: Adapted from Henley WL: Hypersensitivity reactions and tissue injury. Pediatr Ann 16:422–436, 1987.
Bochner B, Lichtenstein LM: Anaphylaxis. N Engl J Med 324:1785–1790, 1991.

HYPERTENSION

Common Causes

Agitation
Anxiety
Coarctation of the aorta
Essential hypertension
Immobilization
Obesity
Pain
Renal causes
  Acute tubular necrosis
  Congenital anomalies
    Hydronephrosis
    Nephrophthisis
    Polycystic kidneys
    Renal aplasia/hypoplasia/ dysplasia
    Segmental hypoplasia
  Glomerulonephritis (acute and chronic)
    Membranoproliferative, etc.
    Postinfectious
  Liddle's syndrome
  Miscellaneous nephropathy
    Amyloidosis
    Diabetes mellitus
    Gout
  Nephrolithiasis
  Nephrotic syndrome
    Idiopathic
    Minimal change disease

Renal causes *(Cont.)*
  Obstructive uropathy
  Other nephritides
    Familial nephritis
    Hemolytic-uremic syndrome
    Henoch-Schönlein purpura
    Hypersensitivity/transfusion reaction
    Periarteritis nodosa
    Radiation
    Systemic lupus erythematosus
  Pyelonephritis
  Renal failure (acute and chronic)
  Renal transplantation
  Renal vascular disease
    Renal artery
      Aneurysm
      Arteritis
        Embolic disease
        External compression
      Fibromuscular dysplasia
      Fistula
      Stenosis
      Thrombosis
      Trauma
    Renal vein thrombosis
  Retroperitoneal fibrosis
  Trauma

Renal causes *(Cont.)*
    Tumors
        Extrinsic tumors
            Adrenal carcinoma
            Neuroblastoma
    Small pressure-cuff size

        Renin-secreting tumors
           (J-G cell)
        Wilms' tumor

Uncommon Causes

Cardiovascular etiologies
    Anemia
    Aortic aneurysm/thrombosis
    Arteriovenous fistula
        Aortic insufficiency
        Aorticopulmonary window
        Patent ductus arteriosus
    Bacterial endocarditis
    Iatrogenic hypervolemia
    Polycythemia
    Pseudoxanthoma elasticum
    Radiation aortitis
    Takayasu's arteritis

Drugs and chemicals
    Glucocorticoids
    Glycyrrhizic acid (licorice)
    Heavy metals (lead, cadmium,
        mercury)
    Methysergide
    Mineralocorticoids
    Monoamine-oxidase inhibitors
    Oral contraceptives
    Phencyclidine
    Sodium salts
    Sympathomimetics (decongestants)
    Tricyclic antidepressants

Rare Causes

Burns
Central nervous system
    Dysautonomia (Riley-Day
        syndrome)
    Encephalitis
    Guillain-Barré syndrome
    Increased intracranial pressure
    Poliomyelitis
    Neurofibromatosis
Collagen vascular
    Dermatomyositis
    Scleroderma
Cystinosis
Endocrine
    Congenital adrenal hyperplasia
        $11\text{-}\beta$-hydroxylase deficiency
        17-hydroxylase deficiency
    Cushing's syndrome

Endocrine *(Cont.)*
    Hyperaldosteronism
        Primary
            Conn's syndrome
            Dexamethasone-suppressible
            Idiopathic nodular hyperplasia
        Secondary
    Hyperthyroidism
    Pheochromocytoma
Fabry's disease
Hypoxia
Malignant hyperthermia
Metabolic
    Hypercalcemia
    Hypernatremia
    RTA with nephrocalcinosis
Sickle-cell anemia
Stevens-Johnson syndrome

Malignant Hypertension in Children

    The crisis of hypertension, or a hypertensive emergency, is heralded by a blood pressure high enough to cause damage to such target organs as the brain (hypertensive encephalopathy), eye (retinopathy, infarction of anterior visual pathways), kidneys (renal failure), and the heart (left ventricular hypertrophy and subsequent failure). Longstanding hypertension can also yield these effects but over a much longer time period. Severe hypertension in the pediatric age range has an incidence of 1 out of 1000 and is usually secondary to renal disease (e.g., renal scarring from chronic pyelonephritis or obstructive uropathy, glomerulo-nephritis, and renovascular disease). Nonrenal etiologies include coarctation of the aorta and catecholamine-excess states. In tertiary medical centers, some of the most frequent and severe cases of hypertension are a result of complications from end-stage renal disease and postrenal transplantation.

Given the child or infant with an exceedingly high blood pressure, whether symptomatic or not, the following data collection may be useful in elucidating the etiology and duration of the hypertension. Intravenous hypertensive therapy, in the case of a hypertensive crisis, should be initiated quickly to prevent end-organ damage. If no hypertensive crisis exists and hypertension has been documented on at least three different occasions, maintenance therapy with oral hypertensive agents should be initiated.

1. Key Historical Data

History	Significance
a. Neonatal umbilical artery catheterization	Renal artery stenosis
b. History of unexplained fever, urinary tract infection, failure to thrive	Reflux nephropathy
c. Nocturia, peripheral edema, hematuria, failure to thrive	Renal disease
d. Joint pain and swelling, rash	Connective tissue disease
e. Palpitations, flushing, sweating, fever, weight loss	Pheochromocytoma
f. Weakness, muscle cramps	Hyperaldosteronism
g. Ingestion of drug	Drug-induced hypertension
h. Family history of hypertension, renal disease	Inherited renal disease

2. Physical Findings

a. Short stature, peripheral edema, pallor	Renal disease
b. Cafe-au-lait spots	Neurofibromatosis
c. Tachycardia, increased sweating at rest, flushing	Pheochromocytoma
d. Moon facies, truncal obesity, striae	Cushing syndrome; steroid abuse
e. Absent or delayed femoral pulses, leg pressure significantly lower than arm pressure	Coarctation of the aorta
f. Abdominal bruit	Renovascular disease
g. Tachycardia, tachypnea, hepatomegaly, rales	Congestive heart failure secondary to severe or longstanding hypertension

2. Physical Findings *(Cont.)*

h. Hypertensive fundoscopic changes — Chronic severe hypertension

i. Bell's palsy — Chronic severe hypertension

j. Neurologic deficit (e.g., absent pupillary reflex, hemiparesis) — Side-effect of chronic or severe acute hypertension

3. Initial Laboratory Examination

Test	Possible Significance
a. Complete blood count	Low hemoglobin—chronic renal disease Low platelets and white cell count—connective tissue disease
b. Urinalysis	Renal disease
c. Urea, creatinine	Renal disease
d. Sodium, potassium, blood gases	Renal disease; mineralocorticoid excess
e. Renin	Renovascular disease
f. Chest x-ray	Evidence of cardiac failure
g. ECG	Hypertensive cardiomyopathy

Reference: Adapted from Farine M, Arbus GS: Management of hypertensive emergencies in children. Pediatr Emerg Care 5:51–55, 1989.

HYPOGONADISM

Hypogonadism and Obesity

The association between obesity and gonadal insufficiency or dysfunction has long been noted, yet the exact relationship of these two problems remains unclear. Endocrinologists have subdivided the myriad of syndromes and disease entities into four major categories:

1. **Abnormalities of the peripheral metabolism of sex hormones**

   a. Obese adult men have been noted to have low serum testosterone levels and poorly developed secondary sexual characteristics.

   b. Eunuchoid, hypogonadic males are frequently obese and often lose weight with the exogenous administration of testosterone.

   c. Obesity in adult women is frequently associated with dysfunctional uterine bleeding, amenorrhea, and increased conversion of circulating androgens to estrogens.

2. **Acquired hypothalamic conditions or Frohlich's syndrome** (specifically lesions to the ventromedial nucleus of the hypothalamus)

   a. Craniopharyngioma

   b. Trauma

3. **Extragonadal endocrine disorders**
   a. Hypothyroidism
   b. Cushing's syndrome
   c. Pseudohypoparathyroidism

4. **Genetic syndromes of hypogonadism and obesity**
   a. *Hypogonadotropic hypogonadism*
      i. *Kallmann's syndrome* (anosmia or hyposmia, midline defects including cleft lip and palate, color blindness, neurosensory defects, renal and bone abnormalities)
      ii. *Prader-Willi syndrome* (hypotonia in the newborn period, short stature, mental retardation, diabetes mellitus and insulin resistance, distinctive facial features such as almond-shaped eyes)
      iii. *Laurence-Moon-Bardet-Biedl syndrome* (retinitis pigmentosa, polydactyly, syndactyly, brachydactyly, mental retardation, spastic paraplegia, genitourinary tract anomalies)
      iv. *Biemond syndrome* (iris coloboma, mental retardation, polydactyly)
      v. *Börjeson-Forsman-Lehman syndrome* (severe mental retardation, short stature, coarse facies, microcephaly, seizures, nystagmus, ptosis)
      vi. *Carpenter syndrome* (acrocephalosyndactyly, mental retardation)

   b. *Hypergonadotropic hypogonadism*
      i. *Klinefelter syndrome* (XXY chromosome, small testes, gynecomastia)
      ii. *Alström syndrome* (retinal degeneration, nerve deafness, diabetes mellitus, acanthosis nigricans, nephropathy)

Reference: Castro-Magana M: Hypogonadism and obesity. Pediatr Ann 13:491–500, 1984.

HYPOTONIA—NEONATAL

Common Causes

Asphyxia
Benign, congenital

Sepsis
Trauma

Uncommon Causes

Congenital joint laxity
Down syndrome
"Hypermobility syndrome"
Hypothyroidism

Neonatal myasthenia
Spinal cord injury
Werdnig-Hoffmann disease

Rare Causes

Achondroplasia
Cerebro-hepato-renal syndrome
Congenital lactic acidosis

Congenital myopathies
  Central core disease
  Myotubular myopathy

Congenital myopathies *(Cont.)*
  Nemaline myopathy
Cri du chat syndrome
Ehlers-Danlos syndrome
Familial dysautonomia
Fetal warfarin syndrome
Generalized gangliosidosis
Glycogen storage disease (Type II)
Hyperammonemia
Lidocaine toxicity

Mannosidosis
Maple-syrup urine disease
Marfan syndrome
Myotonic dystrophy
Nonketotic hyperglycinemia
Osteogenesis imperfecta
Prader-Willi syndrome
Trisomy 13 syndrome
William's syndrome (idiopathic
  hypercalcemia)

The Differential Diagnosis of Hypotonia

Hypotonia, or decreased muscle tone, can be a presenting sign in a number of pathologic conditions affecting the central or peripheral nervous system. It is important to distinguish hypotonia from muscle weakness, which is a diminution of muscle power or strength but normal tone. Typically, when decreased muscle strength and tone appear together, diseases of the peripheral nervous system should be suspected; when hypotonia occurs without alterations in muscle strength, a disorder of the central nervous system should be investigated.

Anatomic localization of the process producing hypotonia is useful in generating a differential diagnosis. This can be done easily at the bedside.

1. **Diseases of the central nervous system or upper motor neuron disease** (processes involving the brain and spinal cord but not the anterior horn cells):

    a. Muscle strength is usually preserved and often normal.
    b. Deep tendon reflexes of the affected limbs are *always* preserved. (They may be exaggerated if the disease in question affects the pyramidal tracts.)
    c. Infantile reflexes either persist or, if lost, return (e.g., the Babinski reflex, palmar and plantar grasp, sucking, rooting, and snouting reflexes).
    d. Sensation is generally preserved and normal.
    e. The sign of hypotonia may be associated with dysequilibrium, such as gait imbalance, wide stance, ataxia, or dysmetria with or without a tremor.

2. **Diseases affecting the peripheral nervous system or lower motor neuron disease** (processes involving the anterior horn cell, myoneural junction, and innervation of muscle):

    a. Patients exhibit prominent weakness in concert with hypotonia.
    b. Deep tendon reflexes may be normal or decreased, but they are never hyperreflexive; in diseases involving the anterior horn cells and peripheral motor neurons, deep tendon reflexes are frequently absent.
    c. Primitive or infantile reflexes are absent (with the exception of newborns).
    d. Sensation abnormalities are not present (with the exception of specific disorders that affect both the peripheral motor *and* sensory nerves).
    e. Equilibrium is compromised secondary to impaired muscle strength; the dysequilibrium, therefore, should be in proportion to the associated muscle weakness.

The following two tables list acute and subacute causes and chronic causes of hypotonia.

Acute and Subacute Diseases Producing Hypotonia

BRAIN AND SPINAL CORD	ANTERIOR HORN CELL	PERIPHERAL NERVE	MYONEURAL JUNCTION	MUSCLE

Metabolic Encephalopathy
  Hypoxia/ischemia
  Hypoglycemia
  Bilirubin
  Ammonia
  Acidosis
Toxic Encephalopathy
  Drugs
  Poisons
  Animal bites
    (reptile, insect)
  Vaccinal
Trauma
  Concussion
  Contusion
  Hemorrhage
Infection
  Encephalitis
  Meningitis
  Myelitis (transverse)
Para-Infectious Acute
  Cerebellar Ataxia
Hydrocephalus
Neoplasia
  Posterior fossa tumors
Collagen Vascular
Disease
	Poliomyelitis	Guillain-Barré Syndrome
		Trauma
		Peripheral Neuropathy
		  Vitamin deficiency
		  (B_1, B_6, B_{12}, folate)
		  Drug induced
		  Heavy metal (Pb)
		  Diabetes
		  Uremia
		  Porphyria
		  Diphtheria
		  Vaccinal
		  Collagen vascular
		  disease
			Botulism
			Myasthenic Syndromes
			  Antibiotics
			  Metabolic poisons
			  (organo-
			  phosphates)
				Infectious Myositis
				  Viral
				  Parasitic
				  (trichinosis)
				Endocrine
				  Hypothyroidism
				  Addison's disease
				Collagen vascular
				  disease

From Vannucci RC: Pediatr Ann 18:404–410, 1989, with permission.

Chronic Causes of Hypotonia

BRAIN AND SPINAL CORD	ANTERIOR HORN CELL	PERIPHERAL NERVE	MYONEURAL JUNCTION	MUSCLE

1. Congenital Malformations
  a. Disorders of neurulation
    Anencephaly
    Encephalocele
    Myelomeningocele
  b. Disorders of diverticulation
    Holoprosencephaly
    Arnold-Chiari malformation
    Dandy-Walker syndrome
  c. Disorders of commissuration
    Agenesis of the corpus collosum
    Agenesis or hypoplasia of the septum pellucidum
	1. Spinal muscular atrophy disorders
	2. Werdnig-Hoffmann disease
		1. Congenital motor and sensory neuropathies
		2. Hereditary sensory and motor neuropathies (e.g., Charcot-Marie Tooth, Dejerine-Sottas syndromes)
		3. Inherited recurrent focal neuropathies
		4. Familial dysautonomia
			1. Myasthenia gravis	1. The muscular dystrophy syndromes
				2. Congenital myopathies (e.g., central core disease, minicore disease, nemaline myopathy, severe x-linked myotubular myopathy)
				3. Mitochondrial disorders
				4. Periodic paralyses
				5. Inflammatory myopathies
				6. Myotonic syndromes
				7. Endocrine myopathies
				8. Metabolic myopathies (e.g., Glycogen storage disease of heart and muscle or Pompe's disease)

Table continued on next page.

Chronic Causes of Hypotonia (Cont.)

BRAIN AND SPINAL CORD	ANTERIOR HORN CELL	PERIPHERAL NERVE	MYONEURAL JUNCTION	MUSCLE

d. Disorders of histogenesis
    Microcephaly vera
    Cerebral gigantism
    Cerebellar aplasia
    Neuronal heterotopias
    Lissencephaly
2. Inborn Errors of Metabolism
   (e.g., carbohydrate, amino acid,
   fatty acid)
3. Storage Disorders
   a. Glycogen
   b. Gangliosidosis
   c. Mucopolysaccharidosis
   d. Mucolipidosis
   e. Peroxisomal
4. Toxic encephalopathies
5. Infectious encephalitis
   (e.g., TORCH)
6. Hypothyroidism (congenital)
7. Hydrocephalus				

Reference: Vannucci RC: Differential diagnosis of diseases producing hypotonia. Ped Ann 18:404–410, 1989.

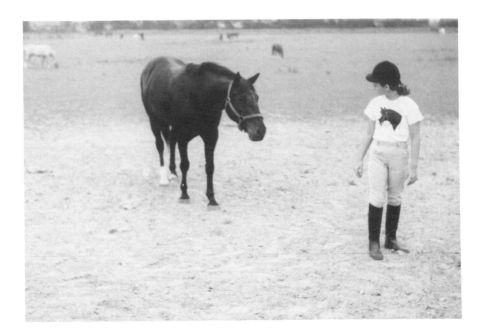

I but use you a minute, then I resign you, stallion,
Why do I need your paces when I myself out-gallop them?
Even as I stand or sit passing faster than you.

Walt Whitman
From *Song of Myself*

I

IDIOPATHIC THROMBOCYTOPENIC PURPURA

Who Needs a Bone Marrow Examination?

Is a bone marrow examination necessary when you are faced with a child with the clinical findings of acute idiopathic thrombocytopenic purpura whose examination results are otherwise normal and whose blood cell count and blood smear reveal only thrombocytopenia?

Naturally the clinician, and the parent, worry that the thrombocytopenia may be a manifestation of leukemia. A study in which the records of 2239 patients with acute lymphoblastic leukemia were reviewed showed that none of these children had significant thrombocytopenia with no other hematologic or physical manifestations of the leukemia.

A bone marrow examination is *unnecessary* in your patient if:

1. No blasts are present in the peripheral blood film;
2. The platelet count is less than 50,000/mm^3;
3. The hemoglobin concentration is more than 11.00 g/dl;
4. The absolute neutrophil count is more than 1500/mm^3; and
5. There is no organomegaly.

Reference: Dubansky AS, et al: Isolated thrombocytopenia in children with acute lymphoblastic leukemia: A rare event in a pediatric oncology study group. Pediatrics 84:1068–1071, 1989.

IMMUNODEFICIENCY

The Humoral Immunodeficiency Syndromes

Humoral immunodeficiency syndromes are characterized by an impairment in the host's capacity to manufacture antibodies. Although the particular syndrome may be congenital or acquired, these patients exhibit little or no immunoglobulin upon serum testing. The typical child with humoral immunodeficiency presents with frequent, recurrent, and persistent bacterial infections in association with low immunoglobulin levels or a particular impairment in the production of a specific antibody.

Children with humoral immunodeficiency are particularly susceptible to infections by encapsulated organisms (e.g., *Streptococcus pneumoniae*, group A streptococci, and *Hemophilus influenzae*) because of an inability to produce opsonizing antibodies. Other pathogens that frequently infect these patients include mycoplasma, *Giardia lamblia, Clostridium difficile,* and *Staphylococcus aureus.* The types of frequently occurring infections include pneumonia, upper respiratory tract infections, otitis media, sinusitis, conjunctivitis, diarrhea, and furunculosis. Children with humoral immunodeficiency, on the other hand, have an intact ability to form T cells, natural killer cells, phagocytic cells, and complement, so that frequent or recurrent viral, fungal, and parasitic infections are not a prominent feature.

The evaluation of a child who presents with frequent infections of the type described above begins with a thorough history, specifically addressing which infections the child has had, the etiologic agents identified, and their natural history in that host. A careful physical examination with attention to particular findings consistent with the humoral immunodeficiency syndromes is also warranted. The laboratory examination should begin with determination of quantitative serum IgG, IgA, and IgM; a functional antibody response to immunization with diphtheria and tetanus; and complete blood count with attention to white cell morphology on the peripheral smear. Further work-up might include quantitative serum isohemagglutinins; a bone marrow biopsy to detect plasma cells; a lymph node biopsy for histologic analysis of primary follicles, germinal centers, and plasma cells; B cell phenotypic markers; IgG subclasses; and salivary IgA. The essential features of the primarily humoral immunodeficiency syndromes are summarized in tabular form, below:

Humoral Immunodeficiency Syndromes

SYNDROME	IMMUNE DEFECT	CHARACTERISTIC FEATURES	CLINICAL ASSOCIATIONS
X-linked agamma-globulinemia (Bruton's)	Block at level of pre-B → B cell	Very low Ig levels No B cells in PB	Echovirus infection Dermatomyositis Lymphoreticular malignancy IVGG indicated
Autosomal recessive agammaglobu-linemia	Very low B cells in PB	Females also affected	Similar to X-linked (Bruton's) IVGG indicated
Transient hypogamma-globulinemia of infancy	Unknown	B cell population normal	Ig ↑ and infections ↓ by age 2 IVGG not indicated
Common variable immunodeficiency	Intrinsic B cell defects T suppressor activity T or B auto-antibodies	B cells present in PB	Autoimmune disease Lymphadenopathy/ splenomegaly Sprue-like syndrome Lymphoreticular malignancy IVGG not indicated
IgA deficiency	Intrinsic B cell defect T suppressor activity	Common May be drug-induced Anti-IgA antibodies common	Autoimmune disease Risk of anti-IgA ana-phylactoid reaction IVGG not indicated
Hyper-IgM syndrome	Defective isotype switch	↑↑ IgM with low IgG, IgA	Autoimmune disease Lymphadenopathy IVGG indicated
Selective or qualitative deficiency	Lack of T cell "help"	IgG2, IgG4 most common Ig levels normal or high	IgA deficiency IVGG used for broadly ↓ response to anti-gen challenge

Reference: Hassett JM: Humoral immunodeficiency: A review. Pediatr Ann 16:404–411, 1987.

IMMUNOLOGY

Nonimmunologic Defense Mechanisms

The human body is blessed with a number of nonimmunologic defense mechanisms that serve as the "first line of defense" in preventing microbial invasion. These include the skin, mucous membranes, and their secretory components. It should also be noted that normal vascular perfusion of tissues, adequate flow of urine, bile and respiratory secretions, and the presence of normal commensal bacterial flora are necessary in the daily prevention of microbial invasion. Indeed, many pediatric patients who suffer from chronic recurrent infections have defects in these anatomic and physical barriers rather than true immunodeficiencies. The workup of such a patient, therefore, should always establish the integrity of such anatomic, nonimmunologic barriers to infection.

Defects in Nonimmunologic Defense Mechanisms Contributing to Recurrent Infections

Abnormal barriers	Microbiologic flora	Foreign bodies
Eczema	Alteration by antibiotic therapy	Pulmonary
Burns	Abnormal drainage	Heart valves
Skull fractures	Ureteral stenosis	Vascular catheters
Sinus tracts	Vesicoureteral reflux	Urinary catheters
Abnormal vascular perfusion	Dysfunction of eustachian tubes	
Angiopathy (e.g., diabetes)	Cystic fibrosis	
Edema (e.g., nephrotic syndrome, congestive heart failure)	Ciliary dysfunction	
Infarction (e.g., sickle cell disease)	Tracheoesophageal fistula	

Reference: Shyur S-D, Hill HR: Immunodeficiency in the 1990s. Pediatr Infect Dis J 10:595–611, 1991.

INBORN ERRORS OF METABOLISM

Inborn Errors of Metabolism Presenting in the Neonatal Period

Inborn errors of metabolism are not as rare as we might believe. Although incidence rates are hard to come by due to undiagnosed cases, the possibility that a healthy full-term neonate who becomes suddenly ill has a treatable metabolic error is nearly as likely as that infant having an acquired infection. The tragedy of inborn errors of metabolism in the neonatal period is that a missed diagnosis can lead to rapidly progressive neurologic deterioration, coma, and death.

The characteristic symptoms of inborn errors are, like those of sepsis, largely nonspecific and variable: lethargy, failure to thrive, vomiting, seizures, and respiratory distress in the immediate neonatal period. Taken as a group, conservative estimates suggest that 20% of disease among full-term neonates without risk factors can be accounted for by metabolic errors. While by no means inclusive, the tables below indicate the more common inborn errors of metabolism that present within the first days of life and the results of appropriate tests.

Early diagnosis and treatment are the keystones to the prevention of neurologic sequelae or death. When presented with a sick, full-term infant, pursue the usual sepsis work-up but do not neglect the evaluation for metabolic disease.

Inborn Errors of Metabolism with Enzyme Deficiencies and Diagnostic Signs (Part I)

DISORDER	DEFICIENT ENZYME	ACID BASE	ANION GAP	PLASMA GLUCOSE	PLASMA LACTATE	PLASMA PYRUVATE	PLASMA AMINO ACIDS
Urea Cycle Disorders							
Carbamylphosphate synthetase (CPS)	CPS I	Respiratory alkalosis	N	N	N	N	Absent citrulline, glutamine, alanine, and arginine
OTC deficiency	OTC	Respiratory alkalosis	N	N	N	N	Same as CPS def.
Citrullinemia	Arginosuccinate synthetase	Respiratory alkalosis	N	N	N	N	Citrulline, glutamine, alanine, arginine
Argininosuccinic acidemia	Argininosuccinase	Respiratory alkalosis	N	N	N	N	Argininosuccinate and its anhydrides, citrulline, and glutamine, and arginine
Disorders of Branched-chain Amino Acid Metabolism and Leucine Degradation							
Maple syrup urine	Branched-chain keto-acid dehydrogenase	Metabolic acidosis	N→↑	N	N	N	Leucine, isoleucine, valine, alloisoleucine present
Isovaleric acidemia	Isovaleryl-CoA dehydrogenase	Metabolic acidosis	N→↑	N	N	N	
Propionic acidemia	Propionyl-CoA dehydrogenase	Metabolic acidosis	N→↑	↓	N→↑	N	Glycine
Methylmalonic acidemia	Methylmalonyl-CoA mutase, adenosylcobalmin synthetic enzyme	Metabolic acidosis	N→↑	↓	N→↑	N	Glycine—one form with homocystine
Disorders of Carbohydrate Metabolism							
Galactosemia	Galactose 1-phosphate uridyltransferase	Hyperchloremic metabolic acidosis	N	N	N	N	
Glycogen storage disease	I:G-6-phosphatase; Ib:G-6-phosphatase translocase	Metabolic acidosis	↑	↓	↑	↑	N to alanine
Others							
Nonketotic hyperglycinemia	Glycine cleavage complex	N to respiratory acidosis	N	N	N	N	Glycine
Multiple carboxylase deficiency	Biotin, holocarboxylase synthetase	Metabolic acidosis	N→↑	N	N→↑	?	
Type II glutaric aciduria	Multiple acyl-CoA dehydrogenase, electron transfer flavoprotein (EFTP)	Metabolic acidosis	N	↓	N→↑	N	Lysine
Congenital lactic acidosis	Pyruvate dehydrogenase (PDH) complex, pyruvate carboxylase, mitochondrial electron transport defect	Metabolic acidosis	↑	N→↓	↑	↑	Alanine

Table continued on next page.

Inborn Errors of Metabolism with Enzyme Deficiencies and Diagnostic Signs (Part II)

DISORDER	PLASMA NH4	URINE DNPH*	URINE KETONES	URINE RS*	URINE ORGANIC ACIDS	OTHER
Urea Cycle Disorders						
Carbamylphosphate synthetase (CPS)	4+	–	–	–	–	
OTC deficiency	4+	–	–	–	Orotic acid	X-linked inheritance
Citrullinemia	4+	–	–	–	–	
Argininosuccinic acidemia	4+	–	–	–	–	
Disorders of Branched-chain Amino Acid Metabolism and Leucine Degradation						
Maple syrup urine	N	+	+	–	2-oxoisovaleric, 2-hydroxyisovaleric, 2-oxoisocaproic, 2-hydroxyisocaproic, 2-oxo-3-methylvaleric,	Odor of maple syrup
Isovaleric acidemia	N→2+	–	+	–	N-isovalerylglycine, 3-hydroxyisovaleric, free isovaleric acid	Odor of sweaty feet
Propionic acidemia	N→4+	–	+	–	3-hydroxypropionic acid, methylcitrate	Neutropenia, thrombocytopenia
Methylmalonic acidemia	N→4+	–	+	–	Methylmalonic acid; may have low concentrations of propionate metabolites	Neutropenia, thrombocytopenia
Disorders of Carbohydrate Metabolism						
Galactosemia	N	–	–	+	May have tyrosine metabolites with liver dysfunction	May present with gram-negative sepsis, cataracts, and hyperbilirubinemia
Glycogen storage disease	N	–	+	–		Cholesterol, triglycerides, and uric acid; may be masked in newborns by frequent feedings
Others						
Nonketotic hyperglycinemia	N	–	–	–		Seizures usually prominent
Multiple carboxylase deficiency	N→2+	–	+	–	3-methylcrotonyl, glycine, 3-hydroxypropionic, 3-hydroxyisovaleric, methylcitrate	
Type II glutaric aciduria	N→2+	–	–	–	Glutaric acid, 2-hydroxyglutaric acid, and ethylmalonic and 2-hydroxyisovaleric dicarboxylic acids	Odor of sweaty feet; dysmorphic features
Congenital lactic acidosis	N→2+	–	–/+	–	Lactic acid	PDH-facial dysmorphology may be present

*DNPH = dinitrophenylhydrazine; RS = reducing substances.

Other Disorders of Inborn Errors of Metabolism
Reported in the Neonatal Period

3-Methylcrotonylglycinuria and 3-hydroxy-
    isovaleric aciduria
2-Methylacetoacetyl-CoA thiolase deficiency
Succinyl-CoA: 3-ketoacid-CoA transferase
    deficiency
D-Glyceric acidemia
5-Oxoprolinuria
Hyperornithinemia-hyperammonemia-
    homocitrullinuria syndrome
5,10-Methylenetetrahydrofolate reductase
    deficiency

Molybdenum cofactor deficiency
Short-chain acyl-CoA dehydrogenase deficiency
Long-chain acyl-CoA dehydrogenase deficiency
2-Ketoadipic aciduria
3-Hydroxy-3-methylglutaryl-CoA lyase deficiency
Fructose 1,6-diphosphatase deficiency
Peroxisomal disorders: Zellweger syndrome,
    neonatal adrenoleukodystrophy, infantile
    Refsum's disease, pseudo-Zellweger syndrome
Hepatorenal tyrosinemia

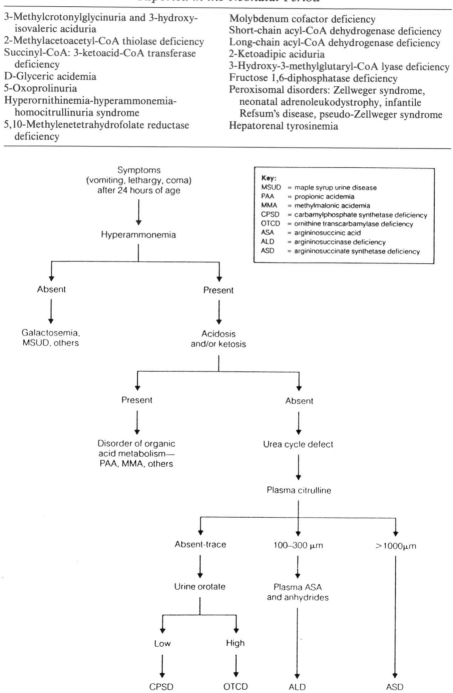

Making the diagnosis when initial tests show hyperammonemia.

General Protocol for Diet-responsive Disorders

1. Discontinue intake of offending compounds and precursors.
2. Correct fluid and electrolyte abnormalities.
3. Institute hemodialysis in cases of progressive hyperammonemia or coma.
4. Provide a minimum of 120 cal/kg/d utilizing intravenous and oral nutrition. Mead Johnson product MJ80056 is a convenient source of nonprotein calories.
5. Institute pharmacologic trial of specific vitamin cofactor.
6. Add minimal amounts of the essential offending compounds, as indicated by careful and frequent monitoring of plasma levels.
7. Adjust calories, fluids, and amounts of offending compounds individually according to growth and plasma concentrations.

From Arn PH, et al: Contemporary Pediatrics 5(Dec):59, 1988, with permission.

Reference: Arn PH, et al: Inborn errors of metabolism: Not rare, not hopeless. Contemporary Pediatrics 5(Dec):47–63, 1988.

Clinical Symptomatology of Inborn Errors of Metabolism in the Neonate or Infant

The newborn or older infant with an acute onset of nonspecific symptoms is an all too frequent dilemma for pediatricians. Along with infections, cardiac defects, gastrointestinal diseases, and insults to the central nervous system, however, an inborn error of metabolism (IEM) must be considered.

Symptoms indicating a possibility of an IEM (one or all):

1. Infant becomes acutely ill after period of normal behavior and feeding; this may occur within hours or weeks.
2. Neonate or infant has seizures and/or hypotonia, especially if seizures are not retractible.
3. Neonate or infant has an unusual odor.

Symptoms indicating strong probability of an IEM, particularly when coupled with the above symptoms:

1. Persistent or recurrent vomiting
2. Failure to thrive (failure to gain weight or weight loss)
3. Apnea or respiratory distress (tachypnea)
4. Jaundice or hepatomegaly
5. Lethargy
6. Coma (particularly intermittent)
7. Unexplained hemorrhage
8. Family history of neonatal deaths, or of similar illness, especially in siblings
9. Parental consanguinity
10. Sepsis (particularly *Escherichia coli*, a common form of sepsis in patients with galactosemia)

Reference: Ward JC: Inborn errors of metabolism of acute onset in infancy. Pediatrics in Review 11(7):205–216, 1990. Adapted from Table 1 of cited paper.

INCIDENCE VS. PREVALENCE

The incorrect use of these two terms is prevalent among clinicians. This is unfortunate both for interpretation of clinical information and statistics, and for the accuracy of personal expression. The correct definitions are:

Incidence: The expression of the rate at which a certain event occurs. In particular, the incidence rate is a rate in which the numerator is the number of new cases of a disease in a population during a specified time and the denominator is the number of the population at risk.

$$\textbf{Incidence rate } = \frac{\text{Number of new cases of a disease}}{\text{Total population at risk}} \text{ (Per unit of time)}$$

Prevalence: The total cases in existence at a certain time in a designated area expressed as a rate.

$$\textbf{Prevalence rate } = \frac{\text{Number of existing cases}}{\text{Total population}} \begin{array}{l}\text{(At a certain time in} \\ \text{a designated area)}\end{array}$$

If the incidence is stable over time,

$$\text{Prevalence = Incidence} \times \text{Average duration of disease.}$$

INJURIES

Is It Possible to Make a Difference?

Sweden has the lowest child injury death rate of any country in the world, 88 deaths in 1988 in a population of 8.5 million. We admit up front the list of caveats needed in comparing the homogeneous society of Sweden with the complex population of the United States. However, notice in the figure the progress in Sweden in lowering childhood injury fatalities since 1957–1959. In 1988 10 Swedish children drowned, compared to 100 in 1954. What happened?

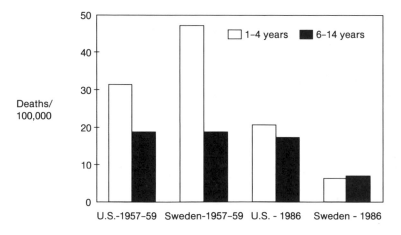

Injury fatalities, Sweden and the United States, 1957 through 1959 and 1986. Data from World Health Organization.

For the past 25 years the task of lowering childhood injuries and deaths in Sweden was the responsibility of the Joint Committee for the Prevention of Childhood Accidents, which embarked on a three-pronged approach that has achieved remarkable results. The three parts of the process were:

1. A system for injury surveillance and prevention research to identify the important problems, to test countermeasures, and to implement better trauma care.
2. The provision of a safer environment for children through legislation and regulation. This included, for example, separating children from hazards such as traffic and making the child's environment safer (windows, stairs, stoves, etc.).
3. Educating the public about injury prevention.

It has made a difference.

Reference: Bergman AB, Rivara FP: Sweden's experience in reducing childhood injury. Pediatrics 88:69–74, 1991.

INTOEING

"Doctor, My Kid Walks Funny," or What to Do About Intoeing

Parents of infants and toddlers just learning how to walk frequently notice the symptom of "toeing-in." Despite frantic expectations of special exercises, braces, or corrective shoes, most conditions that cause an intoed posture are rarely due to a pathologic or orthopedic anomaly and are not much affected by interventions. Indeed, the overwhelming majority of such cases are within the norms of physical development.

A General Game Plan for the Child Who Presents With Intoeing

1. Reassure most parents that the condition of intoeing will resolve on its own as the child progresses in his or her growth and development.
2. Identify those patients within the limits of normal development, explain the condition carefully to the parents, and monitor the child over the course of time to ensure resolution.
3. Avoid unnecessary treatments.
4. Distinguish the rare orthopedic entities from the normal variants in order to provide interventional therapy (see table).

Causes of Intoeing in Childhood

	INITIAL PRESENTATION (NONAMBULATORY CHILD)	NORMAL RESOLUTION (AMBULATORY CHILD)	PROBLEMS REQUIRING CORRECTION
Hips	a. External rotation contracture (positional and not a cause of of actual intoeing)	a. External contracture is lost.	Rotational asymmetries may be the result of hip dislocation.
	b. Minimal or no internal rotation	b. Greater internal rotation as a manifestation of increased femoral anteversion	Dislocation is treated by reduction and retention of the femoral head into the socket.

Table continued on next page.

Causes of Intoeing in Childhood (Cont.)

	INITIAL PRESENTATION (NONAMBULATORY CHILD)	NORMAL RESOLUTION (AMBULATORY CHILD)	PROBLEMS REQUIRING CORRECTION
Femur	High angle of anteversion (40–60° at birth) apparent only after external rotational contractures have been stretched out by ambulation. This angle is a cause of actual intoeing (see figure).	Gradual remodeling of angle in childhood reaching adult configuration of 10–20° between ages 5 and 10 years.	Unresolved femoral anteversion that interferes with function is rare. Correction is by derotational external osteotomy (not recommended for cosmetic purposes)

The **angle of femoral anteversion** is created by the long axis of the neck of the femur and the transcondylar axis of the knee joint and is normally 10° to 20° in adults *(top)*. The angle is higher in newborns (40° to 60°) and young children *(bottom)*, producing intoeing, but usually remodels to the adult angle by age 5 to 8.

Table continued on next page.

Causes of Intoeing in Childhood (Cont.)

	INITIAL PRESENTATION (NONAMBULATORY CHILD)	NORMAL RESOLUTION (AMBULATORY CHILD)	PROBLEMS REQUIRING CORRECTION
Lower Leg	Internal tibial torsion is normal in a nonwalking child and a cause of actual intoeing (see figure).	Tibial torsion gradually unwinds, disappearing between ages 18 months and 4 years.	Unresolved tibial torsion that persists beyond age 6 or 7 is rare. It requires corrective osteotomy.

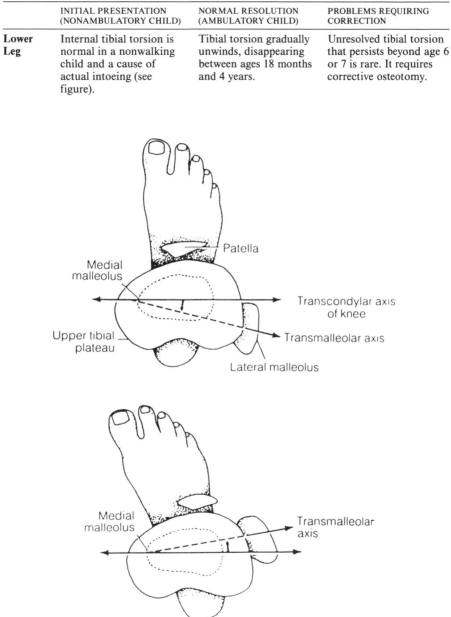

Internal tibial torsion is one cause of intoeing. When the patella is straight and facing forward, the normal position of the lateral malleolus is 10° to 15° posterior to the medial malleolus *(top)*. If the lateral malleolus is on the same level as the medial malleolus, or anterior to it, internal tibial torsion is present *(bottom)*.

Table continued on next page.

Causes of Intoeing in Childhood (Cont.)

	INITIAL PRESENTATION (NONAMBULATORY CHILD)	NORMAL RESOLUTION (AMBULATORY CHILD)	PROBLEMS REQUIRING CORRECTION
Foot	a. Positional varus (the borders of the foot are straight and there is no actual foot deformity)	a. Positional varus disappears with standing, usually between 9 and 14 months. Intoeing caused by internal tibial torsion and increased femoral anteversion ceases as these conditions begin to resolve.	
	b. Metatarsus adductus (a fixed) deformity of the foot in which the forepart of the foot is angled away from the foot's main longitudinal axis toward the midline).		b. Rigid metatarsus adductus requires serial casting followed by the use of a passive holding device.
	c. Equinovarus (or clubfoot)		c. Clubfoot requires correction with casting and surgery.

The physical examination should also include an assessment of the child's spine. A search for spinal curvatures and dermatologic evidence of possible neurologic disease should be made. Minor neural tube defects, for example, may not be obvious in a preadolescent patient, but after the pubertal growth spurt they can present as asymmetrical muscle weakness and rotational weakness of the leg.

Reference: Rosman MA: When parents ask about intoeing. Contemporary Pediatrics 4(1):116–122, 1987.

INTRAOSSEOUS INFUSION

The child presenting emergently with shock secondary to overwhelming sepsis, dehydration, trauma, and life-threatening status epilepticus demands immediate vascular access. This noble goal, unfortunately, is not always easily achieved. The intraosseous infusion of fluids and drugs directly into the bone marrow, however, is an especially useful skill for the pediatrician to acquire for such situations. It should be reserved for the emergencies noted above and employed only when other methods of intravenous access have failed.

Anatomy

The marrow sinusoids of long bones drain into medullary venous channels; nutrient and emissary veins drain into the systemic venous system. Marrow cavities are particularly appealing in patients with severe hypovolemia and peripheral circulatory shock, because they act as rigid and uncollapsable veins. Further, medications injected via intraosseous infusion are absorbed almost immediately into the general circulation. One caveat that needs mentioning is to be aware of the child's age; the soft, vascular red marrow in long bones seen in infants and young children is physiologically replaced by the less vascular yellow marrow at approximately 5 years of age.

Technique (see figure)

1. The patient's leg should be restrained with a small sandbag placed behind the knee for support. The skin should be cleansed with povidone-iodine or alcohol using an aseptic technique. Local anesthetic is optional and may not be necessary in patients with depressed mental status.

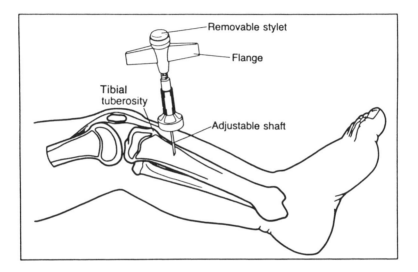

Placement of the Illinois sternal or iliac bone marrow-aspiration needle in the proximal tibial location. The disposable needle has a flange at the top to make it easier to grip, a locking stylet to prevent the needle from being plugged with bone during insertion, and a screw mechanism to adjust the length of the exposed shaft. Depending on the gauge and manufacturer, the length of the shaft can be adjusted from 0.16 to 4.76 cm (1/16 to 1 7/8 in).

2. Disposable sternal or iliac bone-marrow aspiration needles (15 to 18 gauge) are preferable. The shaft should be short with a protective sheath in order to prevent the needle's tip from being forced too deeply into or through the bone.
3. The proximal tibia is the optimal site of insertion, because it precludes interference from ventilation or chest compressions during placement. The site of insertion should be on the midline of the anterior tibia, 1 to 3 cm or two fingers' width below the tibial tuberosity at an angle of 60° to 90° away from the growth plate. Advance the needle using a screwing or boring type of motion.

   [N.B.: alternative insertion sites include the distal tibia and the femur, 2 to 3 cm above the external condyles; the sternum and ileum are less suitable sites and should be avoided.]

4. Entry into the marrow space is confirmed by noting a lack of resistance after the needle has passed through the cortex. Marrow should be easily aspirated into a syringe and fluids should infuse freely. Before injection, hypertonic and alkaline solutions should be diluted.

5. The needle should stand upright without support but must be stabilized and secured by taping the flanges of the needle in order to prevent loss of access.
6. Flush the needle with a heparin-containing saline to prevent clotting before administering a conventional solution.
7. The insertion site must be observed for evidence of extravasation.
8. Once conventional vascular access has been obtained (normally within 1 to 2 hours after establishing the intraosseous infusion), the bone-marrow needle should be removed. Longer intraosseous infusions increase the risk of infectious complications.
9. A sterile dressing should be placed over the dressing site and pressure applied to the dressing for 5 minutes.

Possible Complications

1. Subcutaneous and occasional subperiosteal infiltration of fluid or leakage at the puncture site.
2. Clotting of marrow in the needle, which can impede access.
3. Localized cellulitis and subcutaneous abscesses have been reported in about 0.7% of all cases.
4. Osteomyelitis has been reported in approximately 0.6% of cases.
5. Theoretically, damage to the growth plates and marrow elements can occur, but this is rarely observed. Fat and bone emboli are also of concern but rarely occur.

Contraindications

The procedure is contraindicated in children with osteogenesis imperfecta, osteopetrosis, and an ipsilateral fractured extremity due to risk of subcutaneous extravasation. The risk of infectious complication increases when the needle is introduced through an area affected by cellulitis or burn injuries. The procedure should not be performed in children over the age of 5 years.

Reference: Fisher DH: Intraosseous infusion. N Engl J Med 322:1579–1581, 1990.

INTUSSUSCEPTION

The Need for Prompt Recognition

The pediatrician is usually the first physician to see a child with an intussusception. Prompt recognition of this acute disorder will reduce morbidity and mortality. Remembering the following facts will facilitate early diagnosis and improve management.

Age of Patients	% Presenting at Given Age
Under 12 months	52%
1–2 years	24%
2–3 years	10%
3–7 years	11%
Over 7 years	3%

Signs and Symptoms	% Presenting with Given Sign or Symptom
Pain	94%
Vomiting (at least once)	91%
Gross blood with stool	66%
Abdominal mass	59%

Patients typically are healthy infants and children with no previous history of gastrointestinal disease. Nearly all infants present with recent onset of abdominal pain and at least one episode of vomiting. The pain is characterized by the child's crying and drawing his legs into his abdomen. Males are affected about twice as often as females. The mass is usually sausage-shaped and is palpable along the course of the colon. On occasion one may elicit Dance's sign—an emptiness in the right lower quadrant that reflects the fact that the intussuscepting bowel has moved out of this portion of the abdomen.

Etiology of Intussusception

In less than 10% of patients will an etiologic factor be determined. Specific causes include Meckel's diverticulum (most common), ileal polyp, ileal granuloma, inspissated meconium in patients with cystic fibrosis, Henoch-Schönlein purpura, and lymphosarcoma.

Although the barium reduction will successfully reduce approximately 75% of all intussusception, *it is advisable for all patients over 6 years of age to have elective exploratory laparotomy because of the high probability that intussusception at this age has a specific cause; it is frequently produced by an intestinal lymphosarcoma.*

Reference: Wayne ER, Cambell JB, Burrington JD, Davis WS: Radiology 107:597, 1973.

From McMillan JA, et al: The Whole Pediatrician Catalog. Philadelphia, W.B. Saunders, 1977, p 382, with permission.

IRON DEFICIENCY ANEMIA

A Progression of Findings

Throughout the world anemia is the most common manifestation of nutritional deficiency. In the U.S. iron deficiency is associated with the majority of nutritional anemias.

The onset of iron deficiency anemia is preceded by a sequence of abnormalities that may exist a considerable time before the anemia. Given that iron deficiency is a multisystem problem and that symptoms may occur well in advance of the onset of anemia, screening tests have been devised to detect iron deficiency before anemia is present. The sequential changes are indicated in the table.

Sequential Changes in the Development of Iron Deficiency

		STAGE I IRON DEPLETION		STAGE II IRON-DEFICIENT ERYTHROPOIESIS	STAGE III IRON DEFICIENCY
Serum ferritin	E A R L Y	Decreased levels		Decreased levels	Decreased levels
Bone marrow iron		Decreased staining		Decreased staining	Decreased staining
Total serum iron binding capacity (TIBC)		Normal	I N T E R M E D I A T E	Elevated	Elevated
Serum iron		Normal		Decreased levels	Decreased levels
Erythrocyte proto-porphyrins		Normal		Increased levels	Increased levels
Hemoglobin		Normal		Normal	Low
Hematocrit		Normal		Normal	Low
Mean corpuscular volume (MCV)		Normal		Normal or low	L A T E	Low
Red cell morphology		Normal		Normal	Microcytosis Hypochromia

Reference: Bates HM: Lab Management 18:9, 1980.

Blue Sclerae as a Sign of Iron Deficiency Anemia

In his classic textbook, *The Principles and Practice of Medicine*, Sir William Osler described a common but rarely noted finding among iron-deficient, undernourished teenage girls: the presence of blue sclerae. A group of British gastroenterologists recently studied the presence of blue sclerae in association with iron deficiency anemia and found the sign to be far more sensitive and equally specific for iron deficiency anemia than the presence of mucosal pallor. Further, the search for blue sclerae is easier to confirm, because it is not affected by skin thickness, blood transfusions, pigmentation, or perfusion, which can be confusing in an accurate assessment of mucosal pallor.

The blue sclerae sign in iron deficiency anemia most likely results from impaired collagen synthesis; iron is a vital cofactor in the hydroxylation of proline and lysine residues. The result is a thin sclera that allows greater visibility of the choroid, and a bluish color is observed. Blue sclerae are associated with other diseases, as listed below, but these disorders are extremely rare and certainly less common than iron deficiency anemia in the general population. The presence of blue sclerae, therefore, should prompt the physician to consider a possible underlying iron deficiency.

Disease Entities Associated with Blue Sclerae

Iron deficiency anemia
Anemia secondary to chronic blood loss (e.g., duodenal ulcers, inflammatory bowel disease, gluten enteropathy)
Osteogenesis imperfecta
Inherited connective tissue disorders (e.g., Ehlers-Danlos syndrome, pseudoxanthoma elasticum)

Rheumatologic disorders (e.g., rheumatoid arthritis, systemic lupus erythematosis)
Malignancies of the gastrointestinal tract
Corticosteroid use
Anemia secondary to hookworm infection (ankylostomiasis)
Myasthenia gravis

Reference: Kalra L, Hamlyn AN, Jones BJM: Blue sclerae: A common sign of iron deficiency. Lancet ii:1267–1269, 1986.

Koilonychia—A Sign of Iron Deficiency

Koilonychia, or spooning of the nails, refers to the loss of the longitudinal and lateral convexity of the nail associated with thinning and fraying of its distal portion. The terminal and lateral borders are flared dorsally as the normal convexity is replaced by flattening and concavity of the nail plate.

Although spooning of the nail can be seen as a result of local fungal infections or as a hereditary abnormality, it is also an early sign of iron deficiency in infants and children as well as adults.

The nail of the index finger is more frequently and more severely deformed. The third finger and the thumb are also commonly involved. The spooning occurs symmetrically, which should provide a clue to diagnosis. If still in doubt, then look at the feet. Most infants with spoon nails will also display the same involvement on the nail of the big toe.

This provides a simple way of making a presumptive diagnosis of iron deficiency.

Reference: Hogan GR, Jones B: J Pediatr 77:1054, 1970.
From McMillan JA, et al: The Whole Pediatrician Catalog, Vol. 2. Philadelphia, W.B. Saunders, 1979, p 202, with permission.

IRON OVERDOSE

Iron Poisoning—An Emergency Assessment

Because most patients with serum iron values in excess of 300 μg/dl are likely to develop signs and symptoms of iron overdose, which clinical signs and laboratory determinations do, in fact, predict a serum iron concentration of greater than 300 μg/dl and serve as a guide for admission and therapy?

Five clinical and laboratory findings have been found to be significantly different in patients with serum iron concentrations greater than or less than 300 μg/dl. These five findings are:

1. White cell count $> 15,000/mm^3$
2. Blood sugar > 150 mg/dl
3. Presence of vomiting
4. Presence of diarrhea
5. Radiopaque material visible on flat plate of abdomen.

Vomiting has the highest sensitivity value, as well as the highest negative predictive value. The absence of vomiting makes is highly unlikely that the patient has a serum iron in excess of 300 μg/dl.

Importantly, patients do not develop signs or symptoms of acute iron toxicity more than 6 hours after ingestion. Any patient who remains asymptomatic for 6 hours following ingestion may be discharged with minimal risk of having a dangerously elevated serum iron concentration.

In summary, initial management of iron overdose should consist of induced emesis or lavage with a large bore tube. If any of the five screening tests described above is positive, a serum iron concentration of greater than 300 μg/dl is likely, and a serum iron concentration should be obtained. If a delay in obtaining a serum iron is anticipated, the patient should be given an intramuscular dose of deferoxamine (50 mg/kg up to a maximum of 1 g). If the drug produces a "vin rose" color to the urine, indicating that the serum iron concentration exceeds the total iron-binding capacity, the patient requires treatment. Patients who have negative results for all five tests should be observed for at least 6 hours for symptoms. Those remaining asymptomatic may be discharged.

Reference: Lacouture PG, et al: Emergency assessment of severity in iron overdose by clinical and laboratory methods. J Pediatr 99:89–91, 1981.

Never lend your car to anyone to whom you have given birth.

Erma Bombeck

J

JAUNDICE

Jaundice in Infancy

Visible jaundice occurs at serum bilirubin levels greater than 5 mg/dl. Most infants, full-term and premature, exhibit signs of a transient, unconjugated hyperbilirubinemia during the first week of life. This "physiologic jaundice" is the result of a complex interplay among several factors such as:

1. an elevated bilirubin load secondary to increased red blood cell (RBC) volume, decreased RBC survival, and an increased enterohepatic circulation.
2. defective hepatic uptake of bilirubin from the serum due to diminished levels of ligandin and competition for binding to intracellular proteins.
3. defective bilirubin conjugation caused by decreased UDP-glucuronyl-transferase activity.
4. defective bilirubin excretion.

The National Collaborative Perinatal Project has determined that the majority of infants with physiologic jaundice will not have a serum bilirubin level > 12.9 mg/dl if full term, or 16 mg/dl if premature. Risk factors for developing hyperbilirubinemia during the first week of life include breastfeeding, maternal diabetes, induction of labor with oxytocin, male sex, and Oriental race.

The essential questions to answer, when evaluating a jaundiced newborn, are the severity of the hyperbilirubinemia and the type (conjugated vs. unconjugated). A rapid rise in serum bilirubin, such as an infant who develops hyperbilirubinemia in the first 24 hours of life or a rise in serum bilirubin greater than 5 mg/dl/day, warrants immediate investigation. A jaundiced infant without risk factors or prolonged jaundice (>1 week in a full term; >2 weeks in a premature infant) also needs to be evaluated, as does the infant with conjugated hyperbilirubinemia.

Unconjugated Hyperbilirubinemia

If the fractionation of the serum bilirubin documents as unconjugated hyperbilirubinemia, then the search for its cause should progress as follows (please note that the history, physical examination and clinical course will help guide the extent of the evaluation):

1. Fractionate serum bilirubin
2. Blood type and Rh (mother and infant)
3. Hemoglobin, hematocrit, and reticulocyte count
4. Coombs test (direct and indirect)
5. Peripheral blood smear
6. Prothrombin time/partial thromboplastin time
7. Platelet count

193

8. Alkaline denaturation of hemoglobin test (of emesis)—adult vs. fetal hemoglobin
9. Sepsis work-up (blood, urine, cerebrospinal fluid culture)
10. Thyroid screen thyroxine, triiodothyronine, thyroid-stimulating hormone)
11. Phenobarbitol trial
12. Interruption of breastfeeding

The Differential Diagnosis for Unconjugated Hyperbilirubinemia

1. Physiologic jaundice
2. Hemolysis (e.g., ABO incompatibility; erythroblastosis fetalis; and red blood cell defects such as spherocytosis, elliptocytosis, G-6-PD deficiency, and pyruvate kinase deficiency)
3. Hemorrhage (e.g., birth trauma, cephalohematoma)
4. Breast milk jaundice
5. Swallowed maternal blood
6. Placental dysfunction
7. Sepsis
8. Clotting disorders
9. Infant of a diabetic mother
10. Hypothyroidism
11. Intestinal obstruction (e.g., pyloric stenosis, duodenal stenosis, or atresia)
12. Crigler-Najjar syndrome (an hereditary disorder of glucuronyl transferase resulting in an elevated unconjugated bilirubin level; Type II Crigler-Najjar is distinguished from Type I by a rapid decline in serum bilirubin level with phenobarbital therapy [5 mg/kg/day])
13. Lucey-Driscol syndrome (a syndrome of retention jaundice due to defective bilirubin conjugation in infants resulting from an unidentified factor transmitted by the mother to her infant).

Conjugated Hyperbilirubinemia

Conjugated hyperbilirubinemia is always pathologic in the neonate and its presence demands a diagnostic evaluation. The primary emphasis of this work-up is to identify those infants with treatable infectious and metabolic diseases, recognizable congenital or genetic disorders, or extrahepatic obstruction who would benefit from surgical intervention. This evaluation should begin with a complete history and physical examination, and the laboratory evaluation should proceed as follows:

1. Fractionate serum bilirubin
2. Serum transaminases, alkaline phosphatase (or 5'-nucleotidase), albumin, cholesterol
3. Prothrombin time
4. Stool color
5. Cultures (blood, urine, CSF, etc.)
6. Hepatitis B surface antigen, TORCH titers, VDRL
7. Serum α1-antitrypsin level
8. Metabolic screen (urine/serum amino acids; urine for reducing substances)
9. Thyroid screen
10. Ophthalmologic examination
11. Sweat chloride
12. Skull, long bones, abdominal, and chest x-ray films
13. Abdominal ultrasound
14. Duodenal intubation (string test for duodenal fluid color, bilirubin, bile acids)
15. Hepatobiliary scintigraphy
16. Percutaneous liver biopsy

Differential Diagnosis of Conjugated Hyperbilirubinemia*

1. Extrahepatic obstruction
   a. Infantile obstructive
      cholangiopathy
      Biliary atresia
      Neonatal hepatitis
      Choledocholithiasis
   b. Other causes
      Bile plug syndrome
      Choledocholithiasis
      Spontaneous bile duct
         perforation
      Extrinsic bile duct compression
2. Genetic and metabolic disorders
   a. Disorders of carbohydrate
      metabolism
      Galactosemia
      Fructosemia
      Glycogen storage disease type IV
   b. Disorders of amino acid metabolism
      Tyrosinemia
   c. Disorders of lipid metabolism
      Niemann-Pick disease
      Gaucher disease
      Wolman disease
      Cholesterol ester storage disease
   d. Chromosomal disorders
      Trisomy 18
      Down syndrome
   e. Miscellaneous genetic & metabolic
      disorders
      α_1-Antitrypsin deficiency
      Neonatal hypopituitarism
      Cystic fibrosis
      Zellweger cerebrohepatorenal
         syndrome
      Familial hepatosteatosis
3. Persistent intrahepatic
   cholestasis
   a. Paucity of intrahepatic
      bile ducts
   b. Arteriohepatic dysplasia
   c. Benign recurrent intra-
      hepatic cholestasis
   d. Byler disease
   e. Hereditary cholestasis
      with lymphedema
   f. Trihydroxycoprostanic
      acidemia
4. Acquired intrahepatic
   cholestasis
   a. Infections
      Hepatitis B
         (non-A, non-B?)
      Syphilis
      Toxoplasmosis
      Rubella
      Cytomegalovirus
      Herpes
      Varicella
      Echovirus
      Coxsackievirus
      Leptospirosis
      Tuberculosis
      Bacterial sepsis
   b. Drug-induced
      cholestasis
   c. Cholestasis associated
      with parenteral
      nutrition

*From Rosenthal P, Sinatra F: Pediatrics in Review 11:82, 1989, with permission.

Reference: Adapted from Rosenthal P, Sinatra F: Jaundice in infancy. Pediatrics in Review 11:79–86, 1989.

Progression of Dermal Icterus in the Newborn

The rate of rise of serum bilirubin in the newborn infant who is jaundiced should always be monitored by laboratory determinations. The pediatrician, however, through simple examination of the infant, may make some estimation as to the rate of rise of serum bilirubin.

Dermal icterus has been shown to progress in a cephalopedal fashion; that is, as the infant's bilirubin rises, more of the skin becomes icteric. The icterus begins at the head and neck and progresses caudally to the palms and soles. The following table correlates the level of indirect bilirubin with the area of skin that is icteric in full-term infants whose jaundice is not due to Rh incompatibility.

Area of the Body	Range of Indirect Bilirubin (mg/100 ml)
Head and neck	4–8
Upper trunk	5–12
Lower trunk and thighs	8–16
Arms and lower legs	11–18
Palms and soles	> 15

As icterus progresses, the area that had been jaundiced remains jaundiced, so that the entire body is icteric when the bilirubin rises above 15 mg/100 ml. The fading of the icterus as the bilirubin level falls affects all body areas at the same time, so that the intensity rather than the extent of the staining fades. The staining may progress more rapidly in the low birth weight infant, whereas the infant with Rh disease may demonstrate a relative lag in dermal staining.

Correct estimation of the extent of icterus involves the examination of the completely undressed infant under blue-white fluorescent light. Icterus may be detected by blanching the skin with pressure of the thumb and noting the color of the underlying skin. This is a more difficult determination to make in deeply pigmented black infants, but the palms and soles, at least, may be easily examined even in these patients.

Reference: Kramer LI: Advancement of dermal icterus in the jaundiced newborn. Am J Dis Child 18:454, 1969.

From McMillan JA, et al: The Whole Pediatrician Catalog. Philadelphia, W.B. Saunders, 1977, pp 127–128, with permission.

JOINT PAIN

Common Causes

Chondromalacia patellae
Growing pains
Osteomyelitis
Overuse
Septic arthritis
Sickle-cell disease
Sympathetic effusion
Tietze's syndrome
Transient synovitis
Trauma
  Contusion

Trauma *(Cont.)*
  Fracture
  Hemarthrosis
  Sprain/strain
Viral arthritis
  Adenovirus
  Epstein-Barr virus
  Hepatitis
  Mumps
  Rubella
  Varicella

Uncommon Causes

Attention-seeking behavior
Child abuse
Foreign body
Legg-Calve-Perthes disease
Mycoplasma
Osgood-Schlatter disease
Osteochondritis dissecans
Popliteal cyst
Psoriatic arthritis

Reactive arthritis
  Brucella
  Campylobacter
  Salmonella \
  Shigella
  Yersinia
Referred pain (retroperitoneal/intra-
  peritoneal inflammation)
Slipped capital femoral epiphysis
Subluxation of the patella

Rare Causes

Bone tumors
Carpal-tarsal osteolysis
Congenital joint laxity
  Ehlers-Danlos syndrome
  Marfan syndrome
  Stickler's syndrome
Cystic fibrosis
Fabry's disease
Gaucher's disease
Giardia
Gout
Hyperlipoproteinemia
Hyperparathyroidism
Idiopathic chondrolysis
Immunodeficiency
  Complement deficiency
  Hypogammaglobulinemia
Immunologic
  Acute rheumatic fever
  Ankylosing spondylitis
  Behçet's syndrome
  Dermatomyositis
  Giant-cell arteritis
  Henoch-Schönlein purpura
  Hepatitis
  Inflammatory bowel disease
  Juvenile rheumatoid arthritis

Immunologic *(Cont.)*
  Kawasaki's disease
  Mixed connective tissue disease
  Polyarteritis nodosa
  Reiter's syndrome
  Scleroderma
  Serum sickness
  Sjögren's syndrome
  Systemic lupus erythematosus
Leukemia
Lipogranulomatosis
Lyme disease
Mucopolysaccharidosis
Mycobacterial disease
Psychogenic rheumatism
Reflex sympathetic dystrophy
Rickets
Sarcoidosis
Stevens-Johnson syndrome
Subacute bacterial endocarditis
Syphilis
  Charcot joint
  Infection
Thyroid disease
Villonodular synovitis
Whipple's disease

JUVENILE RHEUMATOID ARTHRITIS
(See also ARTHRITIS)

Features of Juvenile Rheumatoid Arthritis

Juvenile rheumatoid arthritis (JRA) is an entity with protean manifestations. There is a remarkable heterogeneity of JRA, which has been divided into three major categories: (1) systemic, (2) pauciarticular-onset type (in which four or fewer joints are affected), and (3) polyarticular-onset type (the type most similar to typical rheumatoid arthritis). There has been some acceptance among rheumatologists and orthopedists to further subdivide the pauciarticular group. Early-onset pauciarticular JRA primarily affects young girls; chronic iridocyclitis is a common feature, as is the tendency to have positive antinuclear antibody tests. Late-onset pauciarticular JRA, on the other hand, affects mostly older boys; sacroiliitis is a common feature and many patients go on to develop ankylosing spondylitis in adult life.

Features of the Three Major Types of JRA

	SYSTEMIC ONSET	POLYARTICULAR ONSET	PAUCIARTICULAR ONSET
High fever	++++	0	0
Rheumatoid rash	++++	+++	++
Lymphadenopathy	+++	++	+
Splenomegaly	+++	++	++
Hepatomegaly	++	+	+
Pericarditis	+++	+	0
Myocarditis	++	0	0
Pneumonitis, pleuritis	++	+	0
Chronic iridocyclitis	+	+	+++
Subcutaneous nodules	0	++	0
Leukocytosis	+++	0	0
Rheumatoid factor	0	+++	0

++++ = most cases; +++ = many cases; ++ = some cases; + = occasional cases; 0 = rare or no cases.

Reference: Adapted from Tarana A: JRA and red herrings. Hospital Practice 23:129–150, 1988.

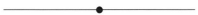

The greatest poem ever known
Is one all poets have outgrown:
The poetry, innate, untold,
Of being only four years old.

Christopher Morley
From *To A Child*

K

KAWASAKI'S DISEASE

Is It Really Kawasaki's Disease?

Kawasaki's disease, also known as mucocutaneous lymph node syndrome, occurs worldwide. It is an acute, febrile, multisystemic disease of children that is usually benign and self-limited. In the United States the annual incidence is 4.5–8.5 cases per 100,000 children below 5 years of age. In an outbreak in a community, the incidence can rise to 150 per 100,000 children.

Every house officer seems to make this diagnosis five times more frequently than that of scarlet fever and other more common red rashes. Is it really Kawasaki's disease? The figure shows us what to expect if and when we are to make this diagnosis, and the list below helps us to distinguish this disorder from its imitators.

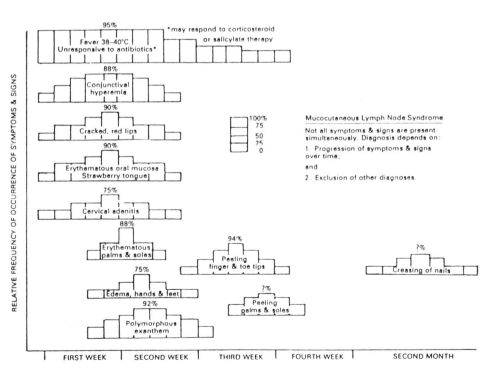

Familiarity with its features will help you to make the diagnosis.

Major Manifestations

Fever in excess of 38.5° C for 5 days
Redness and induration of palms and soles
Desquamation of skin over fingers during convalescence
Polymorphous exanthem over trunk; no vesicles
Conjunctivitis
Redness and fissuring of the lips
Strawberry tongue
Diffuse redness of oropharynx
Acute, nonpurulent swelling of cervical lymph nodes

Other features of the disease may include tachycardia, gallop rhythm, distant heart sounds, heart murmurs, EKG changes, diarrhea, proteinuria, pyuria, leukocytosis, mild anemia, elevated platelet count, increased erythrocyte sedimentation rate, and increasing level of IgE during period of illness.

Less frequent manifestations include arthralgia, arthritis, aseptic meningitis, and mild jaundice.

Mortality is approximately 0.3 to 2%. The most serious complication is vasculitis of the coronary arteries, although early deaths may result from severe myocarditis. Deaths are due primarily to thrombosis of large coronary-artery aneurysms and resultant myocardial infarction, which occurs late in the course of the disease (between the third and fourth week). Coronary angiography during the illness may reveal abnormalities in as many as 60% of patients. These include aneurysms, dilatation, stenosis, tortuosity, and irregularity of arterial vessel walls. These appear to regress with recovery, but at present, the long-term prognosis is unknown.

Age incidence: The incidence is highest in children of 1 year of age and approximately 80% of all patients are under 4 years of age.

Etiology: Unknown. No evidence of point source or person-to-person transmission has ever been documented.

Treatment: Unresponsive to antibiotics. When administered early, high-dose intravenous gamma globulin together with aspirin has been shown to be effective in reducing coronary artery abnormalities.

Recurrences: Rare.

May mimic some of the features of scarlet fever, measles, atypical measles, rubella, Stevens-Johnson syndrome, juvenile rheumatoid arthritis, staphylococcal scalded-skin syndrome, and acrodynia (mercury poisoning).

References: Kawasaki T, Kosaki F, Okawa S, et al: A new infantile febrile mucocutaneous lymph node syndrome prevailing in Japan. Pediatrics 54:271, 1974.

Kawasaki disease (editorial). Lancet i:675, 1976.

Newburger JW, Takahashi M, Beiser AS, et al: A single intravenous infusion of gamma globulin as compared with four infusions in the treatment of acute Kawasaki syndrome. N Engl J Med 324:1633–1639, 1991.

Shackelford PG, Strauss AW: Kawasaki syndrome (editorial). N Engl J Med 324: 1664–1666, 1991.

Gersony WM: Diagnosis and management of Kawasaki disease. JAMA 265(20):2699–2703, 1991.

Clinical Features Associated with Kawasaki's Disease

The clinical features that substantiate a diagnosis of Kawasaki's disease are listed below.

Diagnostic Criteria for Kawasaki's Disease

1. Fever lasting for at least 5 days*
2. Presence of four of the following five conditions:
   a. Bilateral conjunctival injection
   b. Changes of the mucosa of the oropharynx, including injected pharynx, injected and/or dry fissured lips, strawberry tongue
   c. Changes of the peripheral extremities, such as edema and/or erythema of hands and/or feet, desquamation usually beginning periungually
   d. Rash, primarily truncal; polymorphous but nonvesicular
   e. Cervical lymphadenopathy
3. Illness not explained by other known disease process.

Other features of Kawasaki's disease may help establish the diagnosis, may explain complications as they arise, or may allow for anticipatory management of the patient. These associated findings include the following:

Clinical Manifestations Associated with Kawasaki's Diseases

NONCARDIAC MANIFESTATIONS	CARDIAC MANIFESTATIONS
Anterior uveitis	Aortic aneurism
Arthritis/arthralgia	Coronary aneurism
Aseptic meningitis	Late coronary artery occlusion
Hepatic dysfunction	Myocarditis
Diarrhea	Pericardial effusion
Hydrops of the gallbladder	
Pneumonitis	
Sterile pyuria	
Tympanitis	

*Many experts believe that, in the presence of classic features, the diagnosis of Kawasaki's disease can be made (and limited treatment instituted) before the fifth day of fever by experienced individuals.

Reference: Management of Kawasaki syndrome: a consensus statement prepared by North America participants of The Third International Kawasaki Disease Symposium, Japan, December, 1988. Pediatr Infect Dis J 8:663–667, 1989.

Anterior Uveitis and Kawasaki's Disease

Anterior uveitis involves inflammation of the vessels of the anterior uveal tract, including the iris and the ciliary body. Anterior uveitis, also referred to as iridocyclitis, is a common manifestation of Kawasaki's disease, and its detection during the first week of illness may help establish the diagnosis. Slit-lamp examination is required in order to establish the presence of anterior uveitis, and, because the usual symptoms of eye pain and photophobia may be minimal, it has been suggested that ophthamologic examination should be a routine part of the evaluation of patients suspected of having Kawasaki's disease.

Other illnesses that may be associated with conjuncitivitis in the pediatric patient are listed below. Anterior uveitis may be found in some of these conditions.

Streptococcal and staphylococcal
   toxin-mediated diseases
Adenovirus and other viral infections
   (enterovirus, measles*)
Stevens-Johnson syndrome*
Leptospirosis*
Yersinia pseudotuberculosis
   infection
Rickettsial infection
Reiter's syndrome*

Inflammatory bowel disease*
Post-infectious immune
   complex disease* (e.g.,
   post-meningococcal)
Sarcoidosis*
Systemic lupus erythematosus*
Behçet's syndrome*
Juvenile rheumatoid arthritis
   (esp. early-onset pauciarticular-
   type JRA)

---

* May have evidence of anterior uveitis on slit lamp examination.
Reference: Smith LBH, Newburger JW, Burne JC: Kawasaki syndrome and the eye. Pediatr Infect Dis J 8:116–118, 1989.

KIDNEYS

A Technique for the Palpation of the Kidneys of Neonates

Congenital malformations of the urogenital tract occur in approximately 12% of all newborns. In 0.5% of all newborns, significant renal anomalies are present. These should be detected early in life in order to avoid subsequent complications. Almost all significant anomalies can be detected by careful abdominal palpation. A simple technique that will enable you to palpate the kidneys of 95% of all neonates is as follows:

1. Support the infant in a semireclining position facing you by placing your left hand behind the infant's shoulders, neck, and occiput.
2. Place the fingers of your right hand in the infant's left costovertebral angle posteriorly.
3. Use the thumb of your right hand to search the infant's abdomen systematically, at first superficially and then deeply.
4. Deep palpation is performed by applying gentle, steadily increasing pressure subcostally in a posterior and cephalad direction. The thumb can then be slipped downward without reducing the posteriorly directed pressure. Usually, the upper pole of the kidney can be felt trapped between the descending thumb and the posteriorly placed fingers.
5. Next, change hands and examine the opposite side of the abdomen.

After practice on some two dozen infants, this technique can be mastered and subsequently performed in 30 seconds. Because of its high yield, it deserves your optimal skill and attention.

Reference: Perlman M, Williams J: Detection of renal anomalies by abdominal palpation in newborn infants. Br Med J 2:347, 1976.
From McMillan JA, et al: The Whole Pediatrician Catalog. Philadelphia, W.B. Saunders, 1977, with permission.

L

LANGUAGE

Pattern of Normal Language Development—A Summary

Pattern of Normal Language Development

AGE	VOCALIZATION AND SPEECH	RESPONSE COMPREHENSION
1 mo	Much crying and whimpering; produces some vowel and few consonant sounds.	Smiles: decreases activity; startles at loud sounds.
3 mo	Different cries for pain, hunger, and discomfort; decreased crying time; some repetitive sounds ("ga, ga, ga"); coos and sighs.	Vocal gurgle in response to soothing voice; some imitative response to speech.
5 mo	Babbles; vocal play; many repetitive sounds, all vowels, *m, k, g, b* and *p*; laughs out loud.	Imitative response to speech decreased; turns and looks to sound; recognizes familiar voice; vocalizes displeasure.
7 mo	Considerable variety in babbling, loudness and rhythm of all vocalizations; adds *d, t, n* and *w* to repertory of sounds; talks to toys.	Gestures increase as part of vocal responses to stimuli; response to sound is increasingly influenced by visual factors.
9 mo	Cries to get attention; increasing variations in pitch: "mama," "dada" and "baba" part of vocal play but not associated with a person or object.	Retreats from strangers, often accompanied by crying; may imitate hand clapping.
11 mo	May use one word correctly; imitates sounds and correct number of syllables, little crying.	Comprehends "no no"; responds to "bye-bye" or "patty-cake" with appropriate gestures.
1–2 yr	Much unintelligible jargon; all vowels present; improves articulation so that 25% of words intelligible; names many objects by 24 mo; much echolalia.	Recognizes 150–300 words by 24 mo; responds correctly to several commands, e.g., "sit down," "give me that," "stand up," "come here," etc.
2–3 yr	Tries new sounds but articulation lags behind vocabulary; 50–75% of words intelligible; often omits final consonants; jargon nearly absent.	Comprehends 800–1,000 words by 3 yr; responds to many commands using "on," "under," "up," etc.
3–4 yr	Speech nears 100% intelligibility; faulty articulations of *l* and *r* frequent; uses 3–4 words in sentences; uses a few plurals by 4 yr.	Recognizes plurals, sex differences, adjectives and adverbs; comprehends complex sentences.
4–6 yr	Syntax correct by 6 yr, forms 5- or 6-word sentences that are compound or complex with some dependent clauses; fluent; articulation good except for *sh, z, ch* and *j;* can express temporal relations; voice well modulated in conversation.	Understands 2,500–3,000 words; carries out commands involving 3–4 actions; comprehends "if," "because" and "why."

Reference: Adapted from Capute AJ, Accardo PJ: Developmental Disabilities in Infancy and Childhood. Baltimore, Brookes Publishing, 1991.

203

LEUKOKORIA

Leukokoria: A Differential Diagnosis

Leukokoria, or the white pupil, is generally viewed by the examining physician as a sign of ocular disease. It occurs when a lesion interferes with the path of the ophthalmoscope's white light shined into a patient's eyes. Under normal circumstances, the ingoing beam passes through a clear cornea, aqueous humor, pupil, lens, vitreous, and retina to reflect off the vascular choroid. Given the vascularity of the choroid, the light reflected out of the eye appears red in color and is termed the "normal red reflex." While the red reflex is certainly important to document when performing an eye exam, it should be noted that even when it occurs intraocular lesions may be present. Indeed, any lesion not directly in the path of the ingoing beam would not interfere with the red reflex and would subsequently be undiagnosed. Listed below, in order of frequency, are some of the more common causes of leukokoria.

1. Cataracts
2. Persistent hyperplastic primary vitreous
3. Retrolental fibroplasia
4. Retinal dysplasia
5. Retinoblastoma
6. Chorioretinal coloboma
7. Retinal detachment
8. Retinoschisis
9. Congenital retinal folds
10. Persistent pupillary membrane
11. Hyaloid cysts
12. Uveitis
13. Nematode endophthalmitis (toxacara)
14. Panophthalmitis
15. Coats disease (unilateral exudative retinitis)
16. Norrie's disease (sex-linked recessive disorder characterized by bilateral blindness following severe retinal detachments, deafness, and mental retardation)
17. Juvenile xanthogranuloma
18. Ocular tumors
19. Ocular trauma
20. Vitreous hemorrhages
21. Medullated nerve fibers
22. Chorioretinal degeneration
23. Incontinentia pigmenti
24. Phakomatoses
25. High myopia
26. Intraocular foreign body

Reference: Catalono JD: Leukokoria—the differential diagnosis of a white pupil. Pediatr Ann 12:498–505, 1983.

LIMB PAIN

Common Causes

Growing pains
Infection
    Cellulitis
    Osteitis
    Osteomyelitis
    Post-rubella vaccination

Infection *(Cont.)*
    Septic arthritis
    Soft-tissue abscess
    Toxic synovitis
    Viral myositis
Sickle-cell disease-vaso-occlusive crisis

Trauma
  Chondromalacia patellae
  Compartment syndromes
  Dislocation and subluxation
  Fracture
  Hypermobility syndrome
  Joint strain, sprain, internal
    damage
  Myositis ossificans

Trauma *(Cont.)*
  Pathologic fracture
  Postimmunization
  Shin splints
  Soft-tissue contusion or
    hemorrhage
  Stress fracture
  Tendonitis, fasciitis, bursitis
  Traumatic periostitis

Uncommon Causes

Accessory tarsal ossicle
Collagen vascular disease
  (e.g., dermatomyositis, lupus)
Conversion reactions
Henoch-Schönlein purpura
Juvenile rheumatoid arthritis

Legg-Calvé-Perthes disease
Osgood-Schlatter disease
Osteochondritis dissecans
Rheumatic fever
Tarsal coalition

Rare Causes

Bone tumors (osteogenic sarcoma,
  Ewing's sarcoma, chondrosarcoma)
Cushing's syndrome
Familial Mediterranean fever
Hemophilia
Histiocytosis X
Hyperparathyroidism
Hypervitaminosis A
Inflammatory bowel disease
Leukemia
Mucopolysaccharidosis

Myopathies
Neuroblastoma
Osteoporosis
Popliteal cyst
Rickets
Scurvy
Slipped-capital femoral epiphysis
Soft-tissue tumors (rhabdomyo-
  sarcoma, fibrosarcoma)
Sympathetic reflex dystrophy

LIMP

Common Causes

Attention-seeking behavior (usually
  after minor trauma)
Calluses/corn/ingrown toenails
Chondromalacia patellae
Contusion
Foreign body (especially plantar surface)
Fracture (may be occult)
Growing pains
Hemophilia (hemarthrosis,
  soft-tissue bleed)
Immunization (local reaction)
Leg length discrepancy

Mimicry
Myositis (acute viral)
Poorly fitting shoes (tight
  or loose)
Shin splints
Sickle-cell disease (painful
  crisis/infarction)
Soft-tissue/cutaneous infection
Sprain/strain
Tendonitis
Torsion deformities
Transient synovitis

Uncommon Causes

Arthritis (septic)
Baker's cyst
Blount's disease
Bone tumor (benign and malignant)
Calcaneal spurs
Child abuse
Congenital contractures
Coxa vara
Erythema nodosum
Legg-Calvé-Perthes disease
Leukemia
Neuromuscular disease
  Ataxia
  CNS bleed
  CNS infection
  Flaccid paralysis
  Migraine
  Muscular dystrophy
  Peripheral neuropathy
    Causalgia
    Diabetes mellitus
    Guillain-Barré syndrome
    Heavy metal intoxication

Neuromuscular disease *(Cont.)*
  Peripheral neuropathy *(Cont.)*
    Periodic paralysis
    Poliomyelitis
    Tick paralysis
  Radiculopathy
  Spastic paralysis
Osgood-Schlatter disease
Osteochondritis dissecans
Osteomyelitis
Phlebitis
Plantar wart
Referred pain
  Discitis
  Epidural/paraspinal abscess
  Iliac adenitis
  Intraperitoneal infection/inflammation
  Pelvic inflammatory disease
  Retroperitoneal mass
Slipped capital femoral epiphysis
Subluxation of the patella

Rare Causes

Arthritis/arthralgia
  Acute rheumatic fever
  Dermatomyositis
  Henoch-Schönlein purpura
  Inflammatory bowel disease
  Juvenile rheumatoid arthritis
  Kawasaki's disease
  Polyarteritis nodosa
  Serum sickness
  Systemic lupus erythematosus
Brucellosis
Caffey's disease
Congenital joint laxity (Ehlers-Danlos)
Erythromelalgia
Freiberg's disease

Hepatitis
Hypervitaminosis A
Hysteria
Intervertebral disc herniation
Köhler's disease
Larsen-Johansson disease
Neuroblastoma
Pott's disease
Pyomyositis
Rickets
Scurvy
Sever's disease
Sinding-Larsen disease
Trichinosis

LUMBAR PUNCTURE

Estimating Lumbar-Puncture Depth in Children

The lumbar puncture (LP) is a frequently used diagnostic procedure particularly among infants and young children presenting with an acute infectious illness. Yet the procedure can be difficult, particularly for physicians who do not perform LPs with regularity, often resulting in inserting the needle too deeply and disrupting the venous plexus that lies beneath the dura on the anterior wall of the vertebral canal. Such a traumatic lumbar puncture is contaminated with blood, rendering the cerebrospinal fluid white cell count all but useless. Further, a bloody tap may confuse matters if a culture result is positive because the patient is bacteremic but does not have meningitis.

A group of pediatricians at the Medical College of Wisconsin have developed a linear regression analysis of how deep to insert the lumbar puncture needle based upon the child's body surface area in square meters and the depth at where CSF reflux occurred. Each lumbar puncture was performed by positioning the child in the right lateral decubitus position with maximal flexion at the waist and neck. The needle was inserted, perpendicular in relation to the back, at the L_3 or L_4 vertebral interspace. Using the following equation:

$$\text{Depth of lumbar puncture} = 0.77 \text{ cm} + 2.56 \text{ (body surface area in m}^2\text{)}$$

these physicians were able to estimate the depth of lumbar puncture to within approximately 5 mm in most young children without incurring trauma or CSF reflux (see figure).

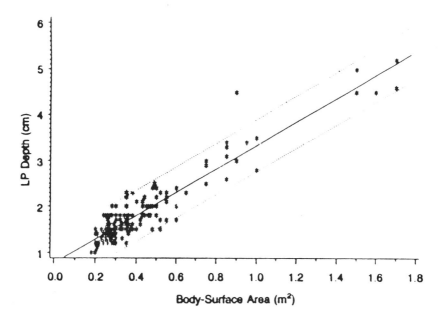

Relation of the depth of lumbar puncture to body-surface area. Dotted lines represent the 95% confidence limits for the predicted depth of lumbar puncture.

Reference: Bonadio WA, Smith DS, Metrou M, Dewitz B: Estimating lumbar puncture depth in children. N Engl J Med 319:952–953, 1988.

How to Interpret the Bloody Tap

Spinal fluid is supposed to be clear. When it isn't, the preliminary information received from the laboratory may be difficult to interpret. The effect of blood on CSF results (usually as a result of inserting the spinal needle too deeply and piercing the vascular plexus ventral to the epidural space) has actually been studied, and these studies make it possible to take a logical approach to the interpretation of the bloody tap.

CSF WBC. The effect of blood on the WBC is the most difficult parameter to calculate. Though it is intuitive that the WBC count would be altered in proportion to the WBC count in the peripheral blood, many studies have demonstrated that it is not this simple. Certainly when the observed CSF WBC is higher than would be predicted from the peripheral WBC/RBC ratio, or when the percentage of PMNs is higher than that in the peripheral blood count, infection involving the central nervous system should be suspected. However, management decisions should not be made based on the CSF WBC alone when the CSF is contaminated with blood.

CSF Glucose. When experiments have been done to determine the effect of mixing blood with CSF, no change in CSF glucose concentration can be demonstrated. Though it has been suggested that hypoglycorrhachia (abnormally low glucose in CSF) may result from RBC contamination, experimental studies have not confirmed this contention, and a low CSF glucose should be regarded as a low CSF glucose.

CSF Protein. There is no question that blood in the CSF raises the protein concentration. The increase in protein has been found to be *approximately* 1 mg/dl for every 1000 RBCs. This is only an approximation, however, and for most purposes the CSF protein concentration is not helpful when the tap is bloody.

Xanthochromia. When hemoglobin from lysed RBCs remains in the CSF for an extended period of time, the breakdown products oxyhemoglobin, methemoglobin, and bilirubin create a yellowish discoloration of the CSF after the specimen is centrifuged. CSF contaminated by fresh blood, as in a traumatic lumbar puncture, remains clear and colorless after centrifugation. The pigmentation that results from RBC breakdown persists for about 7 days after the hemorrhage has stopped. Since RBC lysis occurs in CSF after about 4 hours, specimens that are not analyzed within that time period may be xanthochromic even if the blood resulted from fresh contamination.

Traumatic lumbar puncture occurs in one out of every 5 LP attempts in pediatric patients, and the likelihood of a traumatic tap increases inversely with the age of the patient. Since bleeding usually occurs as a result of introducing the spinal needle too far, a method to avoid this problem has been devised. This method involves removing the spinal needle stylet once the needle has been introduced through the epidermis and the dermis. As the needle is very slowly advanced, the flow of spinal fluid can be seen as soon as the needle tip is in the subarachnoid space. The stylet should be replaced prior to withdrawing the needle to minimize the pressure gradient between the subarachnoid space and the atmosphere as the needle is withdrawn. It is important that the stylet remain in the needle until the epidermis and the dermis are traversed. Implants of small islands of skin during lumbar puncture have been reported to lead to the later development of epidermoid tumors along the needle track.

Reference: Boadio WA: Contemporary Pediatrics, November: 109–116, 1989.

Lumbar Punctures and the Peripheral White Blood Cell Count

As if there weren't enough factors to consider in the performance of a lumbar puncture (LP), a team of Israeli pediatricians have brought up one more: the timing of obtaining the peripheral white blood cell (WBC) in relation to performing the LP. A prospective study of 26 neonates and infants suspected of having meningitis noted a significant increase in the peripheral WBC after the LP was completed (10, 960 $\pm$ 3,500 cells/μl before the LP; 13,300 $\pm$ 3,970 cells/μl after the LP, $p < 0.001$). The greatest increase in white cells was seen in the neutrophil and lymphocyte fraction, presumably because these cells are so quickly released from the marginal granulocyte pool. There were no significant differences, before and after LP, in serum glucose, urea, hemoglobin, and platelet counts. While the LP does not impair interpretation of the CSF glucose to serum glucose ratio, the data depicted below make a strong case for obtaining the peripheral WBC count prior to performing the LP (see figure and table).

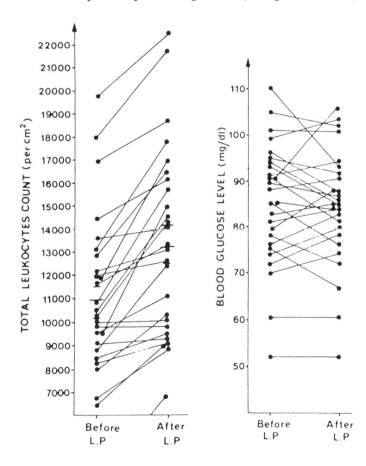

WBC counts *(left)* and serum glucose levels *(right)* before and 10–15 minutes after LP procedure (broad line indicates the change of the mean values, and the 2 pairs of smaller lines the SEM).

Mean ± SD of the Blood Tests Studied Before and 10–15 Minutes After the LP Procedure

	MEAN BLOOD LEVELS	
	BEFORE LP	AFTER LP
WBC count (cells/μl)	10960 ± 3500	13300 ± 3970*
Glucose (mg/dl)	85.3 ± 13.4	84.1 ± 12.6
Hemoglobin (gr/dl)	11.6 ± 2.2	11.7 ± 2.2
Thrombocytes (×10³)	269 ± 113	315 ± 93
Urea (mg/dl)	6.3 ± 2.3	6.5 ± 2.5

*p < 0.001 (T-paired test).

Reference: Shohat M, Goodman Z, Rogovin H, Nitzan M: The effect of lumbar puncture procedure on blood glucose level and leukocyte count in infants. Clin Pediatr 26:477–479, 1987.

LYME DISEASE

Clinical Manifestations of Lyme Disease

Lyme disease is an arthropod-borne infection that is heralded by a distinctive skin eruption (erythema chronicum migrans), followed, in stages, by neurologic or cardiac complications and arthritis. Its vector is the deer tick, *Ixodes dammini*, and the etiologic agent is the spirochete *Borrelia burgdorferi*. Because the clinical manifestations of Lyme disease are so protean in their presentation, with considerable overlap between the three major stages and their time of appearance, the accompanying temporally organized flow chart of its natural history ought to be useful, as well as the table.

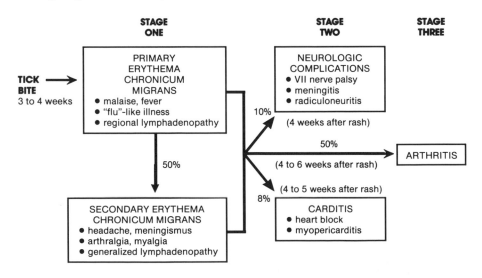

Clinical manifestations of Lyme disease.

Manifestations of Lyme Disease by Stage*

SYSTEM[†]	EARLY INFECTION		LATE INFECTION
	LOCALIZED (STAGE 1)	DISSEMINATED (STAGE 2)	PERSISTENT (STAGE 3)
Skin	Erythema migrans	Secondary annular lesions, malar rash, diffuse erythema or urticaria, evanescent lesions, lymphocytoma	Acrodermatitis chronica atrophicans, localized scleroderma-like lesions
Musculo-skeletal system		Migratory pain in joints, tendons, bursae, muscle, bone; brief arthritis attacks; myositis[‡]; osteomyelitis[‡]; panniculitis[‡]	Prolonged arthritis attacks, chronic arthritis, peripheral enthesopathy, periostitis or joint subluxations below lesions of acrodermatitis
Neurologic system		Meningitis, cranial neuritis, Bell's palsy, motor or sensory radiculoneuritis, subtle encephalitis, mononeuritis multiplex, myelitis[‡] chorea[‡], cerebellar ataxia[‡]	Chronic encephalomyelitis, spastic parapareses, ataxic gait, subtle mental disorders, chronic axonal polyradiculopathy, dementia[‡]
Lymphatic system	Regional lymphade-nopathy	Regional or generalized lymphadenopathy, splenomegaly	
Heart		Atrioventricular nodal block, myopericarditis, pancarditis	
Eyes		Conjunctivitis, iritis[‡], choroiditis[‡], retinal hemorrhage or detachment[‡], panophthalmitis[‡]	Keratitis
Liver		Mild or recurrent hepatitis	
Respiratory system		Nonexudative sore throat, nonproductive cough, adult respiratory distress syndrome[‡]	
Kidney		Microscopic hematuria or proteinuria	
Genitourinary system		Orchitis[‡]	
Constitutional symptoms	Minor	Severe malaise and fatigue	Fatigue

*The classification by stages provides a guideline for the expected timing of the illness's manifestations, but this may vary from case to case.
[†] Systems are listed from the most to the least commonly affected.
[‡] The inclusion of this manifestation is based on one or a few cases.
From Steere AC. N Engl J Med 321:589, 1989, with permission.

Adapted from: Eichenfield AH: Diagnosis and management of Lyme disease. Pediatr Ann 15: 583–594, 1986.
Steere AC: Lyme disease. N Engl J Med 321:586–596, 1989.

What Is the Long-term Course of Lyme Disease in Children?

The natural history of Lyme disease is not yet completely known. In a recent report the authors studied the long-term course of Lyme arthritis in 46 children in whom the onset of the disease occurred between 1976 and 1979 and who received no antibiotic therapy for at least the first 4 years of the illness. Of the 46 children (age range, 2 to 15 years), 33 (72%) initially had erythema migrans, 7 (15%) had influenza-like symptoms, and 6 (13%) had migratory joint pain. These manifestations were followed by brief attacks of arthritis, particularly affecting the knee. The percentage of children with recurrent episodes of arthritis declined each year. By year 4, only 10 children still had a mean of two episodes of arthritis per year; the duration of arthritis was generally longer in older children ($P < 0.05$). During the sixth year of illness, two children had keratitis, and more than 10 years after the onset of disease, a subtle encephalopathy developed in two other children. Of the 39 children whom the authors were able to contact in 1988–1989, 12 (31%) still had occasional brief episodes of joint pain and 1 had marked fatigue. All 46 children had positive IgG antibody responses to *Borrelia burgdorferi* throughout the illness and on long-term follow-up. As compared with those who became asymptomatic, the children with recurrent symptoms more often had IgM responses to the spirochete and had significantly higher IgG titers ($P < 0.05$).

The long-term course of initially untreated Lyme disease in children may include acute infection followed by attacks of arthritis and then over several years by keratitis, subtle joint pain, or chronic encephalopathy. This combination of symptoms in a patient with a high IgG antibody titer to *B. burgdorferi* is of concern, and the appropriate treatment for these patients is not yet certain.

Reference: Szer IS, Tayler E, Steere AC: The long-term course of Lyme arthritis in children. N Engl J Med 325:159–163, 1991.

LYMPHADENOPATHY (GENERALIZED)

Common Causes

Infection (viral, fungal, spirochetal)
Juvenile rheumatoid arthritis
Serum sickness

Uncommon Causes

Drug reactions
   Anticonvulsants, antithyroid,
    isoniazid
Hodgkin's disease
Infection, bacterial
Leukemia
Non-Hodgkin's disease
Systemic lupus erythematosus

Rare Causes

Angioimmunoblastic
   lymphadenopathy
Dysgammaglobulinemia
Gaucher's disease
Hemophagocytic syndromes
Histiocytic medullary reticulosis
Histiocytosis
HIV infection
Hyperthyroidism
Metastatic neuroblastoma
Niemann-Pick disease

A Diagnostic Approach to Lymphadenopathy

Is the lymphadenopathy generalized or localized? Generalized lymphadenopathy is defined as enlargement of more than two noncontiguous node regions. Generalized lymphadenopathy is caused by generalized disease.

Generalized Lymphadenopathy

What are associated signs and symptoms?
Rash?
Hepatosplenomegaly?
Thyroid enlargement?
Joint involvement?
Heart and lung abnormalities?
Pallor?
Easy bruising?

Infections

Exanthems	Pyogenic
Cytomegalovirus	Tuberculosis
Infectious mononucleosis	Syphilis
Infectious hepatitis	Toxoplasmosis
Typhoid fever	Brucellosis
Malaria	Histoplasmosis

Collagen Vascular Disease

Lupus erythematosus
Rheumatoid arthritis

Immunologic Reactions

Serum sickness, drug reactions
Granulomatous disease (sarcoid)

Storage Disease

Gaucher's disease
Niemann-Pick disease

Malignancies

Leukemia
Lymphoma
Histiocytosis
Neuroblastoma, metastatic

Hyperthyroidism

Localized Lymphadenopathy

Signs of infection in the involved node?
Evidence of infection in the drainage area of node?
History of recent antigenic introduction in the node's drainage area?

Supraclavicular — Always consider mediastinal disease (tuberculosis, histoplasmosis, coccidioidomycosis, sarcoidosis). Always consider lymphoma. In absence of evidence of pulmonary infection, early biopsy indicated.

Axillary — Secondary to infections in the hand, arm, lateral chest wall, or lateral portion of the breast. May be result of recent immunization in the arm.

Epitrochlear — Secondary to infections on ulnar side of hand and forearm. Observed in tularemia when bite occurs on finger. Also seen in secondary syphilis.

Inguinal — Infection in lower extremity, scrotum, penis, vulva, vagina, skin of lower abdomen, perineum, gluteal region, or anal canal. May be seen in lymphogranuloma venereum. May represent metastatic disease from testicular tumors or bony tumors of the leg. Immunization in leg.

Cervical — Generally the result of localized infection. See accompanying table for differential diagnosis.

Causes of Cervical Adenitis

CAUSE	COMMENT
Viral upper respiratory infections	Most common cause. Nodes soft, minimally tender, and not associated with evidence of redness and warmth of overlying skin.
Bacterial infection	Streptococcus and staphylococcus most common etiologic agents. Usually secondary to previous or associated infection in drainage area of node. More frequently unilateral. Signs of infection — tenderness, warmth, and redness generally present. Look for primary focus of infection in scalp, mouth, pharynx, and sinuses.
Tuberculosis	*Mycobacterium tuberculosis* infections generally bilateral, involve multiple nodes. Associated with evidence of chest disease and systemic signs. Atypical mycobacteria infections more commonly unilateral initially. Not associated, in general, with other foci of disease. With either agent, evidence of local warmth and redness uncommon.

Table continued on next page.

CAUSE	COMMENT
Infectious mononucleosis	Fever, malaise, preceding upper respiratory infection often noted. Splenomegaly common. Atypical lymphocytes present. Epstein-Barr virus titers required for diagnosis in younger children.
Cytomegalovirus Toxoplasmosis	Indistinguishable clinically from Epstein-Barr virus infections. Requires serologic studies to make the diagnosis.
Cat-scratch disease	History of contact with young cat. May be preceded by history of fever and malaise. Adenopathy restricted to area drained by initial cat scratch.
Sarcoidosis	Disease bilateral. Chest x-ray almost always abnormal. May have keratitis, iritis and evidence of bone disease.
Hodgkin's disease	Common presenting symptom. Frequently unilateral at time of initial manifestation. Node is rubbery, nontender, and not associated with signs of inflammation. Make certain that supraclavicular involvement is not present. When present, strongly suspect lymphoma.
Non-Hodgkin's lymphoma	Bilateral at time of initial presentation in approximately 40% of patients. Cervical and submaxillary nodes commonly involved together.

Algorithm: Generalized Lymphadenopathy

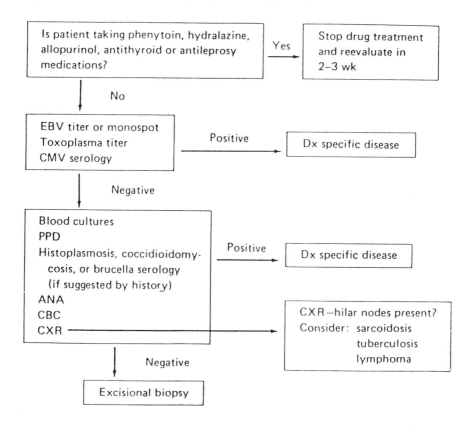

Algorithm: Cervical Lymphadenopathy

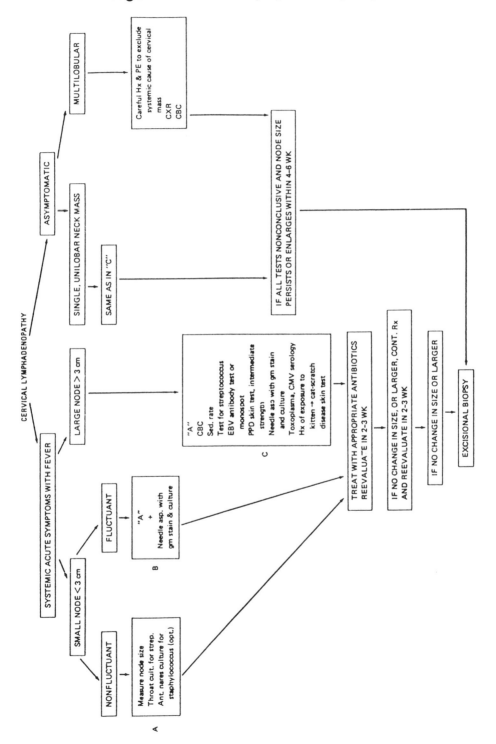

Algorithm: Localized Lymphadenopathy

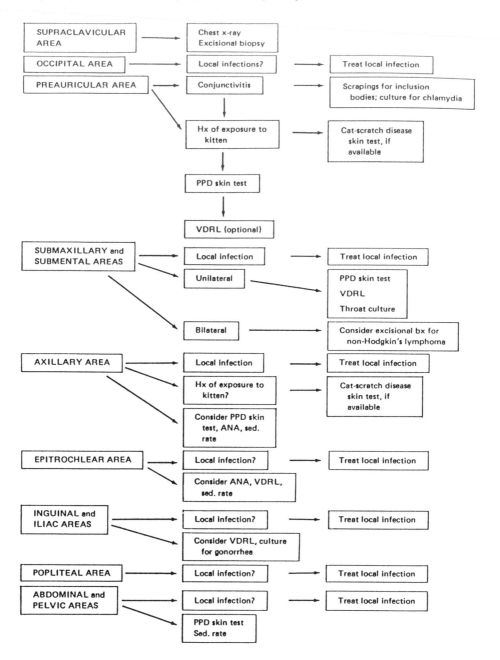

Reference: Bedros AA, Mann JP. Lymphadenopathy in children. Adv Pediatr 28:341, 1981, with permission.

From McMillan JA, et al: The Whole Pediatrician Catalog. Philadelphia, W.B. Saunders, 1977 (Vol 1), pp 30–32, and 1982 (vol 3), pp 9–10, with permission.

M

MAGNESIUM

Magnesium Deficiency: A Common Problem

Magnesium deficiency has a reported incidence of 10% among all patients in tertiary care hospitals. It is frequently associated with hypocalcemia and/or hypokalemia. Despite one's good intentions, dosing the hypomagnesemic, hypokalemic, hypocalcemic patient with large amounts of calcium and potassium salts will do little to correct his or her electrolyte imbalance until the serum magnesium is restored to a normal value. Magnesium deficiency has numerous causes as noted in the table below; nutritional deficiency leads the list. Symptoms of hypomagnesemia are manifested primarily as neuromuscular irritability (e.g., tetany, tremors, and seizures). Changes in personality, anorexia, nausea, abnormal cardiac rhythms and EKG changes can also be seen (see table).

*Causes of Magnesium Deficiency**

Nutritional

Prolonged parenteral fluid administration	Starvation with metabolic acidosis
	Protein-calorie malnutrition
Total parenteral nutrition without magnesium	Kwashiorkor
	Alcoholism

Intestinal

Chronic diarrhea from any cause (e.g., chronic ulcerative colitis, Crohn's disease, laxative abuse, villous adenoma, adenocarcinoma of rectum)	Malabsorption
	Short-bowel syndrome
	Gluten enteropathy
	Pancreatic insufficiency with steatorrhea
	Tropical sprue
	Familial malabsorption of magnesium

Renal

Disease related	Drug related
Renal tubular acidosis	Diuretics (furosemide, ethacrynic acid, thiazides)
Acute tubular necrosis (diuretic phase)	Antibiotics (gentamicin, tobramycin, ticarcillin, carbenicillin, amphotericin B)
Chronic glomerulonephritis	
Chronic pyelonephritis	Antineoplastic drugs (cisplatin, combinations of antibiotics and cytotoxic agents)
Familial and sporadic renal magnesium loss	Cyclosporine

*From Hospital Practice, February 15, 1987, with permission.

Table continued on next page.

Causes of Magnesium Deficiency (Cont.)

Endocrine and Metabolic

Primary and secondary aldosteronism	Primary hyperparathyroidism (due to hyper-
Hyperthyroidism	calcemia; immediately postoperatively in
Excessive lactation	patients with osteitis fibrosa cystica)
Pregnancy (third trimester)	Uncontrolled diabetes with marked glucosuria
Hypercalcemia	Acute intermittent porphyria

Congenital, Neonatal

Maternal diabetes
Maternal hyperparathyroidism or hypoparathyroidism
Exchange transfusions (citrate effect)

Reference: Flink EB: Magnesium deficiency. Causes and effects. Hospital Practice 22:116A–116P, 1987.

MALIGNANT DISEASE

Clues to Malignant Disease

Certain congenital malformations and acquired diseases are recognized to be associated with an increased incidence of malignancy. The conditions listed below should signal a warning and cause a high index of suspicion, regular observation, and appropriate studies for early detection of the associated malignancies.

In addition there are familial associations connected to certain tumors, such as brain tumors, Hodgkin's disease, and Ewing sarcoma, which have been reported in siblings more frequently than chance alone would explain. Awareness of these associations may allow for earlier detection of both malignancies and congenital and other syndromes.

Congenital and Acquired Conditions Associated with Increased Risk of Malignancy in Childhood

CONDITION	ASSOCIATED MALIGNANCY
Agammaglobulinemia	Lymphoma, lymphosarcoma
Albinism	Basal cell carcinoma, squamous cell carcinoma
Aniridia (non-familial)	Wilms' tumor
Ataxia telangiectasia	Leukemia, lymphoma, lymphosarcoma
Beckwith's syndrome	Wilms' tumor, liver carcinoma, adrenal cortical carcinoma, nesidioblastosis of pancreas
Bloom's syndrome	Leukemia
Chédiak-Higashi syndrome	Lymphoma, lymphosarcoma, leukemia
Congenital X-linked immuno-deficiency	Lymphoma, leukemia
D-trisomy	Leukemia
Down syndrome	Leukemia

Table continued on next page.

Congenital and Acquired Conditions Associated with Increased Risk of Malignancy in Childhood (Cont.)

CONDITION	ASSOCIATED MALIGNANCY
11 p syndrome	Wilms' tumor
Familial polyposis of colon	Colonic carcinoma
Family history (first degree) of malignancy	Same or other malignancy
Fanconi anemia	Leukemia, hepatoma
Genitourinary anomalies	Wilms' tumor
Giant cell hepatitis	Carcinoma of liver
Gonadal dysgenesis	Gonadal cancer
Hemihypertrophy	Wilms' tumor, adrenal cortical carcinoma, liver carcinoma, hepatoblastoma
Hippel-Lindau disease	Pheochromocytoma
Horner syndrome	Neuroblastoma
IgM deficiency	Lymphoma
Irradiation:	
in utero	Leukemia
of head and neck in early life	Thyroid carcinoma, brain and parotid tumors
for retinoblastoma	Osteosarcoma
for Wilms' tumor	Osteosarcoma, osteochondroma
for neuroblastoma	Osteosarcoma, osteochondroma
Klinefelter's syndrome	Leukemia
Multiple endocrine adenomatosis I (Wermer syndrome)	Schwannoma
Multiple endocrine adenomatosis II (Sipple syndrome)	Thyroid carcinoma, pheochromocytoma
Multiple mucosal neuromas	Medullary thyroid carcinoma
Maternal stilbestrol during pregnancy	Vaginal adenocarcinoma
Neurofibromatosis	Pheochromocytoma, sarcoma, schwannoma, leukemia
Nevus sebaceous	Basal cell carcinoma
Poland's syndrome	Leukemia
Renal dysplasia	Wilms' tumor
Severe combined immunodeficiency	Lymphoma, leukemia
13 q syndrome	Retinoblatoma
Thyroid cancer (medullary)	Pheochromocytoma
Ulcerative colitis/regional ileitis	Colonic carcinoma
Wiskott-Aldrich syndrome	Lymphoma, lymphosarcoma
Xeroderma pigmentosum	Basal cell or squamous cell carcinoma

References: Craven EM: Pediatric conditions associated with malignancy (letter). JAMA 215:795, 1971.

Feman SS, Apt L: Eye findings associated with pediatric malignancy. J Pediatr Ophthalmol 9:224, 1972.

Leventhal BG, in Behrman RE, Vaughan VC: Nelson Textbook of Pediatrics, 13th ed. Philadelphia, W.B. Saunders, 1987, p 1081.

MAPLE SYRUP URINE DISEASE

What Is the Intellectual Outcome?

Maple syrup urine disease (MSUD) is the most common inborn error of amino acid metabolism and presents acutely in the neonatal period. Classic MSUD is characterized by lethargy, poor feeding, vomiting, and alternating periods of hypertonicity and flaccidity. In untreated disease, progressive neurologic deterioration, seizures, cerebral edema, coma, and death will usually occur within the first month of life.

A recent report of a controlled study of the intellectual outcome in 16 children with MSUD compared the outcome of MSUD diagnosed after symptoms became apparent with that of MSUD diagnosed prospectively and treated presymptomatically. Affected children treated presymptomatically had higher IQ scores than their affected siblings treated after their disease became symptomatic. The authors concluded that early and meticulous treatment of MSUD can result in intellectually normal children.

Therapy for MSUD consists of a diet low in branched-chain amino acids. However, little is known about the long-term clinical course of these patients or their lifespan.

Reference: Kaplan P, Mazur A, Field M, et al: Intellectual outcome in children with maple syrup urine disease. J Pediatr 119:46–50, 1991.

MARFAN'S SYNDROME

Diagnostic Criteria for Marfan's Syndrome

Diagnostic Manifestations

Skeletal

Anterior chest deformity, especially
    asymmetric pectus excavatum
    or carinatum
Dolichostenomelia not due to scoliosis
Arachnodactyly
Vertebral column deformity
Tall stature, especially compared with
    unaffected first-degree relatives
High, narrowly arched palate and
    dental crowding
Protrusio acetabulae
Abnormal appendicular joint mobility
    Congenital flexion contractures
    Hypermobility

Ocular

Ectopia lentis*
Flat cornea
Elongated globe
Retinal detachment
Myopia

Cardiovascular

Dilation of the ascending aorta*
Aortic dissection*
Aortic regurgitation
Mitral regurgitation due to
    mitral valve prolapse
Calcification of mitral annulus
Mitral valve prolapse
Abdominal aortic aneurysm
Dysrhythmia
Endocarditis

* A major manifestation.

Pulmonary

Spontaneous pneumothorax
Apical bleb

Skin and integument

Striae atrophicae
Inguinal hernia
Other hernia

Central nervous system

Dural ectasia*
  Lumbosacral meningocele
  Dilated cisterna magna
  Learning disability (verbal performance
    discrepancy)
  Hyperactivity with or without attention
    deficit disorder

Requirements for Diagnosis

In the absence of an unequivocally affected first-degree relative:
  Involvement of the skeleton and at least two other systems; at least one major
  manifestation.

In the presence of at least one unequivocally affected first-degree relative:
  Involvement of at least two systems: at least one major manifestation preferred, but this will depend on family's phenotype.

Urine amino acid analysis in the absence of pyridoxine supplementation confirms
  absence of homocystinuria.

Conditions Most Often Considered in Differential Diagnosis

Homocystinuria
Familial or isolated mitral valve prolapse
Familial or isolated annuloaortic ectasia (Erdheim disease)
Congenital contractural arachnodactyly
Stickler syndrome

Reference: Beighton P, et al: Internal nosology of heritable disorders of connective
tissue. Am J Med Genet 29:581–593, 1988.

MEAN CORPUSCULAR VOLUME

Causes of Elevated MCV

Normal newborn
Reticulocytosis
Spurious elevations (cold agglutinins)
Hypothyroidism
Liver dysfunction
Down syndrome

Hereditary orotic aciduria
B_{12}/folate deficiency
Aplastic anemia
Preleukemia
Leukemia
Diamond-Blackfan syndrome

Iron Deficiency or Thalassemia Trait?

Children with mild microcytic anemias are commonly encountered in the
practice of pediatrics. Most of these patients have either iron deficiency or

thalassemia trait. The use of red cell indices can provide a simple means of making a presumptive diagnosis without requiring serum iron determinations or hemoglobin electrophoresis.

Two formulas employing these indices have been proposed. They are as follows:

1. The Mentzer formula $= \dfrac{\text{MCV}}{\text{Red cell count}}$

Interpretation: Values in excess of 13.5 strongly suggest that the patient has iron deficiency anemia, whereas values below 11.5 indicate that thalassemia trait is the most likely diagnosis.

2. The discriminant function $= \text{MCV} - \text{RBC} - (5 \times \text{Hb}) - 3.4$

Interpretation: Positive values suggest a diagnosis of iron deficiency, while negative values indicate that thalassemia trait is the cause of the microcytic anemia.

Caution: These formulas are useful only in uncomplicated situations. Confusing answers may be obtained in patients with associated hemolytic anemias or in patients with thalassemia minor who have hemorrhage or are pregnant, or in patients who are polycythemic secondary to chronic hypoxemia.

These formulas are useful in initial evaluation of patients. If iron deficiency is suggested by the formula and the patient does not respond to iron therapy, then further evaluation is indicated. A diagnosis of thalassemia trait should be confirmed in at least one family member.

References: Mentzer WC Jr: Differentiation of iron deficiency from thalassemia trait. Lancet i:882, 1973.

England JM, Fraser PM: Differentiation of iron deficiency from thalassemia trait by routine blood-count. Lancet i:449, 1973.

From McMillan JA, et al: The Whole Pediatrician Catalog. Philadelphia, W.B. Saunders, 1977, with permission.

MENINGITIS

Meningeal Signs

Inflamed meninges of any etiology (i.e., meningitis, intracranial bleeding, exposure to chemical agents, and CNS tumors) will produce the signs of Kernig and Brudzinski. These signs are frequently looked for and mentioned in the physical evaluation of a toddler or child suspected of having meningitis, yet the eponyms are often mixed up or interchanged in the excitement of describing such a patient. This confusion over the meningeal signs would, undoubtedly, inflame Drs. Kernig and Brudzinski, each of whom thought his sign was superior to the other's in diagnosing meningitis. In actuality, as bedside signs of meningeal irritation, both signs are of equal value.

Kernig's sign. This sign is named for the Russian physician Vladimir Michailovich Kernig (1840–1917), who described it in 1884. The examiner should place the patient in a supine position and passively flex the hip to 90° while the knee is also passively flexed to about 90° (see figure below). In a positive Kernig's sign, the patient's knee will resist passive extension and he may complain of intense pain, presumably induced by stretching inflamed sciatic nerve roots. The key here is that <u>K</u>ernig's sign begins with the <u>k</u>nee.

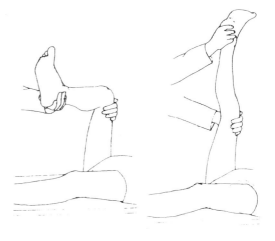

Testing for meningeal irritation (Kernig's sign). (From Macleod J: Clinical Examination, 6th ed. Edinburgh, Churchill Livingstone, 1983, with permission.)

Brudzinski's sign. Several signs are named for the Polish pediatrician Josef von Brudzinski (1874–1917) who described the "neck sign" in 1909. With passive flexion of the patient's neck, the examiner should note a flexion at the knee and hips (see figure below). This sign, like Kernig's sign, is a reflection of the patient's protective response to preventing the eager examining physician from stretching his or her inflamed sciatic and intradural nerve roots.

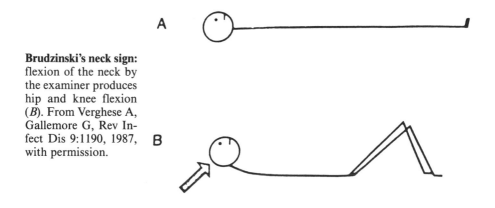

Brudzinski's neck sign: flexion of the neck by the examiner produces hip and knee flexion (*B*). From Verghese A, Gallemore G, Rev Infect Dis 9:1190, 1987, with permission.

Brudzinski's leg signs. Even before describing the neck sign, Brudzinski described contralateral reflex signs (the identical contralateral sign and the reciprocal contralateral sign). They are elicited less often than the neck sign.

As described by Verghese and Gallemore,[4] the identical contralateral reflex sign is elicited in the supine position. When the hip and knee on one side are passively flexed by the examiner, the contralateral leg begins to flex.

The reciprocal contralateral reflex occurs when the leg that has flexed in response to passive flexion of the other leg begins to extend spontaneously. The reciprocal contralateral reflex then follows the identical contralateral reflex and looks like a little kick (see figure below). The contralateral reflex was present in 66% of the cases of meningitis observed by Brudzinski.

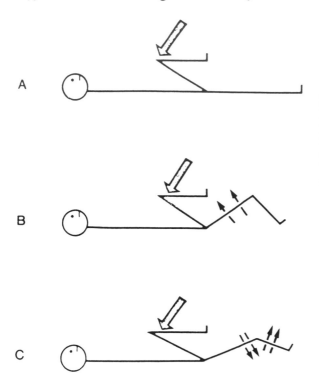

Brudzinski's leg signs. (*A*), Examiner passively flexes patient's leg (*large arrow*). (*B*) The identical contralateral sign: contralateral leg begins to flex (*small arrows*). (*C*) The reciprocal contralateral sign: the same leg that exhibited the active flexion begins to extend spontaneously, a reflex resembling a little kick (*double arrows*). (From Verghese A, Gallemore G: Rev Infect Dis 9: 1191, 1987, with permission.)

References: 1. Kernig W: Ueber ein Wenig Bemerktes Meningitis-Symptom. Berlin Klin Wschr 21:829–832, 1884.

2. Brudzinski J: Un signe nouveau sur les membres inferieurs dans les meningitis chez les enfants (signe de la nunque). Arch Med 12:745–752, 1909.

3. Wilkins RH, Brody IA (eds): Neurological Classics. New York, Johnson Corp, 1973, pp 104–107.

4. Verghese A, Gallemore G: Kernig's and Brudzinski's signs revisited. Rev Inf Dis 9:1187–1192, 1987.

Persistent Pleocytosis

What can be learned from a repeat lumbar puncture in a child with bacterial meningitis? Not very much.

The following table lists the CSF findings in 30 patients with bacterial meningitis who had sequential lumbar punctures. None of the 30 suffered a relapse of meningitis.

Sequential Spinal Fluid Changes in Bacterial Meningitis

	H. INFLUENZAE (21 PATIENTS)				S. PNEUMONIAE (9 PATIENTS)			
Day of Therapy	Cells (mm³)	Glucose (mg/dl)	Protein (mg/dl)	No. of Patients	Cells (mm³)	Glucose (mg/dl)	Protein (mg/dl)	No. of Patients
0	3162 ± 905* (0–15, 250)	36 ± 7 (0–104)	126 ± 22 (20–330)	21	3496 ± 934 (7–7535)	28 ± 10 (0–100)	261 ± 57 (13–530)	9
1	3925 ± 1477 (135–9300)	52 ± 8 (27–76)	88 ± 29 (40–260)	8	6940 ± 6629 (330–13,500)	56 ± 16 (40–71)	—	2
2	1948 ± 732 (162–6100)	45 ± 6 (16–58)	97 ± 16 (70–140)	9	2006 ± 715 (495–3580)	52 ± 6 (42–70)	142 ± 44 (56–196)	3
3	544 ± 252 (51–1368)	50 ± 7 (23–61)	108 ± 37 (34–218)	5	—	—	—	—
4–7	305 ± 164 (48–1617)	42 ± 4 (22–64)	107 ± 22 (42–240)	11	346 ± 208 (65–1172)	58 ± 3 (55–63)	79 ± 12 (56–110)	5
8–10	44 ± 8 (11–77)	47 ± 3 (32–55)	38 ± 3 (29–54)	11	42 ± 6 (5–98)	61 ± 2 (56–65)	42 ± 6 (23–56)	5
11–15	76 ± 10 (3–160)	51 ± 7 (32–63)	51 ± 7 (23–122)	18	17 ± 5 (3–24)	44 ± 3 (38–50)	49 ± 10 (20–66)	4
>15	94 ± 20 (4–176)	48 ± 3 (38–61)	40 ± 3 (22–54)	11	6 ± 1 (5–7)	57 ± 3 (54–60)	10 ± 5 (5–15)	3

Numbers in parentheses represent the range.
*Mean ± standard error.
– = data insufficient.

Reference: Chartrand SA, Cho CT: Persistent pleocytosis in bacterial meningitis. J Pediatr 88:424, 1976.

The Risk for Epilepsy Following Bacterial Meningitis

Most neurologic abnormalities following acute episodes of bacterial meningitis are transient and resolve without permanent loss or subsequent seizures. However, children with persistent neurologic deficits from cerebral injuries sustained during bacterial meningitis are at great risk for seizures, particularly if they had seizures during the acute episode. In most cases the epilepsy that followed occurred within 5 years of the acute illness and the seizures were focal or had a focal onset and therefore were difficult to control.

Children with normal neurologic examinations after the acute episode have an excellent chance of escaping serious neurologic sequelae, including seizures.

Reference: Pomeroy SL, Holmes SJ, Dodge PR, Feigin RD: Seizures and other neurologic sequelae of bacterial meningitis in children. N Engl J Med 323:1651–1656, 1990.

MENINGOCOCCAL INFECTION

Skin Lesions and Prognosis in Meningococcal Infections

The presence, type, and location of skin lesions in meningococcal infections can serve as a useful, immediate indicator of prognosis.

The skin manifestations may be of three types:

1. No lesions or other abnormalities
2. Erythematous, macular, and/or petechial lesions in a generalized distribution over the trunk and extremities.
3. Large purpuric or ecchymotic lesions, usually on the extremities, in association with petechiae.

The clinical manifestations of the disease vary little in groups with no lesions or in those with the generalized macular or petechial eruption, although the incidence of meningitis tends to be increased in those with no skin manifestations.

In contrast, patients with ecchymotic and purpuric lesions have a greater incidence of hyperpyrexia, coagulation abnormalities, shock, and death. The table below illustrates these differences.

Type of Skin Lesions Related to Various Clinical and Laboratory Factors and Mortality

CLINICAL AND LABORATORY FACTORS	SKIN MANIFESTATIONS	
	No Lesion or Generalized Macular/Petechial Lesion (%)	Peripheral Purpuric/Ecchymotic Lesion (%)
Meningitis	54	21
Leukocytosis	85	53
Hyperpyrexia	27	57
Shock	8	62
Bleeding diathesis	7	62
Mortality	3	44

Reference: Toews WH, Bass JW: Skin manifestations of meningococcal infection. Am J Dis Child 127:173, 1974.

From McMillan JA: The Whole Pediatrician Catalog. Philadelphia, W.B. Saunders, 1977, pp 187–188, with permission.

MICROCYTOSIS

Screening Methods in Evaluating Microcytosis

METHOD	FORMULA	THALASSEMIA	IRON DEFICIENCY
Discriminant function	$MCV - (5 \times Hb) - RBC - 8.4$	<1	>1
	$MCH \div RBC$	<3.8	>3.8
	$MCV \div RBC$	<13	>13
	$0.01 \times MCH \times MCV$	$<1,530$	$>1,530$
RBC count		$>5.0 \times 10^{12}/L$	$<5.0 \times 10^{12}/L$
Osmotic fragility	Percent hemolysis	$<95\%$	$>95\%$
Coefficient of variation*	$\sigma/\mu \times 100$	$<14\%$	$>14\%$
Volume distribution curve	EVR_{50}**	<26 fL	>27 fL

*Where μ = median cell volume and σ = standard deviation.
**Estimated volume range for 50% of cells.
Adapted from Johnson CS, Tegos C, Beutler E: Thalassemia minor: Routine erythrocyte measurements and differentiation from iron deficiency. Am J Clin Pathol 80:31, 1983, with permission.

MILESTONES

Milestones of Development—A Summary

Most important milestones in italics

Newborn	Prone—pelvis high, knees under abdomen.
2–4 weeks	Watches mother intently as she speaks to him.
1 month	Ventral suspension (held prone, hand under abdomen)—head up momentarily: elbows flexed: hips partly extended, knees flexed.
4–6 weeks	*Smiles at mother in response to overtures.*
6 weeks	*Ventral suspension—head held up momentarily in same plane as rest of body. Some extension of hips and flexion of knees and elbows.*
	Prone—pelvis largely flat, hips mostly extended. (But when sleeping the baby lies with pelvis high, knees under abdomen, like newborn baby.)
	Pull to sit from the supine—much head lag, but not complete: hands often open.
	Supine—follows object 90 cm away over angle of 90°.
2 months	Ventral suspension—maintains head in same plane as rest of body.
	Hands largely open.
	Prone—chin off couch. Plane of face 45° to couch.
	Smiles and vocalizes when talked to.
	Eyes—follow moving person.
3 months	Ventral suspension—holds head up long time beyond plane of rest of body.
	Prone—plane of face 45°–90° from couch.
	Pulled to sit—only slight head lag.
	Hands loosely open.
	Holds rattle placed in hand.
	Vocalizes a great deal when talked to.
	Follows object for 180° (lying supine).
	Turns head to sound (3 to 4 months) on a level with the ear.
4 months	Prone—plane of face at 90° to couch.
	Hands come together.
	Pulls dress over face.
	Laughs aloud.
5 months	Prone—weight on forearms.
	Pulled to sit—no head lag.
	Supine—feet to mouth. Plays with toes.
	Able to go for object and get it.
6 months	Prone—weight on hands, extended arms.
	Pulled to sit—no head lag.
	Supine—lifts head spontaneously.
	Sits on floor, hands forward for support.

6 months (Cont.)	Held in standing position—full weight on legs. Rolls, prone to supine. Begins to imitate (e.g., a cough). *Chews.* Transfers cube from one hand to another.
7 months	*Sits on floor seconds, no support.* Roll, supine to prone. Held standing—bounces. Feeds self with biscuit. Attracts attention by cough or other methods. Turns head to sound below level of ear.
8 months	Sits unsupported. Leans forward to reach objects. Turns head to sound above level of ear.
9 months	Stands, holding on. Pulls to stand or sitting position. Crawls on abdomen.
9–10 months	*Index finger approach.* *Finger thumb apposition*—picks pellet between tip of thumb and tip of forefinger.
10 months	Creeps, hands and knees, abdomen off couch. Can change from sitting to prone and back. Pulls self to sitting position. *Waves bye.* *Plays patacake.* *Helps to dress*—holding arm out for coat, foot for shoe, or transferring object from one hand to another for sleeve.
11 months	Offers object to mother, but will not release it. One word with meaning. Sitting—pivots round without over-balancing. Walks, holding on to furniture: walks 2 hands held.
One year	2–3 words with meaning. Prone—walks on hands and feet like bear. Walks, one hand held. Casting objects, one after another, begins. *Gives brick to mother.*
13 months	*Walks, no support.* Mouthing of objects stopped. Slobbering largely stopped.
15 months	Creeps up stairs. Kneels. Cubes—tower of two. Takes off shoes. *Feeds self, picking up an ordinary cup, drinking, putting it down.* Imitation of mother in domestic work ('Domestic mimicry'). Jargon.
18 months	*No more casting.* Gets up and down stairs, holding rail. Jumps, both feet.

18 months (Cont.)		Seats self in chair.
		Cubes—tower of 3–4.
		Throws ball without falling.
		Takes off gloves, socks, unzips.
		Manages spoon well.
		Points to 3 parts of body on request.
		Books—turns pages, 2 or 3 at a time.
		Points to some objects, on request.
		Toilet control—tells mother that he wants potty. Largely dry by day.
21–24 months		*Spontaneously joins 2 or 3 words together to make sentence.*
2 years		Picks up object from floor without falling.
		Runs.
		Kicks ball without overbalancing.
		Turns door knob, unscrews end.
		Cubes—tower of 6 or 7.
		Puts on shoes, socks, pants: takes off shoes, socks.
		Points to 4 parts of body on request.
		Pencil—imitates vertical and circular strokes.
		Book—turns pages singly.
		Mainly dry at night.
		Climbs stairs, two feet per step.
24 months	*Motor: Gross*	Runs well, no falling.
		Walks up and down stairs alone.
		Kicks large ball on request.
	Fine Adaptive	Turns pages of book singly.
		Builds tower of 6–7 cubes.
		Aligns cubes for train.
		Imitates vertical and circular strokes.
	Language	Uses pronouns.
		Three-word sentences; jargon discarded.
		Carries out 4 directions with ball ("on the table," "to mother," "to me," "on the chair").
	Personal-social	Verbalizes toilet needs consistently.
		Pulls on simple garment.
		Inhibits turning of spoon in feeding.
		Plays with domestic mimicry.
30 months	*Motor: Gross*	Jumps up and down.
		Walks backward.
	Fine Adaptive	Holds crayon in fist.
		Copies crude circle, closed figure.
		Names some drawings: house, shoe, ball, dog.
	Language	Refers to self as "I".
		Knows full name.
	Personal-social	Helps put things away.
		Unbuttons large buttons.

3 years	Motor:Gross	Alternates feet going upstairs.
		Jumps from bottom step.
		Rides tricycle, using pedals.
	Fine	Holds crayon with fingers.
	Adaptive	Builds tower of 9–10 cubes.
		Imitates 3-cube bridge.
		Names own drawing.
		Copies circle and imitates cross.
	Language	Uses plurals.
		Gives action in picture book.
		Gives sex and full name.
		Obeys 2 prepositional commands ("on," "under").
	Personal-social	Feeds self well.
		Puts on shoes.
4 years	Motor	Walks downstairs alternating feet.
		Does broad jump.
		Throws ball overhand.
		Hops on one foot.
	Adaptive	Draws man with 2 parts.
		Copies cross.
		Counts 3 objects with correct pointing.
		Imitates 5-cube gate.
		Picks longer of two lines.
	Language	Names 1 or more colors correctly.
		Obeys 5 prepositional commands ("on," "under," "in back," "in front," "beside").
	Personal-social	Washes and dries face and hands; brushes teeth.
		Distinguishes front from back of clothes.
		Laces shoes.
		Goes on errands outside of home.
5 years	Motor	Skips, alternating feet.
		Stands on 1 foot more than 8 seconds.
		Catches bounced ball.
	Adaptive	Builds 2 steps with cubes.
		Draws unmistakable man with body, head, etc.
		Copies triangle.
		Counts 10 objects correctly.
	Language	Knows 4 colors.
		Names penny, nickel, dime.
		Descriptive comment on pictures.
		Carries out 3 commissions.
	Personal-social	Dresses and undresses without assistance.
		Asks meaning of words.
		Prints few letters.
6 years	Motor	Advanced throwing.
		Stands on each foot alternately, eyes closed.
		Walks line backward, heel-toe.
	Adaptive	Builds 3 steps with blocks.
		Draws man with neck, hands, and clothes.

6 years (Cont.)	*Adaptive* (Cont.)	Adds and subtracts within 5. Copies diamond.
	Language	Uses Stanford-Binet items (vocabulary). Defines words by function or composition, e.g., "house is to live in."
	Personal-social	Ties shoelaces. Differentiates A.M. and P.M. Knows right from left. Counts to 30.

Reference: Adapted from Palmer FB: Streams of development. In Oski FA, et al (eds): Principles and Practice of Pediatrics. Philadelphia, J.B. Lippincott, 1990, pp 606–615.

MONONUCLEOSIS

"Alice in Wonderland" Syndrome and Infectious Mononucleosis

Central nervous system involvement is estimated to occur in anywhere from 0.7 to 20% of patients with infectious mononucleosis. The 20% figure includes electroencephalographic abnormalities as a sole manifestation of central nervous system disease. The neurologic abnormalities may range from acute meningoencephalitis to facial diplegia, retinal abnormalities, mononeuritis, and the Guillian-Barré syndrome.

To this list of neurologic complications should be added the presence of metamorphopsia or the "Alice in Wonderland" syndrome. Metamorphopsia refers to the complaints of distortions in the apparent sizes, shapes, and spatial relations of objects seen. This symptom has previously been recognized in some patients with migraine, epilepsy, or drug-induced hallucinations.

When it occurs in infectious mononucleosis, as a manifestation of central nervous system involvement, it may last from three weeks to three months.

When the patient begins to see things peculiarly, be sure you see correctly the peripheral blood smear, the Mono Spot Test, and, if necessary, the Epstein-Barr virus titers.

References: Copperman SM: "Alice in Wonderland" syndrome as a presenting symptom of infectious mononucleosis in children. Clin Pediatr 16:143, 1977.

Schnell RG, et al: Infectious mononucleosis: Neurologic and EEG findings. Medicine 45:51, 1966.

From McMillan JA, et al: The Whole Pediatrician Catalog, Vol. 2. Philadelphia, W.B. Saunders, 1979, p 172, with permission.

Complications of Infectious Mononucleosis

Most children with infectious mononucleosis experience a typical episode without complications. However, complications, when they do occur, may be so dramatic that they become the principal manifestation of the disease. Among the most severe complications, and one perhaps most feared by clinicians, is splenic rupture, which can occur with minor trauma. Also, swelling of the upper airway may be very severe and cause occlusion. It is obviously important to recognize the many complications of this common disease. They include the following:

Neurologic

Encephalitis
Guillain-Barré syndrome
Facial nerve palsy
Meningoencephalitis
Aseptic meningitis
Transverse myelitis
Seizures
Peripheral neuritis
Mononeuritis multiplex
Optic neuritis
Acute psychosis
Diplopia
Reye's syndrome
Subacute sclerosing panencephalitis
Perceptual distortions (Alice
    in Wonderland syndrome)

Cardiac

Pericarditis
Myocarditis

Hematologic

Hemolytic anemia
Thrombocytopenia
Granulocytopenia
Aplastic anemia
Hemolytic-uremic syndrome
Disseminated intravascular
    coagulation

Pulmonary

Airway obstruction
Interstitial pneumonitis
Pulmonary infiltration

Hepatic

Hepatitis
Multiple granulomas

Other

Splenic rupture
Glomerulonephritis

Reference: Karzon DT: Infectious mononucleosis. Adv Pediatr 22:231, 1976.

MOVEMENT DISORDERS

Disorders of Movement

The patient is observed to be making unusual involuntary movements. Is it a tic, a tremor, chorea, athetosis, or some other involuntary movement? The recognition and classification of the movement disorder is essential for the establishment of a correct diagnosis.

Athetosis refers to a writhing, irregular movement associated with increased tone in the distal extremities. These movements are primarily around the long axis of the limb. Hyperextension of the digits is common. The movements are often continuous, with the amplitude increased by volition or excitement. It is usually the result of birth injury or kernicterus.

Ballismus refers to rapid movements occurring usually at the shoulder, but they may also be observed at the hip. They are irregular and consist of violent hurling, flinging, and throwing in the upper extremity and kicking or circumduction in the lower extremity. It is usually unilateral (hemiballismus). In the adult the lesion in the contralateral subthalamic nucleus is of vascular origin, while in children it represents a severe form of chorea.

Chorea, Greek for dance, may seem an incongruous term for these rapid, involuntary, nonrhythmic jerks of various parts of the body. They involve both proximal and distal portions of the limbs but may involve the face and trunk as well.

Dystonia refers to a movement disorder characterized by simultaneous contraction of agonist and antagonist muscles. The muscular contraction occurs prior to the onset of movement, leading to a tightening and stiffening of the affected parts of the anatomy. The end position, following a movement, is maintained for a prolonged period.

Myoclonus is an involuntary, repetitive, instantaneous, irregular contraction of a group of muscles, or more rarely, a single muscle.

Tremor is a rhythmic, oscillatory movement of a body part. It may be distinguished from myoclonus and tics by the regularity and the equal force and speed of the movement in both directions.

Tic, the most common movement disorder, consists of rapid stereotyped movements in areas about the face, neck, and shoulder that are usually directed away from the midline. They occur irregularly and last less than a second or may occur repetitively over several minutes. They are most obvious during excitement or emotional stress.

The table below summarizes the characteristic features of these movement disorders:

Characteristics of Abnormal Movements

MOVEMENT	SPEED	LOCATION	DIRECTION	STEREOTYPE	RHYTHMICITY	INTERVAL
Athetosis	Slow	Most prominent in distal limbs	Axial rotations (writhing) and hyper-extension	Common; continuous movement in extremity	Not rhythmic	Continuous, amplitude increased by excitement
Ballismus	Rapid	Proximal, especially at shoulder; also at hip; sometimes trunk, face, and muscles of respiration	Hurling, flinging, throwing, kicking, circumducting	Constant location; movements vary	Not rhythmic	0.5 to 120 seconds
Chorea	Rapid	Generalized; may be unilateral	Primarily at right angles to axis; also facial grimacing; flexion and extension	None; movements generally dance from joint to joint; when proximal and severe may appear semi-purposeful	Not rhythmic	0.5 to 5 seconds
Dystonia	Rapid; slow; very slow relaxation	Trunk, head, extremities	Any, often twisting	Common; because of location of movements, relative strength of contracting muscles	Irregular	Irregular

Table continued on next page.

Characteristics of Abnormal Movements (Cont.)

MOVEMENT	SPEED	LOCATION	DIRECTION	STEREOTYPE	RHYTHMICITY	INTERVAL
Mycoclonus	Very rapid	Localized or generalized	Any	Stereotyped	Irregular	0.5 to 5 seconds
Tic	Rapid	Usually in area supplied by motor cranial nerve (face, shoulder, neck)	Rotational; away	Stereotyped	Irregular	1 second to minutes
Tremor	Variable	Usually localized, often in hand	Complex or simple	Extreme stereotype	Very rhythmic; may be irregular	0.1 to 1 second

Reference: Swaiman KF (ed): Pediatric Neurology: Principles and Practice, St. Louis, C.V. Mosby, 1989.
From McMillan JA: The Whole Pediatrician Catalog, Vol. 2. Philadelphia, W.B. Saunders, 1979, pp 269–270, with permission.

MURPHY'S LAW (MEDICAL MURPHOLOGY)

Spitzer's Laws of Neonatology (Abridged)

1. The more stable a baby appears to be, the more likely he will "crump" that day.
2. The distance that you have to go for a transport is directly proportional to the degree of illness of the baby.
3. The nicer the parents, the sicker the baby.
4. The incidence of neonatal problems increases dramatically if either parent is a physician or a nurse.
5. Endotracheal tubes are designed to fall out (become plugged, etc.) at the most critical moment.
6. The milder the RDS, the sooner the infant will find himself in 100% oxygen and maximal ventilatory support.
7. The longer a patient is discussed on rounds, the more certain it is that no one has the faintest idea what's going on or what to do.
8. The sickest infant in the nursery can always be discerned by the fact that he is being cared for by the newest, most inexperienced nursing orientee.
9. The surest way to have an infant linger interminably is to inform the parents that death is imminent.
10. The probability of infection is directly proportional to the number of antibiotics that an infant is already receiving.
11. Lasix® (vitamin L) will squeeze urine out of bricks. Unfortunately, it doesn't always work as well in babies.
12. Antibiotics should always be continued for _____ days. (Fill in the blank with any number from 1 to 21.)
13. If you can't figure out what's going on with a baby, call the surgeons. They won't figure it out either, but they'll sure as hell do something about it.

Reference: Spitzer A: Spitzer's laws of neonatology. Clin Pediatr 20:733, 1981, with permission.

Six Variations for Patients

1. Just because your doctor has a name for your condition doesn't mean he knows what it is.
2. The more boring and out-of-date the magazines in the waiting room, the longer you will have to wait for your scheduled appointment.
3. Only adults have difficulty with child-proof bottles.
4. You never have the right number of pills left on the last day of a prescription.
5. The pills to be taken with meals will be the least appetizing ones.

   ### Corollary
   Even water tastes bad when taken on doctor's orders.

6. If your condition seems to be getting better, it's probably your doctor getting sick.

Matz's Warning

Beware of the physician who is great at getting out of trouble.

Erma Bombeck's Rule

Never go to a doctor whose office plants have died.

Cochrane's Aphorism

Before ordering a test, decide what you will do if it is (1) positive or (2) negative. If both answers are the same, don't do the test.

Bernstein's Precept

The radiologist's national flower is the hedge.

Lord Cohen's Comment

The feasibility of an operation is not the best indication for its performance.

Telesco's Laws of Nursing

1. All the IVs are at the other end of the hall.
2. A physician's ability is inversely proportional to his availability.
3. There are two kinds of adhesive tape, that which won't stay on and that which won't come off.
4. Everybody wants a pain shot at the same time.
5. Everybody who didn't want a pain shot when you were passing out pain shots wants one when you are passing out sleeping pills.

Reference: Bloch A: Murphy's Law, Book Two. Los Angeles, Price/Stern/Sloan Publishers, 1980, pp 62–64.

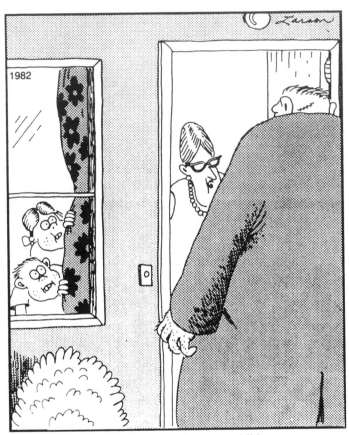

"Why, yes... we do have two children
who won't eat their vegetables."

THE FAR SIDE cartoon by Gary Larson is
reprinted by permission of Chronicle Features,
San Francisco, CA.

N

NEUROFIBROMATOSIS

Diagnosing Neurofibromatosis in Children Under 6

One of the most common single gene disorders is neurofibromatosis, which occurs in 1 of 4000 live births. There is virtually a complete dominant penetrance of the gene for von Recklinghausen's neurofibromatosis (neurofibromatosis-1) localized at the centromeric region of chromosome 17. Yet the diagnosis, particularly in young children, is difficult because there exists so much variation in gene expression with age. Indeed, without a positive family history—which only occurs in 50% of all the cases—the diagnosis is based solely upon clinical signs. The need to commit to memory these signs often occurs to a pediatric intern the morning after admitting a child with café-au-lait spots. Fortunately a recent National Institutes of Health Consensus Conference has delineated the diagnostic guidelines for neurofibromatosis-1 and -2.

Criteria for Diagnosis of Neurofibromatosis-1
(von Recklinghausen's Neurofibromatosis)

Two or more of the following criteria are required for diagnosis:

1. Six or more café-au-lait macules larger than 5 mm in greatest diameter in prepubertal individuals and larger than 15 mm in postpubertal individuals.
2. Two or more neurofibromas of any type, or one plexiform neurofibroma.
3. Freckling in the axillary or inguinal region.
4. Optic glioma.
5. Two or more Lisch nodules (pigmented hamartomas of the iris).
6. A distinctive osseous lesion, e.g., sphenoid dysplasia or thinning of the long bone cortex with or without pseudarthrosis.
7. A first-degree relative (parent, sibling, or offspring) with neurofibromatosis-1 according to the above criteria.

Criteria for Diagnosis of Neurofibromatosis-2
(Bilateral Acoustic or Central Neurofibromatosis)

1. Having a bilateral eighth nerve mass that can be seen with appropriate imaging techniques (e.g., computed tomography, magnetic resonance imaging).
2. Having a first degree relative with neurofibromatosis-2 and either
   a. an eighth nerve mass or
   b. two of the following:
      i. neurofibroma
      ii. meningioma
      iii. glioma
      iv. schwannoma
      v. juvenile posterior subcapsular lenticular opacity

References: 1. Obringer AC, Meadows AT, Zackai EH: The diagnosis of neurofibromatosis-1 in the child under the age of 6 years. Am J Dis Child 143:717–719, 1989.

2. National Institutes of Health: Neurofibromatosis: National Institutes of Health Consensus Development Conference Statement. Bethesda, MD, National Institutes of Health, July 1987, p 6.

NEUROLOGIC DEVELOPMENT

Neurologic Signs of Infancy

A good pediatrician should know the time of appearance and the time of disappearance of the normal reflexes observed during infancy. If your patient displays alterations from the sequence described in the accompanying table, it should alert you to the possibility of neurologic dysfunction.

Normal Reflexes Appearing in Infancy

RESPONSE	AGE AT TIME OF APPEARANCE	AGE AT TIME OF DISAPPEARANCE
Reflexes of position and movement		
Moro reflex	Birth	1–3 months
Tonic neck reflex (unsustained)	Birth	5–6 months (partial up to 2–4 years)
Neck righting reflex	4–6 months	1–2 years
Landau response	3 months	1–2 years
Palmar grasp reflex	Birth	4 months
Adductor spread of knee jerk	Birth	7 months
Plantar grasp reflex	Birth	8–15 months
Babinski response	Birth	Variable
Parachute reaction	8–9 months	Variable
Reflexes to sound		
Blinking response	Birth	
Turning response	Birth	
Reflexes of vision		
Blinking to threat	6–7 months	
Horizontal following	4–6 weeks	
Vertical following	2–3 months	
Optokinetic nystagmus	Birth	
Postrotational nystagmus	Birth	
Lid closure to light	Birth	
Macular light reflex	4–8 months	
Food reflexes		
Rooting response—awake	Birth	3–4 months
Rooting response—asleep	Birth	7–8 months
Sucking response	Birth	12 months
Handedness	2–3 years	
Spontaneous stepping	Birth	
Straight line walking	5–6 years	

Reference: Children Are Different. Columbus, Ohio, Ross Laboratories, 1967, p 67.

NEUTROPENIA

What to Look for When the Pregnancy Is Complicated by Hypertension

The association between maternal hypertension and neutropenia of the newborn had been recognized for some time. What remained a mystery was the etiology, the mechanism of neutropenia, and whether any clinical consequences existed. A 1989 study from the University of Utah removed the shroud from some of the questions and advanced hypotheses regarding the etiology (Table 1).

Table 1. Apparent Risk Factors for Neutropenia in the Newborn Period in Association with Maternal Hypertension

Intrauterine growth retardation
Premature birth
Severe pregnancy-induced hypertension (BP > 160/110 c̄/proteinuria > 5 g/24 h)
Maternal HELLP syndrome (hemolysis, elevated liver enzymes, low platelets)

The Utah study documented neutropenia (duration of 1 h to 30 d) in nearly 50% of the infants of mothers with maternal hypertension. Nosocomial infections occurred in 23% of those infants as opposed to 3% of healthy, non-neutropenic controls. The prevalence of neutropenia differed with respect to the type of hypertension (Table 2).

Table 2. Characteristics of Infants with Neonatal Neutropenia and Their Mothers

	NEUTROPENIA (N = 35)	NO NEUTROPENIA (N = 37)	P VALUE*
Infants			
Birth weight (g)[†]	1550 ± 770	2530 ± 880	<0.001
Gestational age (wk)[†]	31.5 ± 3.5	36.0 ± 3.7	<0.001
Intrauterine growth retardation (n = 12)	10	2	<0.01
Mothers			
Age (yr)[†]	25.8 ± 4.7	24.4 ± 5.7	NS
Race			
Nonwhite	4	7	
White	29	28	NS vs. nonwhite
Hypertension			
Pregnancy-induced			
Mild	5	18	
Severe	13	5	<0.002 vs. mild
HELLP syndrome	8	3	<0.01 vs. mild

*The comparisons of birth weight, gestational age, maternal age, and the interval from membrane rupture to delivery were made according to Student's t-test; the other comparisons were made with Fisher's exact test. NS denotes not significant.
[†] Mean ± SD.

Table continued on next page.

*Table 2. Characteristics of Infants with Neonatal Neutropenia
and Their Mothers (Cont.)*

	NEUTROPENIA (N = 35)	NO NEUTROPENIA (N = 37)	P VALUE*
Hypertension *(Cont.)*			
Chronic			
Mild	2	2	
Severe	5	8	NS
HELLP syndrome	2	1	NS
Delivery			
Cesarean	32	13	
Vaginal	3	24	<0.001 vs. cesarean
Interval between membrane rupture and delivery (hr)[†]	12 ± 6	11 ± 6	NS
Medications			
Magnesium sulfate	14	25	
Magnesium + antihypertensives	10	7	NS
Concurrent illness			
Infection	3	9	
Diabetes mellitus	3	4	NS

[†] Mean ± SD.

Kinetic studies performed on cord blood of the neutropenic infants revealed diminished neutrophil production as opposed to accelerated destruction or excessive margination. The authors proposed two hypotheses to explain the diminished production: (1) deficiency of neutrophil-specific growth factors or (2) inhibition of neutrophil differentiation. The molecular mechanism remains unknown. Until the mechanism is elucidated, therapy rests in recognition of the phenomenon and prophylactic antibiotic use as indicated.

Reference: Koenig JM, Christensen RD: Incidence, neutrophil kinetics, and natural history of neonatal neutropenia associated with maternal hypertension. N Engl J Med 321:557–562, 1989.

NORMOBLASTEMIA

The Cause of Nucleated Red Blood Cells in the Peripheral Blood in Children (Normoblastemia)

Childhood Diseases Associated with Normoblastemia

1. Hematologic/Oncologic
Severe anemia of any cause	Myelofibrosis
Hemolytic anemias	Preleukemia
Iron deficiency	Leukemia
Blood loss	Lymphoma
Megaloblastic anemia	Myeloproliferative disorders
Histiocytosis	Solid tumor invasion of bone marrow

Table continued on next page.

Childhood Diseases Associated with Normoblastemia (Cont.)

2. Infections
   Bacterial infection (especially sepsis)   Osteomyelitis
   Tuberculosis   Fungal

3. Hypoxia
   Congestive heart failure   Asthma and other respiratory
   Cyanotic heart disease   disease

4. Other
   Collagen vascular diseases   Diabetic ketoacidosis
   Sarcoidosis   Thermal injury
   Inflammatory bowel disease   Vinca alkaloids
   Osteopetrosis   Asplenia
   Gaucher's and other storage diseases   Newborn (physiologic)
   Uremia   ??Normal finding

From this long list the most common disorders include cardiac disease, hemolytic disorders, pulmonary disease, and bone marrow replacement.

Reference: Sills RH, et al: Am J Pediatr Hem Onc 5:173, 1983, with permission.

NURSEMAID'S ELBOW

Reducing Nursemaid's Elbow to Simple Terms

Subluxation or partial dislocation of the head of the radius is affectionately termed "nursemaid's elbow," because it typically arises subsequent to a sudden jerk or pull of a toddler's arm. Such a maneuver can be seen at any park, playground, or shopping mall on an hourly basis! More specifically, 90% of all cases of nursemaid's elbow are due to the sudden longitudinal pull or traction at the wrist when the elbow is fully extended and the forearm is pronated. It is typically seen in toddlers between the ages of 1 and 5 years, with a peak incidence among children aged 15 to 30 months.

The child with nursemaid's elbow also tends to hold the arm slightly flexed at the elbow and slightly pronated in order to avoid pain. Typically, the child who has incurred such an injury will refuse to move the affected arm and complains vociferously and painfully at any such attempt to manipulate the elbow, particularly in supination and pronation.

The Anatomy of Nursemaid's Elbow

Dislocation of the head of the radius is best understood by reviewing its anatomy (see figure). The radial head is wrapped by a cuff-like annular ligament. The annular ligament attaches the radius to the ulna but also allows rotary motion of the radial head. These ligamentous fibers combine with other ligaments of the elbow at the radiohumoral joint. Sudden longitudinal traction, when applied to a toddler's pronated forearm, stretches and tears the annular ligament at its distal attachment on the radial neck. With continued traction, the annular ligament slips over the radial head and, once the traction is released, these fibers can become caught between the articular surface of the radial head and the capitellum. The result is pain.

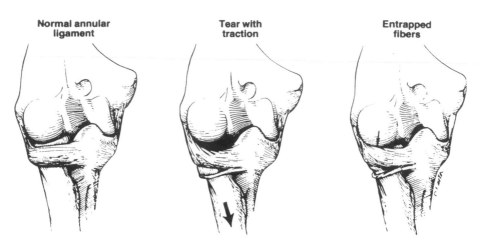

Normal annular ligament   Tear with traction   Entrapped fibers

The annular ligament covers the radial head and attaches the radius to the ulna. With sudden longitudinal traction, the ligament stretches and tears. Fibers of the ligament are then caught between the radial head and the capitellum.

A Prescription for Reducing Nursemaid's Elbow to a Mere Memory

X-rays are rarely indicated in this type of injury. Instead, following the maneuvers illustrated in the figure below should correct the problem quickly and simply.

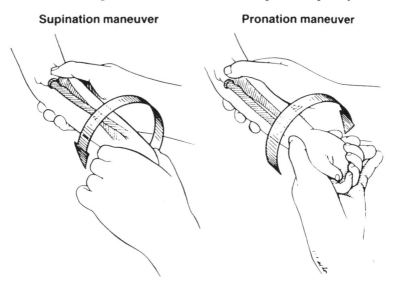

Supination maneuver   Pronation maneuver

To reduce the injury, hold the elbow slightly flexed. Apply pressure over the radial head with the thumb, then hold the child's wrist with the other hand and quickly move the forearm to either a supine or pronated position.

References: Nichols HH: Nursemaid's elbow: Reducing it to simple terms. Contemporary Pediatrics 5(5):50–57, 1988.

Quan L, Marcuse E: The epidemiology and treatment of radial head subluxation. Am J Dis Child 139:1194, 1985.

NUTRITION

Infant Foods—Calories and Their Distribution

When the infant is ready for strained or junior foods, it is important to be aware of the number of calories being provided and their source. The accompanying table lists estimated calories derived from analysis of a variety of products in each category.

Strained Foods

CATEGORY	KCAL/100 GM	PERCENTAGE OF CALORIES		
		Protein	Fat	Carbohydrates
Juices	65 (45–98)	2	2	96
Fruits	85 (79–125)	2	2	96
Vegetables				
Plain	45 (27–28)	14	6	80
Creamed	63 (42–94)	13	13	74
Meats	106 (86–194)	53	46	1
Egg yolks	192 (184–199)	21	76	3
High meat dinner	84 (63–106)	29	45	29
Desserts	96 (71–136)	4	7	89
Cereal	360 (349–393)	39	12	49
Cereal-fruit	85 (76–98)	18	6	76

Junior Foods

Fruits	85 (69–116)	2	2	96
Vegetables				
Plain	46 (27–71)	12	7	81
Creamed	64 (45 72)	13	17	70
Meats	103 (88–135)	56	43	1
Soup-dinner	61 (39–100)	15	27	58

Reference: Fomon SJ: Infant Nutrition, 2nd ed. Philadelphia, W.B. Saunders Company, 1974, p 410, with permission.

Are We Eating the "Wrong" Fruits & Vegetables? (Or What Could Be More Nutritious Than a Fresh Orange?)

Eighteen common fruits and vegetables are listed here, first in order of their nutrient density and a second in order of their total nutrient contribution to the U.S. diet (density times tonnage). Our diets would improve considerably if we ate more from the top of the lefthand list than from the bottom. There is nothing "wrong" with lettuce and oranges, of course, but notice how far down they are in nutritional value. Note too how much more nutritious vegetables are than fruits.

NUTRIENT CONCENTRATION			CONTRIBUTION OF NUTRIENTS TO DIET	
CROP	RANK		CROP	RANK
BROCCOLI	1		TOMATOES	1
SPINACH	2		ORANGES	2
BRUSSELS SPROUTS	3		POTATOES	3
LIMA BEANS	4		LETTUCE	4
PEAS	5		SWEET CORN	5
ASPARAGUS	6		BANANAS	6
ARTICHOKES	7		CARROTS	7
CAULIFLOWER	8		CABBAGE	8
SWEET POTATOES	9		ONIONS	9
CARROTS	10		SWEET POTATOES	10
SWEET CORN	12		PEAS	15
POTATOES	14		SPINACH	18
CABBAGE	15		BROCCOLI	21
TOMATOES	16		LIMA BEANS	23
BANANAS	18		ASPARAGUS	25
LETTUCE	26		CAULIFLOWER	30
ONIONS	31		BRUSSELS SPROUTS	34
ORANGES	33		ARTICHOKES	36

—Prof. M. Allen Stevens, University of
California, Davis (Rick 1978: 78)

The "Skinniest" Cuts of Beef

For those patients who have been placed on a low fat, low cholesterol diet but still insist "real people eat beef," here are some of the "skinniest" cuts of beef you can recommend:

Lean Beef

CUT OF BEEF*	EYE OF ROUND	TOP LOIN	ROUND TIP	ROUND TIP	TENDERLOIN	TOP SIRLOIN
Calories	143 cal	176 cal	157 cal	153 cal	179 cal	165 cal
Total Fat	4.2 g	8.0 g	5.9 g	4.2 g	8.5 g	6.1 g
Saturated Fat	1.5 g	3.1 g	2.1 g	1.4 g	3.2 g	2.4 g
Cholesterol	59 mg	65 mg	69 mg	72 mg	72 mg	76 mg

*Figures for a cooked and trimmed 3 oz serving; 4 oz uncooked beef yields a 3 oz cooked portion.

References: USDA Handbook 8-13, 1990 (revised): U.S.R.D.A. National Research Council, 10th ed, 1989.

Stockman J: Journal Club Newsletter of the Northwestern Memorial Children's Hospital 4(3):9, 1989.

O

OBSESSIVE-COMPULSIVE DISORDER

Step on a Crack and You'll Break Your Mother's Back

Obsessive-compulsive disorder is a significant disturbance of childhood that has not been well studied until recent years. The disorder appears to occur with greater frequency than previously thought, usually in adolescence, and it is more common in boys than girls by at least 2 to 1. It has a presentation very similar to adult OCD. Common obsessional thoughts concern contamination (e.g., feces, dirt, disease) and fears of wrongdoing; common compulsions are hand-washing rituals, grooming, and checking rituals.

Major Presenting Symptoms in 70 Consecutive Children and Adolescents with Severe Primary Obsessive-Compulsive Disorder

COMPULSIONS	REPORTED SYMPTOM AT INITIAL INVERVIEW NO. (%) OF PATIENTS*
Excessive or ritualized hand washing, showering, bathing, tooth brushing, or grooming	60 (85)
Repeating rituals (e.g., going in/out door, up/down from chair)	35 (51)
Checking (doors, locks, stove, appliances, emergency brake on car, paper route, homework, etc.)	32 (46)
Rituals to remove contact with contaminants	16 (23)
Touching	14 (20)
Measures to prevent harm to self or others	11 (16)
Ordering/arranging	12 (17)
Counting	13 (18)
Hoarding/collecting rituals	8 (11)
Rituals of cleaning household or inanimate objects	4 (6)
Miscellaneous rituals (e.g., writing, moving, speaking)	18 (26)
Concern with dirt, germs, or environmental toxins	28 (40)
Something terrible happening (fire/death/illness of self or loved one, etc.)	17 (24)
Symmetry, order, or exactness	12 (17)
Scrupulosity (religious obsessions)	9 (13)
Concern or disgust with bodily wastes or secretions (urine, stool, saliva)	6 (8)
Lucky/unlucky numbers	6 (8)

*Obsessions or compulsions are totaled, so the total exceeds 70.

Table continued on next page.

Major Presenting Symptoms in 70 Consecutive Children and Adolescents with Severe Primary Obsessive-Compulsive Disorder (Cont.)

COMPULSIONS	REPORTED SYMPTOM AT INITIAL INVERVIEW NO. (%) OF PATIENTS*
Forbidden, aggressive, or perverse sexual thoughts, images, or impulses	3 (4)
Fear might harm others/self	3 (4)
Concern with household items	2 (3)
Intrusive nonsense sounds, words, or music	1 (1)

From Swedo, et al: Arch Gen Psychiatry 46:337, 1989, with permission.

References: Swedo SE, Rapoport JL, Leonard H, et al: Obsessive-compulsive disorder in children and adolescents. Arch Gen Psychiatry 46:335–341, 1989.

Riddle MA, Scahill L, King R, et al: Obsessive compulsive disorder in children and adolescents: Phenomenology and family history. J Am Acad Child Adolesc Psychiatry 29:766–772, 1991.

Oski FA: Principles and Practice of Pediatrics. Philadelphia, J.B. Lippincott, 1990, pp 656–657.

OCCAM'S RAZOR

A Diagnostic Principle—Occam's Razor

Without knowing it many clinicians apply Occam's razor to their diagnostic thinking. Occam's razor is a logical principle attributed to William of Occam, although it was used by some scholastic philosophers prior to him. The principle states that a person should not increase, beyond what is necessary, the number of entities required to explain anything, or that the person should not make more assumptions than the minimum needed. This principle is often called the Law of Parsimony. Since the Middle Ages it has played an important role in eliminating unnecessary elements from explanations. Remember William of Occam when you attempt to explain multiple symptoms in your patient with a single diagnosis.

ODORS OF DISEASE

Unusual Odor as a Clue to Diagnosis

Can you smell a rat or sniff out a diagnosis? The sense of smell is not used enough as part of the physical examination. Listed below are diseases associated with unusual odors.

Diseases Associated with Unusual Odors

DISEASE	ENZYME DEFECT	ODOR	CLINICAL FEATURES	TREATMENT
Diabetes mellitus	Lack of insulin or insulin activity	Acetone on breath, fruity	Polyuria, polyphagia, polydipsia, weight loss, acidosis, coma	Insulin administration

Table continued on next page.

Diseases Associated with Unusual Odors (Cont.)

DISEASE	ENZYME DEFECT	ODOR	CLINICAL FEATURES	TREATMENT
Phenyl-ketonuria	Phenylalanine hydroxylase	Musty, "mousy," "horsey"	Progressive mental retardation, eczema, decreased pigmentation, seizures, spasticity	Diet low in phenyl-alanine
Maple syrup urine disease	Branched chain decarboxylase	Maple syrup	Marked acidosis, seizures, coma leading to death in first year or two of life or mental subnormality without acidosis or intermittent acidosis without mental retardation	Diet low in branched chain amino acids; protein restriction and/or thiamine in large doses
Oasthouse urine disease	Defective transport of methionine, branched chain amino acids, tyrosine, and phenylalanine	Yeast-like; dried-celery-like	Mental retardation, spasticity, hyperpnea, fever, edema	Restrict methionine in diet
Odor of sweaty feet, Syndrome I	Isovaleryl CoA dehydrogenase	Sweaty feet	Recurrent bouts of acidosis, vomiting, dehydration, coma, aversion to protein foods	Restrict leucine in diet
Odor of sweaty feet, Syndrome II	Green acyldehydrogenase	Sweaty feet	Onset of symptoms in first week of life with acidosis, dehydration, seizures, and death	High CHO diet (?) Low fat diet (?)
Odor of cats syndrome	Beta-methyl-crotonyl-CoA carboxylase	Cat's urine	Neurologic disorder resembling Werdnig-Hoffmann disease, ketoacidosis, failure to thrive	Leucine restriction (?) Biotin administration
Fish odor syndrome	Unknown	Like dead fish	Stigmata of Turner's syndrome, neutropenia, recurrent infections, anemia, splenomegaly	Unknown
Fish odor syndrome	Trimethylamine oxidase	Like dead fish	Unusual odor of sweat, skin and urine. Normal development	Elimination of fish from the diet
Odor of rancid butter syndrome	Unknown	Rancid butter	Poor feeding, irritability, progressive neurologic deterioration with seizures and death; hepatic dysfunction; possibly same as acute tyrosinosis	Response to decreased phenylalanine and tyrosine intake (?)

Reference: Mace JW, Goodman SI, Centerwall WR, et al: The child with an unusual odor. Clin Pediatr 15:57–62, 1976.

OSMOLALITY

Serum Osmolality

It is often important to estimate serum osmolality before the laboratory measurement becomes available. The following formula will make that estimation more accurate.

The short cut approach is

$$\text{Serum osmolality} = \{Na(mEq/L) = K\ (mEq/L)\} \times 2 + \frac{Glucose}{18} + \frac{BUN}{3}$$

The normal value is 280.

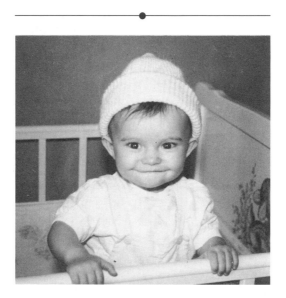

I know a baby
Who smells like fresh muffins
Wrapped in warm linen
Just dried by the breezes
Blown over the lilacs
Brought out by the spring sun
And back from the oceans
With Orient spices

P

PAIN

The Precordial Catch Syndrome

In 1955 Miller and Texidor first described an entity in young adults they termed "precordial catch." It has proven to be a common entity. Perhaps as many as 50% of older adolescents and young adults will experience this sensation of a sudden, brief, nonradiating, periapical pain that is unrelated to exercise or exertion. Both patients and their parents are naturally concerned about heart disease, but you can reassure them that the pain is of no cardiac significance. The precise cause of this painful sensation of "something being caught" and being forced to "freeze" in place is still unknown. The characteristics are described in the list below.

The Pain Itself

Onset:	Sudden, unexpected, unprovoked.
Location:	Left lower anterior aspect of chest; typically infra-apical at the sternal border.
Duration:	Brief ($<$3 minutes, usually 1 minute or less).
Description:	Variable but superficial, knife- or needle-like, burning, stabbing, shooting, sharp, something catches.
Localization:	Site often localized by patient using one or more fingers.
Radiation:	Nonradiating.

Related Factors

Respiration:	Taking a deep breath accentuates pain and makes patient "freeze." Forced inspiration, if possible, relieves pain.
Exertion:	Unrelated to strenuous activity; usually occurs at rest.
Posture:	Pain sometimes occurs when patient bends over or is slouched. Pain is relieved by stretching and straightening if possible.

References: Reynolds JL: Precordial catch syndrome in children. South Med J 82: 1228–1230, 1989.

Miller AJ, Texidor TA: "Precordial catch," a neglected syndrome of precordial pain. JAMA 159:1364–1365, 1955.

PALSY

Neonatal Phrenic Nerve Palsy—The "Belly Dancer's Sign"

Unilateral diaphragmatic paralysis with or without brachial plexus injury may present in neonates as "respiratory distress." The chest roentgenogram may be

249

misleading unless obtained in deep inspiration. Fluoroscopy is required to demonstrate paradoxical motion of the diaphragm on the involved side.

It should be remembered that the existence of diaphragmatic paralysis can be recognized by merely observing the movement of the umbilicus during the respiratory cycle. To perform this maneuver, note the position of the umbilicus at full expiration. Mark this position by placing your pen at the spot. During inspiration, the umbilicus can be seen to shift upward and toward the side of the paralyzed diaphragm. Other suggestive physical findings include unexplained tachypnea without dyspnea, slightly decreased breath sounds on the paralyzed side, fine inspiratory rales on the paralyzed side if atelectasis is present, widening of the subcostal angle on the affected side during inspiration, and flattening of the epigastrium on the side of the paralyzed diaphragm during inspiration. The movement of the umbilicus is the sign most easily identified.

References: Nichols MM: Shifting umbilicus in neonatal phrenic palsy (the belly dancer's sign). Clin Pediatr 15:342, 1976.

Light JS: Respiratory shift in epigastric abdominal wall—a physical sign seen with complete unilateral paralysis of the diaphragm in infants and children. J Pediatr 24:627, 1944.

From McMillan JA, et al (eds): The Whole Pediatrician Catalog. Philadelphia, W.B. Saunders, 1977, p 122, with permission.

PANCREATITIS

Acute Pancreatitis in Children

Pancreatitis is an acknowledged but infrequently recognized cause of abdominal pain in children. The diagnosis is sometimes difficult. The following clinical description may help.

Etiology

Drugs/toxins
  Thiazides
  Steroids
  Azathioprine
  Alcohol
  Tetracycline
  Salicylazosulfapyridine
  Chlorthalidone
  Furosemide
  L-asparaginase
  Oral contraceptives
Trauma/surgery/child abuse
Biliary tract disease
  Choledochal cyst
  Stricture of the common bile duct
  Congenital stenosis of the ampulla of Vater
  Anomalous insertion of the common bile duct
  Cholelithiasis/cholecystitis

Infection
  Mumps (even in the absence of parotitis)
  Hepatitis B virus
  Coxsackie B5
  Epstein-Barr virus
  Mycoplasma
  Influenza B
Diabetes mellitus (ketoacidosis)
Perforated duodenal ulcer
Miscellaneous
  Hyperparathyroidism
  Septic shock
  Cystic fibrosis
  Pregnancy
  Acute porphyria
  Kwashiorkor
  Hyperlipoproteinemia I and V
  Scorpion bites
Idiopathic

Signs and Symptoms

1. *Abdominal pain.* Children may not localize the pain very well. It is usually noted to be in the upper quadrants or the periumbilical area. The pain is usually constant, but it may be intermittent, and it may be made worse by eating. The knee-chest position will usually relieve the pain.

2. *Vomiting.* Vomiting is aggravated by eating or drinking. It does not relieve the pain.

3. *Abdominal tenderness.* Tenderness may be accompanied by guarding and rebound. Maximal tenderness is usually in the midepigastric region. Bowel sounds may be normal, hypoactive, or absent.

4. *Fever.*

5. *Upper gastrointestinal hemorrhage.* The hemorrhage is thought to result from stress and may originate in the stomach, duodenum, or be caused by penetration of an ulcer into the head of the pancreas.

Laboratory Evaluation

1. *Elevated bilirubin.* This may be due to a stone in the common duct or to edema in the head of the pancreas.

2. *X-ray changes.* X-rays may document pleural effusion (most commonly on the left side) and/or ascites. There may also be a dilated segment of small bowel adjacent to the inflamed pancreas (sentinel loop). Isolated gaseous distention of the ascending colon and hepatic flexure may be present (colon cutoff sign). A CT of the pancreas often reveals the presence of a boggy, swollen organ.

3. *Hyperglycemia.* Diabetes mellitus may or may not follow pancreatitis.

4. *Hypocalcemia.*

5. *Elevated serum amylase.* The serum amylase usually begins to rise within hours of the onset of symptoms. It usually peaks within the first 24 hours of illness and returns to normal within 48 to 72 hours. Daily amylase determinations are helpful in following patients. If the amylase remains elevated for over two weeks, a pseudocyst should be suspected. Amylase values may be normal in patients with acute hemorrhagic pancreatitis.

6. *Elevated serum lipase.* These values tend to follow those of the serum amylase.

7. *Elevated urinary diastase.* Timed urine collections are necessary for this determination.

8. *Amylase clearance test.* Amylase clearance may be elevated in patients with severe burns or diabetic ketoacidosis, as well as in those with pancreatitis. It is calculated from the following formula:

$$\frac{\text{Cam (clearance of amylase)}}{\text{Ccr (clearance of creatinine)}} = \frac{\text{Amylase (urine)}}{\text{Amylase (serum)}} \times \frac{\text{Creatinine (serum)}}{\text{Creatinine (urine)}} \times 100$$

Treatment

1. *Relief of pain.* This is best accomplished with meperidine given every three hours. Its effect may be potentiated by promethazine.

2. *Reduction of exocrine pancreatic secretion.* The patient should fast, and intravenous fluids should be supplied. If intravenous fluids are required for more than five days, parenteral alimentation should be initiated. A nasogastric tube should be placed if the patient is nauseated or vomiting, or has an ileus.

When oral feedings are initiated, they should consist of carbohydrates alone initially, because they cause the least stimulation to the pancreas.

Feedings should be restarted when abdominal tenderness has disappeared, any ileus has resolved, and urinary diastase or amylase clearance has become normal.

3. *Treatment of shock and electrolyte abnormalities.*

Although anticholinergic drugs and antibiotics have been used in the treatment of pancreatitis, their use has not improved the prognosis. Mortality may range from about 20% with acute interstitial pancreatitis to about 80% with hemorrhagic pancreatitis.

Reference: Jordan SC, Ament ME: Pancreatitis in children and adolescents. J Pediatr 91:211, 1977.

From McMillan JA, et al (eds): The Whole Pediatrician Catalog, Vol. 2. Philadelphia, W.B. Saunders, 1979, pp 240–243, with permission.

PANNICULITIS

What Do Popsicles and Horses Have in Common?

Both are associated with forms of cold-exposure panniculitis, characterized by single or multiple crops of tender nodules in the subcutaneous fat. Blood vessels also are usually affected, resulting in a histologic picture of fat-cell necrosis. The nodules can be of a size less than 1 cm to over 10 cm across. The clinical picture is one of reddish-purple discoloration and erythematous, enlarging nodules that are often painful to palpation. The lesions are most obvious 24 to 48 hours after the cold injury. They are commonly confused with a cellulitis. The patients are afebrile and feel well, and the lesions subside without treatment in 2 to 3 weeks, leaving no permanent injury.

The popsicle form of panniculitis is produced by sucking on cold objects, such as popsicles and ice cubes, or the lengthy application of the popsicle to any area of the skin.

In equestrian cold panniculitis, the lesions appear on the outer thighs as a result of prolonged horseback riding in freezing weather.

PARASITES

Sushi Eaters Beware!

H. L. Mencken used his father's method of separating the world's population into two groups: those who pay their bills and those who do not. An equally all-encompassing method might be those who eat sushi (the Japanese delicacy of raw fish) and those who don't. Recently, however, a report in the *New England Journal of Medicine* appeared that might diminish the legions of raw fish eaters. The report noted a patient who presented with mild abdominal distension, direct and rebound tenderness in the right lower quadrant, and an elevated white blood cell count. After 6 hours observation, the patient's right lower quadrant tenderness worsened, and she was taken to the operating room for emergency appendectomy. At operation the appendix appeared grossly normal and a pinkish-red, sinuous worm was found moving onto the surgical drapes just prior to surgical closure of the wound. The worm was identified as an early 4th stage larva of the genus *Eustrongylides*, a nematode parasite of fish-eating birds that is frequently found in raw fish. The patient's medical history was remarkable for eating sushi, prepared at her friend's house, the day before.

This case only adds to the growing list of parasitic diseases that can be acquired by ingesting infected fish that is raw or insufficiently cooked, smoked, salted, or marinated. The clinical presentation varies depending upon where the parasite has localized (e.g., the stomach or the intestines). Dominating features of these parastic infections include acute abdominal symptoms such as discomfort, guarding, nausea, severe epigastric pain, and rebound tenderness. An elevated eosinophil count (30 to 40%) is also suspicious for a parasitic infection.

There are a number of parasites that have been reported to be indigenous to many marine fish typically caught off the coasts of the U.S., Japan, and Europe (e.g., salmon, cod, whiting, herring, and haddock). They include:

Anisakis simplex, the most common parasitic disease of sushi eaters.
Pseudoterranova (formerly *Phocanema*) *decipiens*
Contracecum species
Heterophyes heterophyes
Diphyllobothrium latum (broad or fish tapeworm)
Nanophyetus salmincola
Eustrongylides
Gambierdiscus toxicus (ciguatera fish poisoning)

In order to avoid these parasitic infections, the CDC in Atlanta suggests that you cook seafood before consuming it; heating fish to 65°C for 10 minutes appears to kill most worms. Freezing fish for a minimum of 5 days at 20°C (–4°F) also kills most parasitic species. Other methods of preparing raw fish, such as brining or marinating, cannot be relied upon to destroy helminths. Visual inspection and candling (holding the fish up to light) seem to be most reliable in the hands of an experienced sushi chef.

Other fish-related diseases include scombroid (histamine fish poisoning) and a number of viral and bacterial infections from raw shellfish ingestion.

References: Wittner M, Turner TW, Jacquette G, et al: Eustrongylidiasis—a parasitic infection acquired by eating sushi. N Engl J Med 320:1124–1126, 1989.
Schantz PM: The dangers of eating raw fish. N Engl J Med 320:1143–1145, 1989.
Eastaugh J, et al: Infectious and toxic syndromes from fish and shellfish consumption. Arch Intern Med 149:1735–1740,1989.
Morrow JD, et al: Evidence that histamine is the causative toxin of scombroid-fish poisoning. N Engl J Med 324:716–720, 1991.

PARVOVIRUS

Beyond Fifth Disease: The Clinical Spectrum of Parvovirus B19

Once the viral etiology of erythema infectiosum, or fifth disease, was determined to be human parvovirus B19, the true clinical spectrum of B19 infection could be investigated. We now know that B19 infection in healthy children can occur without the usual facial ("slapped cheek") rash or subsequent reticular rash on the extremities and trunk. We also know that B19, when it infects certain populations, may result in prolonged disease with significant consequences. It is the ability of parvovirus B19 to infect and lyse red blood cell precursors that underlies its more serious effects among these patients. The following table lists the patient populations likely to suffer complicated infection with parvovirus B19.

Patient Populations with Complicated Parvovirus B19 Infections

PATIENT POPULATION	MANIFESTATION OF B19 INFECTION
Healthy adults	Arthropathy, with or without rash
Chronic hemolytic anemia	Transient aplastic crisis
Immunodeficiency or immunosuppression	Chronic, persistent, anemia
Fetus	Fetal death associated with hydrops fetalis

It is important to remember that 40–60% of U.S. adults are immune to parvovirus B19 by virtue of previous infection. Thus many women of child-bearing age are not susceptible, even if exposed while pregnant. In addition, fetal hydrops and subsequent death result in less than 10% of pregnancies during which the mother is known to have been infected. Congenital anomalies among infants born to mothers infected with B19 during pregnancy have not been identified.

There is no specific therapy available for parvovirus B19 infection, although intravenous immunoglobulin has been used successfully to control persistent infection in immunocompromised patients.

Reference: Anderson LJ: Human parvovirus B19. Pediatr Ann 19:509–513, 1990.

PELVIC INFLAMMATORY DISEASE

The Importance of the Pelvic Examination in Separating PID from Urinary and Gastrointestinal Disorders

Pelvic inflammatory disease (PID) is a serious problem among sexually active adolescent women. Over 1,000,000 women of reproductive age contract PID each year; teenagers make up 20% of these cases. The incidence of PID among adolescents rises each year as more and more teenagers become sexually active and engage in unprotected sexual intercourse. The short-term complications of PID include perihepatitis (Fitz-Hugh–Curtis syndrome) and tubo-ovarian abscesses, while long-term sequelae include an increased incidence of infertility and ectopic pregnancies. For example, women with a history of one or more episodes of PID were found to have an involuntary infertility rate of 21% (compared to 3% in controls) and a sixfold increase in ectopic pregnancies even with antimicrobial intervention. In light of these complications the successful PID intervention that minimizes the patient's risk must include (1) early recognition, (2) the use of broad spectrum antibiotics to treat the polymicrobial nature of the disease, (3) an emphasis on careful clinical reevaluation of the suspected PID patient within 24 hours to detect antibiotic failure or a misdiagnosis, and (4) evaluation and treatment of the patient's sexual partners.

Unfortunately, the most frequently occurring symptoms of PID lack specificity in their delineation from other disease processes involving the reproductive, urinary, and gastrointestinal tracts, as depicted in the table below:

Common Clinical Symptoms of PID by Organ System

SYMPTOM	REPRODUCTIVE	URINARY	GASTROINTESTINAL
Lower abdominal pain	+	+	+
Urinary symptoms	+	+	+
Intermenstrual bleeding	+	±	±
Dysmenorrhea	+	−	−
Secondary amenorrhea	+	±	±
Nausea/vomiting	+	+	+
Fever	+	+	+
Malaise	+	+	+
Dyspareunia	+	+	+

The history alone will lead the physician potentially to misdiagnose many women with acute PID, and this can put them at great risk for the short-term and long-term sequelae. Although laparoscopy is the definitive means of determining the presence of acute PID, it is not feasible to perform the procedure on every adolescent with lower abdominal pain because of its risks, costs, and the availability of manpower. The performance of a careful pelvic examination, however, in context with the patient's history and chief complaints, can be useful in at least separating reproductive tract disease from urinary and gastrointestinal complaints.

Common Clinical Signs in Acute Lower Abdominal Pain
Among Adolescent Females by Organ System

SYMPTOM	REPRODUCTIVE	URINARY	GASTROINTESTINAL
Lower abdominal tenderness	+	+	+
Perineal rash	+	−	−
Vaginal discharge	+	−	−
Cervical mucopus	+	−	−
Uterine bleeding	+	−	−
Cervical motion tenderness	+	−	+
Uterine tenderness or mass	+	−	−
Adnexal tenderness or mass	+	−	−

Reference: Shafer MA, Sweet RL: Pelvic inflammatory disease in adolescent females. Pediatr Clin North Am 36:513–532, 1989.

The Criteria for the Diagnosis of Acute PID

Given the limitations of history-taking, the pelvic examination, and laparoscopy for PID, the following clinical diagnostic criteria are offered:

All three should be present:

1. Lower abdominal tenderness
2. Cervical motion tenderness
3. Adnexal tenderness (may be unilateral),   plus (*see following list*)

One of the following should be present:

1. Temperature $\geq 38°$ C
2. White blood cell count $\geq 10,500/$mm^3
3. Purulent material obtained by culdocentesis
4. Inflammatory mass present on bimanual exam $\pm$ sonogram
5. ESR > 15 mm/hr
6. Evidence of *N. gonorrhoeae* and/or *C. trachomatis* in the endocervix.
   a. Gram stain with gram-negative diplococci
   b. Monoclonal antibody for *C. trachomatis*
7. > 5 white blood cells per oil-immersion field on Gram's stain of endocervical discharge.

Reference: Sweet RC: Pelvic inflammatory disease and infertility in women. Infect Dis Clin North Am 1:199–215, 1987.

PERTUSSIS

Whooping Cough and the White Blood Cell Count

The white blood cell count can often be helpful in diagnosing pertussis. A marked leukocytosis (WBC $> 25,000/$mm^3) with a differential demonstrating the presence of 50 to 90% lymphocytes is usually considered presumptive evidence of pertussis in infants and children with a cough. (Definitive diagnosis is made by recovery of *B. pertussis*, *B. parapertussis*, or *B. bronchiseptica* from a Dacron or calcium alginate nasopharyngeal swab.)

Despite the availability of vaccines, pertussis is unfortunately still very much with us. It is not generally appreciated that infants under 6 months of age often do not display the aforementioned degree of leukocytosis and that the white cell count may be normal during the prodromal phase of the illness.

The table below illustrates the range of white cell counts by age in patients with pertussis.

White Cell Counts by Age in Patients with Pertussis

TOTAL WBC	0 TO 6 MONTHS %	6 MONTHS TO 2 YEARS %	2 TO 5 YEARS %	5 YEARS %	TOTAL GROUP %
5,000 to 15,000	38	6	14	31	23
15,000 to 25,000	31	49	32	31	36
25,000 to 50,000	29	33	45	31	34
>50,000	2	12	9	7	7

The percentage of lymphocytes in this group of patients varied from 27 to 99% with a mean of 70.4%.

Patients with a leukemoid reaction (WBC $> 50,000$) are more likely to have pulmonary complications such as atelectasis and pneumonia.

The relation of the total white cell count to the stage of the illness is illustrated in the following table.

Relation of the Total White Cell Count to the State of the Illness

WHITE CELL COUNT	CATARRHAL STAGE (WEEKS 1–2) (%)	PAROXYSMAL STAGE (WEEKS 3–5) (%)
5,000 to 15,000	28	12
15,000 to 25,000	42	34
>25,000	30	54

Reference: Brooksaler F, Nelson JD: Pertussis. Am J Dis Child 114:389, 1967.

PHAGOCYTES

Congenital and Acquired Phagocytic Defects

Phagocytic cells are required to destroy microorganisms that would otherwise lead to disease in the host. The functions of these polymorphonuclear cells may be divided as follows: (1) adherence to the vascular endothelium; (2) chemotaxis or the recognition of and migration to a specific chemical stimulus; (3) phagocytosis; and (4) the killing of the ingested microorganism. Deficiency in serum opsonins (antibody or complement) or a deficiency in the number of phagocytes (neutropenia or asplenia) can also yield phagocytic dysfunction. Defects in one or more of these roles can lead to recurrent and severe infections. The phagocytic defects can either be congenital or acquired (in association with another disease). The congenital causes, which are extremely rare in frequency, include defects of cell movement (e.g., hyperimmunoglobulinemia E syndrome, actin dysfunction, and glycoprotein deficiency) and defects of microbial activity (e.g., chronic granulomatous disease, glucose 6-phosphate dehydrogenase deficiency, myeloperoxidase deficiency, and Chédiak-Higashi syndrome). Acquired or secondary phagocytic defects are far more common as detailed in the table below:

Acquired or Secondary Phagocytic Defects

PRIMARY DISEASE OR CONDITIONS	ASSOCIATED CELLULAR DEFECT
Malnutrition	Chemotaxis, phagocytosis, killing
Hypophosphatemia	Phagocytosis, killing
Diabetes mellitus	Chemotaxis, adherence
Leukemia	Adherence, chemotaxis, phagocytosis, killing
Acute alcohol intoxication	Chemotaxis
Thermal injury	Chemotaxis, killing
Rheumatoid arthritis	Chemotaxis, phagocytosis, opsonins
Systemic lupus erythematosis	Chemotaxis
Inflammatory bowel disease	Chemotaxis, phagocytosis, opsonins
Systemic infections	Chemotaxis
Iron deficiency	Chemotaxis, killing
Pregnancy	Chemotaxis, killing
Steroids	Chemotaxis, opsonization
Viral infection	Chemotaxis, killing

Reference: Bell JB, Dougals SD: Phagocyte functions and defects: A ten-year update. Pediatr Ann 16:379–389, 1987.

PHOBIAS

Needle Phobia

A recent case report of a physician who displayed an involuntary fear of receiving injections and having his blood drawn reminds us of the distinct entity psychiatrists call "needle phobia." (The 5-dollar word is belonephobia, from the Greek *belone*, meaning needle.)

Typically, phobias manifest themselves with the physical sign of transient tachycardia. Patients with needle or blood injury phobias, on the other hand, experience a diphasic cardiovascular response: tachycardia followed by bradycardia, hypotension, nausea, diaphoresis, vertigo, and syncope. On rare occasions, shock and death have been reported.

It is difficult to ascertain just how many children and adults have bona-fide needle phobia as opposed to simply not liking needles inserted into their bodies. Some experts estimate it at 5% of the population. Whether or not patients with true needle phobia will even present to a medical clinic or simply avoid all forms of health care is a different question.

Psychiatrists and evolutionary biologists have hypothesized that needle phobia may have a selective value over more traditional "fight or flight" responses to bodily harm. This is to say, there may be protective benefits in a fainting response or adverse cardiovascular reflex when confronted with an aggressive intern armed with a needle. On the other hand, a fainting toddler might be preferable to a screaming one, especially when one is compelled to obtain blood!

References: Ellinwood EH, Hamilton JG: Case report of a needle phobia. J Family Prac 32:420–422, 1991.

Marks I: Blood-injury phobia: A review. Am J Psychiatry 145:1207–1213, 1988.

Photophobia

Photophobia is an abnormal intolerance for light, usually a result of inflammation of the iris and ciliary body. It is not to be confused with photosensitivity, which is also associated with a long list of diseases, usually with skin signs. A better term for photophobia is *photodysphoria*, but the latter is seldom used.

Although the diseases associated with photophobia are often obvious and relatively easily diagnosed (e.g., viral conjunctivitis, measles, or bacterial meningitis), there are other, more subtle conditions that must be considered when the primary diagnosis is not so obvious. Some of these associations are listed below.

More Common Associated Infections

Measles	Viral conjunctivitis
Coxsackie B infection	Arbovirus infection
Lymphocytic choriomeningitis	Bacterial meningitis

Less Common Associated Infections

Phlyctenular conjunctivitis	Rickettsial infections
Yellow fever	(Rocky Mountain spotted fever,
Psittacosis infections	murine typhus)

Noninfectious Associations

Infantile glaucoma	Migraine
Albinism	Corneal ulcer
Vitamin A deficiency	Hysteria (in older child)
Keratitis (e.g., Reiter's syndrome)	Arsenic poisoning
Erythropoietic porphyria	Mercury poisoning
Acute cerebellar ataxia	Drug toxicity
Chédiak-Higashi syndrome	Trimethadione
Aniridia	Ethosuccimide
Cystinosis	PAS

References: Wilson JD, et al (eds): Harrison's Principles of Internal Medicine, 12th ed. New York, McGraw Hill Book Company, 1991.

Illingworth RS: Common Symptoms of Disease in Children, 8th ed. Oxford, Blackwell Scientific Publications, 1984.

Rudolph AM (ed): Pediatrics, 19th ed. New York, Appleton-Lange, 1991.

School Phobia

Vague physical complaints are frequently heard in the pediatrician's office. When combined with normal physical and laboratory findings *and* poor school attendance because of the complaints, the child is often found to have "school phobia," a descriptive term for anxiety over leaving home in the 6 to 10 year old group.

Once a significant child-teacher conflict or fear of harassment by other children has been ruled out, the physician's immediate goal should be the return of the child to full school attendance. Steps in this direction to be discussed during the visit are listed below.

1. Do a thorough physical examination and pertinent laboratory studies as soon as possible. The child should then be given an unequivocal "clean bill of health." The findings should be conveyed to the parents along with a brief but sympathetic explanation about the reality of symptoms caused by anxiety or depression.

2. The parents should be gently but firmly convinced that *immediate* return of the child to school is essential. The parents must insist on the child's return to school for this step to be effective. Delay in return to school makes it increasingly difficult for the child to go back.

3. What to expect and what to do on school mornings should be reviewed with the mother. She should *not* ask the child how he feels. If he is up he should go to school, even if he is late or has missed the school bus. If he comes home at lunch he should be returned. If the child says he is ill, the mother should do one of two things. If questionably or mildly ill, he can be sent to school. If the mother feels the child is truly ill, he should be seen by the physician *early that same morning. The child is not to stay at home without seeing a physician.*

4. The person to be in charge of taking the child to school if he refuses to go should be clarified. This may be one of the parents, another relative, school social worker, or other responsible adult.

5. The school principal should be contacted by the physician, who can ask the school's cooperation in helping the child return to school. This is especially important if the child has a real or imaginary fear regarding some condition at school. The school nurse should also be contacted if she has been sending the child home for minor illness. She should be asked to have the child rest in her office for a time rather than send him home

6. Weekly visits for several weeks are important for follow-up. A final visit several months later will allow long-term assessment.

Failure of this program, if conscientiously carried out by parents, physician and school personnel, suggests the necessity of psychiatric referral to explore the severe dependency problems that are often present.

Prevention of school phobia and related dependency problems can be aided by the encouragement of independence at appropriate times during infancy and preschool problems. The following milestones of independence may be useful guidelines.

WHEN	CHILD SHOULD
By 6 months	be left with baby sitter while parents have evenings out.
By 2 years	be left home, while awake, with baby sitter.
By 3 years	experience being left somewhere other than his home.
As soon as ready	be allowed to feed, dress, and wash himself.
By 3–4 years	be allowed to play in yard by himself.
By 4–5 years	be allowed to play in neighborhood by himself.

Reference: Schmitt BD: Pediatrics 48:433, 1971.
From McMillan JA, et al: The Whole Pediatrician Catalog, Vol. 1. Philadelphia, W.B. Saunders, 1977, pp 44–45, with permission.

PIGMENTURIA

Myoglobinuria, Hemoglobinuria, or Porphyria?

The passage of large quantities of pigment in the urine often produces diagnostic confusion. Many substances may color the urine, but few mimic the appearance of hemoglobin. Hemoglobinuria must be distinguished from myoglobin or porphyrin compounds. Both myoglobin and hemoglobin will give positive results on the commonly employed dipstick (Labstix) for heme. The following table should provide a guide in the initial differential diagnosis of the three major causes of pigmenturia.

Physical and Biochemical Features of the Pigmenturias

PHYSICAL EXAMINATION	MYOGLOBINURIA	HEMOGLOBINURIA	PORPHYRIA
Muscles			
Weakness	+	−	±
Pain	±	−	±
Edema	+	−	−
Neuropathy (peripheral and autonomic)	−	−	+
CNS dysfunction	−	−	±
Skin lesion	−	−	±
Abdominal pain	Rare	−	+

Table continued on next page.

Physical and Biochemical Features of the Pigmenturias (Cont.)

PHYSICAL EXAMINATION	MYOGLOBINURIA	HEMOGLOBINURIA	PORPHYRIA
LABORATORY TESTS			
Urine			
Color	Brown	Red-brown	Burgundy
Benzidine	+	+	−
Hematest-orthotoluidine	+	+	−
80% $(NH_4)_2SO_4$PPT	−	+	?
80% $(NH_4)_2SO_4$SUPER	+	−	?
Porphobilinogen	−	−	+
Spectrophotometry (α band)	582 (oxymyo)	577 (oxyhemo)	594 to 624*
Taurine	Increased	Normal	?
Immunodiffusion	Specific	Specific	−
Serum			
Appearance	Clear	Pink	Clear
Haptoglobin	Normal	Low	Normal
Creatine phosphokinases	Marked increase	Normal	Normal
Carnitine	Increased	Normal	Normal
Immunodiffusion	Specific	Specific	−
Triglycerides	↑ In specific defects	−	−

*Varies with type.

The clinical circumstances may provide the most help in defining the cause of pigment in the urine. The following conditions are associated with myoglobinuria.

Causes of Myoglobinemia and Myoglobinuria

Trauma and ischemic disease
  "Crush" syndrome
  Arterial ischemia of extremities, myocardial infarction
  Pressure necrosis (comatose states)
  Surgical procedures (orthopedic, vascular, cardiac)

Exertional states
  Exertion in otherwise normal individuals (military recruits)
  Convulsive disorders

Metabolic disorders
  Alcoholic myopathy
  Anesthetic associated syndromes (malignant hyperthermia)
  Defects in carbohydrate metabolism (McArdle's disease, phosphofructokinase deficiency, syndrome of abnormal glycolysis)
  Defect in lipid metabolism (deficiency of carnitine, palmityl transferase)
  Hypokalemia
  Toxins (heroin user's rhabdomyolysis, quail eater's disease, Haff disease, snake and hornet venoms)

Hereditary myopathies of unknown cause

Myositis syndromes
  Dermatomyositis, polymyositis, systemic lupus erythematosus

Other factors
  Infections?

Idiopathic rhabdomyolysis

Most hospital laboratories will make a definitive differentiation between myoglobin and hemoglobin by performing a cellulose acetate electrophoresis. Unfortunately, if it is not between 8:00 A.M. and 5:00 P.M., you may be out of luck getting the laboratory to perform this test. An alternative test, which is presumptive of the presence of myoglobin, is based on differential solubility in ammonium sulfate. This is based on the principle that myoglobin is soluble in 80% saturated ammonium sulfate solution, whereas hemoglobin is not.

The test is performed as follows:

1. Clear the urine specimen by centrifugation or filtration.
2. Add 2.8 gm of $(NH_4)_2SO_4$ to 5 ml of urine, making an 80% saturated solution of $(NH_4)_2SO_4$. Allow the solution to stand for 5 minutes, then filter.
3. If myoglobin is in the urine, it will remain in solution. If hemoglobin is in the urine, it will precipitate and will be detected on the filter paper.

A presumptive positive test should be followed by an electrophoresis when available. Whatever test is used, the urine must be absolutely fresh.

References: Robotham JL, Haddow JD: Rhabdomyolysis and myoglobinuria in childhood. Pediatr Clin North Am 23:279, 1976.

Cifuentes E, Norman ME, Schwartz MW, et al: Myoglobinuria with acute renal failure in children. Clin Pediatr 15:63, 1976.

Rosse WF. In Williams WJ, Beutler E, Erslev AJ, Rundles RW (eds): Hematology, 2nd ed. New York, McGraw-Hill, 1978, p 613.

From McMillan JA, et al: The Whole Pediatrician Catalog. Philadelphia, W.B. Saunders, 1977, p 310, with permission.

PLEURAL EFFUSION

Pleural Effusions: Exudates or Transudates?

It seems the question always comes up. Is it a transudate or an exudate? Only an analysis of the fluid obtained by a thoracentesis can answer the question and even then you can't always be certain.

A transudate occurs when the mechanical factors influencing the formation or reabsorption of pleural fluid are altered. Decreased plasma oncotic pressure, and elevated systemic or pulmonary hydrostatic pressure are alterations that commonly produce transudates. In contrast, an exudate results from inflammation or other diseases of the pleural surface. Common conditions producing an exudate include: pneumonia, tuberculosis, pancreatitis, pulmonary infarction, and systemic lupus erythematosus.

Reliance on a single test to distinguish an exudate from a transudate will frequently be misleading. In the past, the measurement of pleural fluid protein, or specific gravity, or cell count has been employed as a diagnostic aid. Any single test will give unacceptably high "false positive" or "false negative" results.

The use of the following three tests will enable you to correctly classify virtually all pleural effusions:

1. $\dfrac{\text{Pleural fluid protein}}{\text{Serum protein}}$ ≥ 0.5 (suggests exudate)

2. Pleural fluid LDH ≥ 200 IU (suggests exudate)

3. $\dfrac{\text{Pleural fluid LDH}}{\text{Serum LDH}}$ ≥ 0.6 (suggests exudate)

The presence of two of these criteria strongly suggests a diagnosis of exudate—the presence of all three virtually assures it.

Some other helpful facts include:

About 80% of transudates will have a white cell count of less than 100/mm³, while 80% of exudates will have white cell counts above 1000/mm³.

Pancreatitis often produces a left-sided pleural effusion.

If congestive heart failure is associated with a unilateral effusion, it is usually right-sided.

Reference: Light RW, MacGregor MI, Luchsinger PC, Ball WC Jr: Pleural effusions: The diagnostic separation of transudates and exudates. Ann Intern Med 77:507, 1972.

Adapted from McMillan JA, et al: The Whole Pediatrician Catalog, Vol. 2. Philadelphia, W.B. Saunders, 1979, pp 221–222.

POISONING

An Unknown Poison

It is axiomatic that the most useful information in an accidental poisoning is the label on the container. In over 90% of poisonings, the poison is known from the label or other source. However, situations sometimes arise where a possible poisoning has occurred, but the amount and nature of the ingested substance are unknown. Features that should suggest poisoning in an ill child include:

1. Abrupt onset of illness
2. Child's age 1 to 4 years
3. History of previous ingestion
4. Multiple organ system involvement that does not fit single disease

A combination of symptoms will sometimes suggest the drug or poison involved:

Symptoms and Signs	Possible Poison
Agitation, hallucinations, dilated pupils, bright red color to the skin, dry skin, and fever	Atropine-like agents LSD
Marked activity, tremors, headache, diarrhea, dry mouth with foul odor, sweating, tachycardia, arrhythmia, dilated pupils	Amphetamines
Slow respirations, pinpoint pupils, euphoria, or coma	Opiates
Salivation, lacrimation, urination, defecation, miosis, and pulmonary congestion	Organic phosphates or poison mushrooms
Sleepiness, slurred speech, nystagmus, ataxia	Barbiturates or tranquilizers
Hypernea, fever, and vomiting	Salicylates
Oculogyric crisis, ataxia, and unusual posturing of head and neck	Phenothiazines
Nausea, vomiting, sweatiness, and pallor are early manifestations; late manifestations include stupor and signs of liver failure	Acetaminophen

The following list expands on signs and symptoms and the toxins with which they may be associated.

Ataxia

Alcohol
Barbiturates
Bromides
Carbon monoxide
Diphenylhydantoin

Hallucinogens
Heavy metals
Organic solvents
Tranquilizers

Convulsions and muscle twitching

Alcohol
Amphetamines
Antihistamines
Boric acid
Camphor
Chlorinated hydrocarbon
    insecticides (DDT)
Cocaine
Cyanide

Lead
Organic phosphate insecticides
Plants (lily of the valley, azalea,
    iris, water hemlock)
Salicylates
Strychnine
Withdrawal from barbiturates,
    benzodiazepine (Valium,
    Librium), meprobomate

Coma and drowsiness

Alcohol—ethyl
Antihistamines
Barbiturates and other hypnotics
Carbon monoxide

Cocaine
Narcotic depressants (opiates)
Salicylates
Tranquilizers

Paralysis

Botulism
Heavy metals

Plants (conium in poison hemlock)
Triorthocresyl phosphate

Pupils

Pinpoint
    Mushrooms (muscarine type)   Organic phosphate insecticides
    Narcotic depressants (opiates)

Dilated
    Amphetamines   Ephedrine
    Antihistamines   LSD
    Atropine   Methanol
    Barbiturates (coma)   Withdrawal-narcotic depressants
    Cocaine

Nystagmus on lateral gaze
    Barbiturates
    Minor tranquilizers (meprobamate, benzodiazepine)

Pulse rate

Slow   *Rapid*
    Digitalis   Alcohol   Atropine
    Lily of the valley   Amphetamines   Ephedrine
    Narcotic depressants

Respiratory alterations

Rapid
Amphetamines
Barbiturates (early)
Carbon monoxide
Methanol
Petroleum distillates
Salicylates

Slow or depressed
Alcohol
Barbiturates (late)
Narcotic depressants (opiates)
Tranquilizers

Wheezing and pulmonary edema
Mushrooms (muscarine type)
Narcotic depressants (opiates)
Organic phosphate insecticides
Petroleum distillates

Paralysis
Organic phosphate insecticides
Botulism

Mouth

Salivation
Arsenic
Corrosive
Mercury
Mushrooms
Organic phosphate insecticides
Thallium

Dryness
Atropine
Amphetamines
Antihistamines
Narcotic depressants

Breath odor

Acetone: acetone, alcohol (methyl, isopropyl), phenol, salicylates
Alcohol: alcohol (ethyl)
Bitter almonds: cyanide
Coal gas: carbon monoxide

Garlic: arsenic, phosphorus, organic phosphate insecticides, thallium
Oil of wintergreen: methyl salicylate
Petroleum: petroleum distillates
Violets: turpentine

Skin color

Jaundice (hepatic or hemolytic)
Aniline
Arsenic
Carbon tetrachloride
Castor bean
Fava bean
Mushroom
Naphthalene
Yellow phosphorus

Cyanosis
Aniline dyes   Nitrites
Carbon monoxide   Strychnine
Cyanide

Red flush
Alcohol   Carbon monoxide
Antihistamines   Nitrites
Atropine   Rifampin
Boric acid

Violent emesis often with hematemesis

Acetaminophen
Aminophylline
Bacterial food poisoning
Boric acid
Corrosives

Fluoride
Heavy metals
Phenol
Salicylates

Abdominal colic

Black widow spider bite
Heavy metals
Narcotic depressant withdrawal

Oliguria-anuria

Carbon tetrachloride
Ethylene glycol
Heavy metals
Hemolytic poisons (naphthalene,
plants)

Methanol
Mushrooms
Oxalates
Petroleum distillates
Solvents

Reference: Mofenson HC, Greensher J: The unknown poison. Pediatrics 54:336, 1974.

Carbamate and Organophosphate Poisoning

Despite many parents' valiant attempts, "Mr. Yuk" does not always deter curious children. Carbamates and organophosphates remain ubiquitous components of insecticides, and their toxic effects can reach the nervous sytem through inhalation, absorption, and ingestion.

The carbamates and organophosphates are anticholinesterases that lead to the accumulation of unhydrolyzed acetylcholine at the receptors. The result is continued stimulation and, ultimately, paralysis of cholinergic transmission. The organophosphates penetrate the central nervous system and will show central effects that the carbamates do not.

Clinical Features of Carbamate and Organophosphate Insecticide Poisoning

Muscarinic	Nicotinic	Central nervous system (organophosphates)
"Sludge"	Muscle symptoms	
Salivation	Fasciculations	Severe headache
Lacrimation	Cramps and fatigue	Tremor
Urination	Loss of deep tendon	Ataxia
Defecation	reflexes	Restlessness
Gastrointestinal pain	Paralysis	Slurred speech
& cramping	Tachycardia	General weakness
Emesis	Hypertension	Seizures
Miosis: if present, look for		Coma
hyperactive bowel sounds		Cardiorespiratory depression

Recognition and Treatment

The muscarine effects generally precede the nicotinic effects. If you have a case of suspected carbamate or organophosphate poisoning, the patient will be atropine-refractory: atropinization should occur in the nonpoisoned patient within 5–20 minutes after a dose of 0.05 mg/kg for a child, or 1–2 mg for an adult.

Prior to the atropine test, the ABCs of Basic Life Support are mandatory. The patient should be thoroughly disrobed and cleansed due to possible continued absorption through dermal contact. If ingestion occurred, initiate ipecac/lavage and charcoal.

Atropine is the cornerstone of therapy. Give the child 0.05 mg/kg as needed; give the adult 0.4 to 2.0 mg IV every 15–30 minutes until the patient cannot spit. In general, a 6–12 h course of atropine is necessary. With carbamate poisoning, the cholinesterase complex is reversible. This is not the case with organophosphates, so additional therapy with pralidoxime, a cholinesterase regenerator, is necessary.

Reference: Mack RB: Carbamate poisoning: A Kafkaesque nightmare. Contemp Peds October:89–91, 1985.

POLYPOSIS

Familial Polyposis

Familial polyposis is an autosomal dominant disorder notable for development of multiple adenomatous polyps in the colon and rectum. The polyps usually do not become apparent until after puberty. The incidence of familial polyposis ranges from 1 in 7,000 to 1 in 10,000 births. The risk of developing colon cancer in affected individuals approaches 100% by age 55. Patients with familial polyposis tend to seek medical attention because of either a family history of polyposis or symptoms of abdominal discomfort, rectal bleeding, and diarrhea. Frequently, the abdominal symptoms do not appear until 10 years after the development of polyps.

Clinical Features

1. Autosomal dominant inheritance (rare spontaneous mutations have been reported).
2. Onset in adolescence
3. Onset of symptoms begin about 10 years after appearance of polyps.
4. Multiple colonic adenomatous polyps
5. Associated extracolonic lesions
   a. Epidermoid cysts (usually on head, neck, and trunk)
   b. Subcutaneous fibromas (usually on the scalp, shoulders, arms and back)
   c. Desmoid tumors of the abdominal wall, mesentary, and retroperitoneum
   d. Osteoma (symptoms a–d in association with polyposis is also known as Gardner syndrome).
   e. Sebaceous cysts
   f. Gastric and duodenal polyps
   g. Congenital hypertrophy of the retinal pigment epithelium (multiple pigmented patches on one or both fundi)
   h. Abnormal dentition (including odontomas, dentigenous cysts, and unerupted, missing, or supernumerary teeth)
6. High risk of colon cancer
   a. 100% risk in untreated patients
   b. Early age of onset (median age is 39 years)
   c. Cancers arise from adenomatous polyps
   d. Synchronous colon carcinomas are common.
   e. Metachronous colon carcinomas are common.

Protocol for Screening Patients at Risk of Familial Polyposis

AGE	ASYMPTOMATIC	SYMPTOMATIC
≤ 13	None	Flexible sigmoidoscopy
14–10	Annual flexible sigmoidoscopy	Colonoscopy or double-contrast barium enema
20–45	Annual flexible sigmoidoscopy, baseline colonoscopy, or double-contrast barium enema at age 20, repeated every 3 years	Colonoscopy or double-contrast barium enema each year

Surgical Management of Familial Polyposis Patients

COLONIC POLYPS	PROCEDURE	POSTOPERATIVE FOLLOW-UP
≤ 10	Endoscopic removal	Every 6 months
Multiple polyposis with <20 rectal polyps	Colectomy with ileorectal anastomosis, or colectomy with mucosal proctectomy and reservoir ileonal anastomosis	Every 6 months Annual
Multiple polyposis with >20 rectal polyps	Total proctocolectomy with ileostomy	Annual

Reference: Boman BM, Levin B: Familial polyposis. Hospital Practice 21(May 15): 155–170, 1986.

POLYURIA

Common Causes

Diabetes mellitus
Diuretic abuse
  Alcohol
  Caffeine
  Medications
Iatrogenic
  Aggressive parenteral hydration
  Diuretic use
Psychogenic polydipsia
Renal failure
Sickle-cell anemia
Urinary tract infection

Uncommon Causes

Diabetes insipidus (central)
Interstitial nephritis
  Analgesic abuse
  Diphenylhydantoin
  Mercury poisoning
  Methicillin reaction
  Sulfonamides
Renal calculi/hypercalcemia
Renal tubular acidosis

Rare Causes

Bartter's syndrome
Cystinosis
Medullary cystic disease of the kidney
Nephrogenic diabetes insipidus
Neuroblastoma/ganglioneuroblastoma
Pheochromocytoma

PORPHYRIAS

Which Type Is Present?

It is important to distinguish porphyrias from simple porphyrinuria, which is associated with a number of common conditions. It is also possible to have some notion of the various forms of porphyrias by clinical signs and routine laboratory results.

In general, of the porphyrias that are associated with excretion of excessive amounts of porphyrin precursors, only acute intermittent porphyria is associated with abdominal pain. Those porphyrias in which the latter part of the heme synthesis pathway is affected are associated with excretion and accumulation of porphyrins. These forms of the disease include congenital erythropoietic porphyria, erythropoietic protoporphyria, and porphyria cutanea tarda. Dermatologic manifestations predominate in these forms.

The forms of the disease in which both porphyrias and their precursors are excreted are associated with both abdominal pain and dermatologic manifestations. These forms include porphyria variegata and hepatic coproporphyria.

The two most common forms of porphyria encountered in clinical practice in the U.S. are porphyria cutanea tarda, with cutaneous signs, and acute intermittent porphyria, with neurologic symptoms, usually occurring in acute episodic attacks.

References: Wappner RS, Brandt IK: In Oski FA, et al (ed): Principles and Practice of Pediatrics. Philadelphia, J.B. Lippincott, 1990, p 132.

Kushner JP: Laboratory diagnosis of the porphyrias (editorial). N Engl J Med 324:1432–1434, 1991.

POTASSIUM: HYPERKALEMIA

Hyperkalemia is defined here as a serum potassium level higher than 5.5 mEq/L.

Common Causes	Uncommon Causes	Rare Causes
Acidosis	Excessive potassium	Addison's disease (adrenal
Renal failure	infusion	insufficiency)
Severe dehydration	Shock	Cell lysis syndromes

POTASSIUM: HYPOKALEMIA

Hypokalemia is defined here as a serum potassium level lower than 3.5 mEq/L.

Common Causes	Uncommon Causes	Rare Causes
Chronic diarrhea	Excessive corticoids	Amphotericin B therapy
Diuretics	Renal tubular disorders	Bartter's syndrome
Malnutrition		Cushing's syndrome
Metabolic alkalosis		Familial periodic paralysis

Fist Clenching Pseudohyperkalemia

There are some lessons in medicine that must be learned over and over. The causes of pseudohyperkalemia appear to be one of those lessons.

When a non-hemolyzed specimen results in a laboratory report of hyperkalemia in the absence of excessive intake or decreased renal excretion, question yourself or question the phlebotomist. Did the adolescent clench his or her fist or use an isometric handgrip? Did the infant or child struggle or resist during blood drawing? Muscular contractions cause local release of potassium and can cause false elevations in serum values (1 to 2 mmol per liter). Do not get caught in the grip of pseudohyperkalemia!

Causes of Hyperkalemia (Serum (K^+) > 4.9 mmol/L)

1. Pseudohyperkalemia
   a. Local release due to muscular contraction
   b. Hemolyzed specimen
   c. Severe thrombocytosis (pH > 10^6 ml)
   d. Severe leukocytosis (WBC > 10^5/ml)

2. Excessive intake
   a. Potassium replacement therapy
   b. Potassium salts of antibiotics
   c. Salt substitutes
   d. High-potassium diet: bananas, orange juice, carrots, celery, broccoli

3. Decreased renal excretion
   a. Potassium-sparing diuretics (e.g., triamterene, spironolactone, amiloride)
   b. Renal insufficiency
   c. Mineralocorticoid deficiency
   d. Hyporeninemic hypoaldosteronism (diabetes mellitus)
   e. Tubular unresponsiveness to aldosterone (e.g., sickle cell disease, SLE)
   f. Heparin administration

4. Redistribution (excessive cellular release)
   a. Acidemia (each 0.1 decrease in pH, 0.4–0.6 mmol/L increase in K^+)
   b. Insulin deficiency
   c. Hypertonicity
   d. Hemolysis
   e. Tissue necrosis, rhabdomyolysis, burns
   f. Hyperkalemic periodic paralysis

Reference: Don BR, et al: Pseudohyperkalemia caused by fist clenching during phlebotomy. N Engl J Med 322:1290–1292, 1990.

PROCEDURES

Site and Depth of Heel Skin Punctures in the Newborn

Every day, including Sundays, literally thousands of newborn infants have heel punctures performed in order to obtain blood samples.

Many of these punctures are badly performed. Little attention is paid to normal anatomy. Serious complications of heel punctures in newborns include calcaneal osteomyelitis and necrotizing chondritis.

The skin's primary arterial blood supply comes from an arterial network at the junction of the lower dermis and upper subcutaneous tissue. Branches from one side of this network supply blood to the subcutaneous tissue, and those from the other side supply the dermis. A large network of veins is also present at the dermal subcutaneous junction. Because of the anatomy, most of the blood obtained from a skin puncture flows from vessels at the dermal subcutaneous junction, and for this reason it is not necessary to extend the puncture any deeper to obtain adequate blood flow.

How deep is this junction? The accompanying figure (below right) illustrates the distance from the skin to the subcutaneous junction (S–S) and the distance from the skin to the periosteum of the calcaneus (S–P) as a function of body weight. A lancet puncture of 2.4 mm will extend below the dermal subcutaneous junction but will not penetrate the perichondrium in even the smallest infants. Do not go deeper than 2.4 mm.

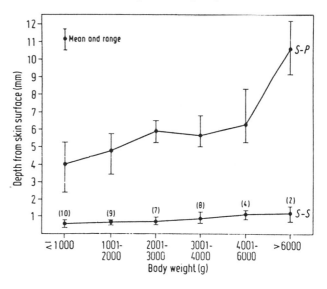

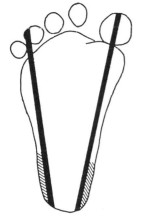

The side-to-side limits of the calcaneus are illustrated in the drawing (left). A line extending posteriorly from a point between the fourth and fifth toes and running parallel to the lateral aspect of the heel, and another line extending posteriorly from the middle of the big toe and running parallel to the medial aspect of the heel, serve as useful guidelines. Heel punctures should be performed on the plantar surface of the heel and beyond the lateral and medial limits of the calcaneus. These safe areas are marked by the hatched lines in the illustration. Don't be responsible for bone spurs.

Reference: Blumenfeld TA, Turi GK, Blanc WA: Recommended site and depth of newborn heel skin punctures based on anatomical measurements and histopathology. Lancet i:230, 1979.

From McMillan JA, et al: The Whole Pediatrician Catalog. Philadelphia, W.B. Saunders, 1977, with permission.

PROTEINURIA

Common Causes

Chronic pyelonephritis
Isolated transient/intermittent
    proteinuria
    Cold exposure
    Congestive heart failure
    Exercise
    Febrile illness
    Idiopathic proteinuria
    Orthostatic proteinuria
    Pregnancy
    Trauma
    Urinary tract infection

Uncommon Causes

Nephritis sediment
    Membranoproliferative glomerulo-
      nephritis
    Postinfectious glomerulonephritis
Nephrotic sediment
    Minimal change disease
    Preeclampsia
Tubular proteinuria
    Acute tubular necrosis
    Obstructive uropathy
    Polycystic kidney disease

Rare Causes

Drugs
    Captopril
    Fenoprofen
    Gold
    Penicillamine
    Probenecid
Nephritic sediment
    Hereditary nephritis
    IGA nephropathy
    Mixed cryoglobulinemia
    Rapidly progressive glomerulo-
      nephritis
    Subacute bacterial endocarditis
    Systemic lupus erythematosus
Nephrotic sediment
    Amyloidosis
    Diabetes mellitus

Nephrotic sediment *(Cont.)*
    Focal glomerulonephritis
    Membranous nephropathy
    Miscellaneous infections
      Hepatitis B
      Malaria
      Syphilis
Overflow proteinuria
    Bence Jones proteinuria
    Lysozymuria (in leukemia)
Tubular proteinuria
    Analgesic abuse
    Chronic hypertension
    Hypercalciuria
    Hyperuricemia
    Radiation nephritis

PRURITUS

Common Causes

Atopic dermatitis
Cholestasis of pregnancy
Contact allergens (plants, cosmetics,
    dyes, medications)
Contact irritants (soaps, chemicals,
    excrement, wool)
Dermatitis herpetiformis

Drugs
    Aminophylline
    Aspirin
    Barbiturates
    Erythromycin
    Gold
    Griseofulvin

Drugs *(Cont.)*
    Isoniazid
    Opiates
    Phenothiazines
    Vitamin A
Dry skin
    Advanced age
    Excess bathing/strong detergents
    Low humidity
Foreign body
Hepatitis
Herpes gestationis
High humidity

Insect bites/infestations
    Fleas, mosquitos, scabies miters,
        lice mites, chiggers
Iron-deficiency anemia
Parasitic infection
    Pinworms
    Toxocara canis
Pityriasis rosea
Psoriasis
Seborrheic dermatitis
Skin infections (bacterial/viral/fungal)
Urticaria
Water contact (aquagenic)

Uncommon Causes

Biliary obstruction
    Drug induced
    Extrahepatic biliary obstruction
    Primary biliary cirrhosis
Chronic renal failure
Hematopoietic malignancies
    Hodgkin's disease
    Leukemia

Hematopoietic malignancies *(Cont.)*
    Lymphoma
Neurodermatitis
Parasitic infection
    Cercaria
    Hookworms
    Trichinosis

Rare Causes

Autoimmune (SLE, JRA)
Congenital ectodermal disorders
Endocrine disorders
    Carcinoid syndrome
    Diabetes mellitus
    Hyper/hypothyroidism
    Hypoparathyroidism
Erythropoietic protoporphyria

Hematopoietic malignancies
    Mastocytosis
    Multiple myeloma
    Polycythemia vera
Malignant solid tumors
Neurologic syndromes
Psychosis

Relieving the Sting or the Itch

Although a number of drugs and lotions are available for the treatment of bites and rashes, home remedies are often as good or even better in producing relief. Here are some tried and true home remedies:

Home Remedies for the Treatment of Bites and Rashes

FOR	TRY
Bee stings, wasp stings, and jellyfish bites	Adolph's meat tenderizer. Add a little water to the powder and rub into the bite. Expect relief in minutes.
Poison ivy	Ban roll-on deodorant. Just rub on the rash and rub away the itch.

Table continued on next page.

Home Remedies for the Treatment of Bites and Rashes (Cont.)

FOR	TRY
Chickenpox	Spray starch. Just spray the lesions with this laundry starch.
Chigger bites	Clear nail polish. Paint each bite with nail polish. The chigger suffocates and the itch disappears.

Reference: From McMillan J, et al (eds): The Whole Pediatrician Catalog, Vol. 3. Philadelphia, W.B. Saunders, 1982, with permission.

PUBERTY

Delayed Puberty and the Adolescent Female

Surely none of us can forget the emotional and physiologic complexities of puberty. The adolescent female who believes her development is delayed can be caught in a maelstrom of anxiety. For the majority of girls with "delayed" puberty, the cause is none other than normal variance. In these cases, the pediatrician is the perfect person to provide the needed reassurance that development will occur. For the minority of females with a pathologic cause of pubertal delay, diagnosis and, in some cases, treatment, are within reach. The tables and evaluation plan that follow will help you and your patient in this delicate matter.

Late, Delayed or Arrested?

"Late" defines the onset of puberty at an age older than the average but within 2 standard deviations of the mean.

"Delayed"—when *no signs* of sexual development have begun by the age of *13*.

"Arrested"—when more than 5 years have passed between adrenarche or thelarche and menarche.

Tanner Stages and Their Mean Age of Appearance

STAGE	BREAST DEVELOPMENT		PUBIC DEVELOPMENT	
	MEAN AGE (YR)	RANGE (YR)	MEAN AGE (YR)	RANGE (YR)
Tanner I (prepubertal)				
Tanner II	11.2	8.0–13.0	11.7	9.3–14.1
Tanner III	12.2	10.0–14.3	12.4	10.2–14.6
Tanner IV	13.1	10.8–15.3	13.0	10.8–15.1
Tanner V	15.3	11.9–18.8	14.4	12.2–16.8
Menarche	12.6	10.0–16.0		

Causes of Delayed Puberty

Constitutional Delay in Growth and Development (CD GD): Family History

Hypogonadotrophic hypogonadism

Hypothalamic-pituitary disorders
Isolated deficiency of GnRH
Isolated deficiency of LH, FSH, or both
Panhypopituitarism
Associated abnormalities
    Kallman syndrome (anosomia)
    Prader-Willi syndrome
    Bardet-Biedl syndrome
Postinflammatory
    Autoimmune (hypophysitis)
    Infectious (meningitis,
      encephalitis)
Trauma
Infiltration
    Histiocytosis X
    Hemochromatosis
Irradiation
Tumor
    Craniopharyngioma
    Optic glioma
    Adenoma

Functional gonadotropin deficiency
Chronic systemic or endocrinologic
    disease
    Cardiovascular (congenital
      or acquired)
    Pulmonary (asthma, cystic fibrosis)
    Hematologic (sickle cell disease)
    Gastrointestinal (celiac disease,
      chronic inflammatory bowel
      disease, other causes
      of malabsorption)
    Renal (renal tubular acidosis,
      renal failure)
    Immunologic (chronic/persistent
      infection, immunocompromise)
    Collagen-vascular (SLE, JRA)
    Endocrine (hypothyroidism,
      glucocorticoid excess,
      hyposomatotropism, IDDM)
Psychiatric (emotional stress)

Hypogonadotropic hypogonadism *Cont.)*

Weight loss
Anorexia nervosa
Malabsorption
Exercise

Hyperprolactinemia
Prolactinoma

Hypergonadotrophic hypogonadism

Primary gonadal abnormalities
Gonadal dysgenesis and its variants
Insensitivity to gonadotropins
Defects in steroidogenesis

Acquired gonadal failures
Postinflammatory
    Autoimmune
    Infectious
Posttraumatic
    Vascular
    Surgical
Infiltration
    Galactosemia
    Myotonic dystrophy
    Ataxia-telangiectasia
Toxic
    Irradiation
    Chemotherapy
Tumor

Hyperandrogenism

Polycystic ovary syndrome (PCOS)
Nonclassical congenital adrenal
    hyperplasia (CAH)

Anatomic genital abnormalities

Rokitansky syndrome (congenital
    absence of uterus and vagina)
Transverse vaginal septum and/or
    imperforate hymen
End-organ insensitivity to androgens
    (testicular feminization)

Reference: Schwartz ID, Root AW: Puberty in girls: Normal or delayed? Contemp Peds Nov:83–104, 1989.

Evaluating Delayed Puberty in Girls

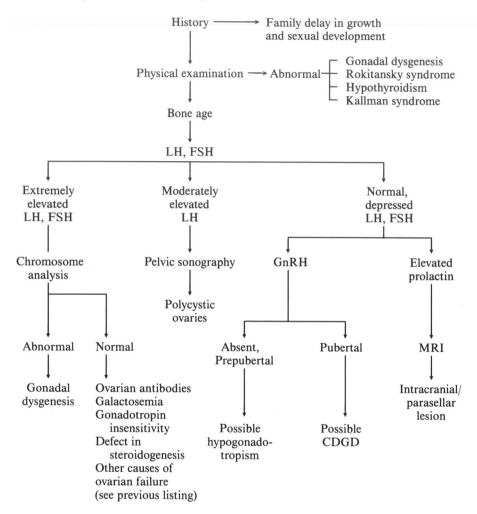

Precocious Puberty: The Other Side of the Coin

Like delayed puberty, precocious puberty can cause significant emotional trauma in the preadolescent female. Unlike delayed puberty, precocious puberty is more often a sign of underlying disease with possible long-term consequences. Since precocious puberty is 4 to 8 times more common in girls, the following differential and algorithm are directed to the evaluation of the female patient.

By definition, isosexual precocious puberty in girls is the appearance of secondary sexual characteristics before the child's eighth birthday. An oft-confused phenomenon is that of "early adolescence" where signs of puberty appear between the ages of 8 and 10. The subsets of girls that are prone to "early adolescence" include those with simple obesity, advanced bone age, or increased body mass index. Below is a differential for each of the three categories of precocious puberty and a recommended work-up.

Categories of Precocious Puberty (True and Complete)

1. **Central isosexual precocity**
   Idiopathic, often familial
   CNS anatomic defects
     Septo-optic dysplasia
     Hydrocephalus
     Cysts
   Postinflammatory
     Meningitis
     Encephalitis
     Brain abscess
   Trauma
   Irradiation
   Tumor
     Hamartoma
     Neurofibroma
     Optic glioma
     Astrocytoma
     Ependymoma
     Dysgerminoma
     Craniopharyngioma
   Postpseudiososexual
     precocity

2. **Pseudoisosexual precocity**
   Gonadotropin-dependent
     HcG secreting tumors (very rare)
     LH&FSH secreting tumors (very rare)
   Gonadotropin-independent
     Ovarian estrogen
       Granulosa cell tumor
       Follicular cysts
     McCune-Albright syndrome
       (irregularly contoured café au lait
       spots, polyostotic fibrous dysplasia,
       and precocious puberty)
     Adrenal estrogen
       Feminizing tumors
     Exogenous estrogen or estrogen-
       like substances
       Oral contraceptives
       Topical estrogen
       Cimetidine
       Cannabis
       Spironolactone
       Digitalis

3. **Primary hypothyroidism**

Incomplete Isosexual Precocity

Premature thelarche, with or without galactorrhea: peak incidence 6 m–2 y; persists from birth in 23% of girls.

Premature menarche: any vaginal bleeding in prepubertal females should alert the pediatrician to possible sexual abuse or trauma, vaginal infection, tumors, foreign body, or urethral prolapse.

Premature adrenarche: incidence higher in African Americans. Congenital adrenal hyperplasia variants.

Algorithm (see top of next page.)

Treatments exist to "turn off" the hypothalamic-pituitary ovarian axis through pharmacologic or surgical therapies. The long-term consequences of precocious sexual development include compromise of final adult stature, possibly increased risk of cervical and breast cancers due to extended exposure to unopposed estrogen, and psychological trauma. When precocious puberty is suspected, a referral to a pediatric endocrinologist is suggested.

Reference: Schwartz ID, Root AW: Puberty in girls: Early, incomplete or precocious? Contemp Peds Jan:147–156, 1990.

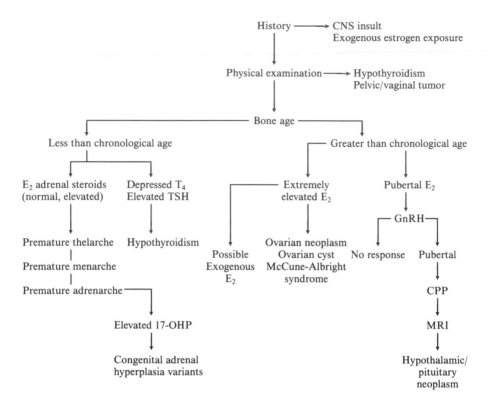

Timing of Puberty and Its Biopsychosocial Correlates

Research on the timing of maturation, precocious puberty, and environmental change has reported fairly consistent findings. The influence of puberty and its timing appear to have the greatest effects in the areas of self-conceptions (body image and self-esteem), developmental needs (heterosexual relationships, peer affiliations, family independence), school performance (academic performance and problem behaviors), and environmental responses (peer, parental, and teacher expectations). These effects vary as a function of:

1. gender,
2. the relationship of the individual's pubertal status to that of his or her peers,
3. definitions of early and late timing, and
4. the behavior under investigation.

In general, the most negative effects have been reported for early-maturing females. Some recent work has shown that the effects of early maturation may be detrimental for both sexes, with early maturation in males being associated with the early initiation of sexual activity and other risk behaviors.

References: Irwin CE Jr: The theoretical concept of at-risk adolescents. Adolescent Medicine: State Art Rev 1:1–14, 1990.

Irwin CE Jr, Millstein SG, Turner R: Pubertal timing and adolescent risk taking: Are they correlated? Pediatr Res 25:8A, 1989.

PUPILS

Abnormal Pupils

DESCRIPTION	NAME	DIFFERENTIAL DIAGNOSIS
Shape		
Absent iris	Aniridia	Wilms' tumor
Scalloped or asymmetric retraction	Irregular iris	Adhesions, old iritis, persistent pupillary membrane, trauma
Tearing the root of the iris from ciliary attachment	Iridodialysis	Trauma
Loss of circular shape	Coloboma	Congenital or operative
Movement and Size		
Loss of light reflex, preservation of accommodation, miosis	Argyll Robertson pupil	Syphilis, also seen occasionally in encephalitis, multiple sclerosis, CNS tumor
Very slow light reflex, preservation of accomodation, mydriasis	Adie's pupil	Benign
Preservation of light reflex, loss of accommodation	Reverse Argyll Robertson pupil	Bilateral: Diabetes mellitus, syphilis, basilar meningitis, tumor of the corpora quadrigemina Unilateral: Diphtheria, intoxication (alcohol), syphilis
Loss of all reflex movements of the pupil	Ophthalmoplegia interna	Third nerve nucleus damage, diabetes mellitus, syphilis, diphtheria, tumor, trauma
Loss of ipsilateral light reflex, loss of contralateral consensual reflex	Optic nerve lesion	Lesion between chiasma and globe
Loss of psychic or sensory mydriasis (may be associated with Horner's syndrome	Sympathetic pupil	Syringomyelia, paralysis of cervical sympathetic nerve
Miosis, preservation of light and accommodation reflexes	Miotic, reactive pupil	Neonates, the elderly, stimulation of pupillary sphincter, paralysis of dilator pupillae (encephalitis, syringomyelia, CNS abscess), tumor or hemorrhage irritating the center for constriction. Opiates, organic phosphates, pilocarpine.
Mydriasis,* preservation of light and accommodation reflexes	Mydriatic, reactive pupil	Mania, schizophrenia, irritation without destruction of cervical sympathetics (i.e., aneurysm, tumor, blood infection), LSD

*The atropines cause cycloplegia: dilatation and *paralysis* of the iris.

Table continued on next page.

Abnormal Pupils

DESCRIPTION	NAME	DIFFERENTIAL DIAGNOSIS
Movement and Size (Cont.)		
Pupils alternately dilate and contract rapidly ("tremor of the iris")	Hippus	Multiple sclerosis, drug/alcohol overdose, homocystinuria, central scotoma with macular damage or disease or injury to axial fibers of optic nerve
More than one pupil in an eye	Polycoria	Congenital, traumatic, surgical
Inequality of size of pupils	Anisocoria	Variation of normal, iritis, diabetes mellitus, cervical sympathetic lesion, eye drops, glaucoma, unilateral damage to third nerve fibers, syphilis, trigeminal neuralgia, carotid or aortic aneurysm, cranial lesion, cerebral herniation, artificial eye
Pupils dilate under light stimulus	Parodoxical pupil (rare)	Syphilis
With strong deviation of the eyes, the pupil of the abducted eye is larger than that of the adducted eye	Tournay's sign	Normal

From Gottlieb AJ, Zamkoff KW, Jastremski MS, Scalzo A, Imboden KJ: The Whole Internist Catalog. Philadelphia, W.B. Saunders Co., 1980, pp 120–121, with permission.

PURPURA (PETECHIAL AND ECCHYMOSES)

Common Causes

Thrombocytopenia
Trauma
Viral infections

Uncommon Causes

Abnormal platelet function
Child abuse
Cupping and coin rubbing
Drug ingestion (aspirin)
Factitious
Henoch-Schönlein purpura
Hereditary coagulation disturbance
Infection
Septic emboli
Uremia
Vasculitis
Violent coughing

Rare Causes

Autoerythrocyte sensitization
Bernard-Soulier (giant platelet) syndrome
Cushing's syndrome
Dysproteinemias
Glanzmann's thrombasthenia
Hereditary hemorrhagic telangiectasia
Macular cerulae
Marfan's syndrome
May-Hegglin anomaly
Osteogenesis imperfecta
Osteopetrosis
Platelet storage pool disease
Protein C deficiency
Protein S deficiency
Purpura fulminans
Schamberg's disease
Scurvy
Vitamin K deficiency

Purpura and Petechiae—Interpreting the Sign

Every little bruise can have a meaning all its own. It is important to look carefully at a hemorrhagic lesion for the clue to its underlying disease. Listed below are some guides to the interpretation of this sign.

Thrombocytopenic purpura	Petechiae are *nonpalpable*. Platelet count $< 20,000/\text{ml}$.
Thrombocytopathic purpura	Easily bruised. Petechiae are *rare*.
Vasculitic purpura (+/– thrombocytopenia)	Petechiae are *palpable*.
Drug purpura (+/– thrombocytopenia)	Often associated with *hemorrhagic bullae* in the mouth.
Allergic purpura (Henoch-Schönlein)	*Pruritic* crops of symmetrical purpura on proximal extremities (4+ lower) associated with *urticarial* and erythematous lesions.
Purpura fulminans (skin manifestations of DIC)	Large symmetrical ecchymoses, particularly on distal extremities, complicated by *acral gangrene*. Petechiae are *rare*.
"Devil's pinches" (autoerythrosensitization vs. factitious)	Females. "Spontaneous" *painful* ecchymoses (+/– erythematous base) on anterior-lateral aspect of thigh and abdomen in a stepladder distribution.
Hyperglobulinemic purpura	Lower extremities (after exercise or prolonged standing). Tendency for skin to develop *brownish pigmentation*. Identical to idiopathic nonhyper-globulinemic syndrome, called Schamberg's disease, except that the latter has normal serum globulin levels.
Cryoglobulinemic purpura	Purpura (+/– gangrene) on *exposed acral areas* (fingers, nose, ears, face).
Amyloid purpura	Spontaneous *periorbital* purpura (usually post Valsalva maneuver). "Touch purpura."
Scorbutic purpura	Purpura around hair *follicles* (perifollicular petechiae). Characteristically associated with corkscrew hairs. Saddle distribution.
Senile purpura	Purple *flat* ecchymotic spots on extensor surface of *forearms*, dorsum of *hands*, and neck in the *elderly*. Identical lesions are found in *cachetic states* and chronic *hypercortisonism*.
Embolic purpura	A. Septic embolic *White centered* petechial lesion often located on mucous membrane and conjunctivae (e.g., bacterial endocarditis). B. Fat emboli Petechiae limited to upper one-half of the body, particularly to *anterior chest*. *Never seen on the face or back* (skimming effect).
Palatine petechiae	Infectious mononucleosis. Sepsis. Trauma (e.g., dentures).

Petechiae	Almost always indicates a disturbance of platelets or a
(lesion ≤ 3 mm)	vasculopathy. Rarely do they indicate an abnormality of coagulation.

Reference: From McMillan JA, et al (eds): The Whole Pediatrician Catalog, Vol 2. Philadelphia, W.B. Saunders, 1979, pp 211–212, with permission.

PYURIA AND BACTERIURIA

Does pyuria always signify the presence of bacteriuria? Is bacteriuria always associated with the presence of pyuria? The answer to both questions is "no." Pyuria in the absence of bacteriuria can be seen:

1. In dehydration
2. In trauma
3. In the presence of an irritating agent in the renal pelvis, bladder, or ureter.
4. In renal tuberculosis
5. In acute and chronic glomerulonephritis
6. After administration of oral polio vaccine
7. After administration of intramuscular iron
8. In renal tubular acidosis
9. In association with a variety of viral infections
10. In Kawasaki disease

Listed below is a comparison between urine bacterial counts and leukocyte counts. Urines were collected by a clean voiding technique, and 5 ml was centrifuged for 3 minutes at 3000 RPM.

COLONY COUNT (BACTERIA/ml)	UNCENTRIFUGED		CENTRIFUGED
	10 or more WBC/mm^3	100 or more WBC/mm^3	5 or more WBC/HPF
10^5	61%	23%	43%
10^4–10^5	28%	0%	14%
10^3–10^4	23%	0%	6%
10^2–10^3	21%	1%	2%
Sterile	10%	1%	1%

Reference: Pryles CV, Lustik B: Pediatr Clin N Amer 18:233, 1971.
From McMillan JA, et al: The Whole Pediatrician Catalog, Vol. 2. Philadelphia, W.B. Saunders, 1979, p 255, with permission.

Q

QUALITY TIME

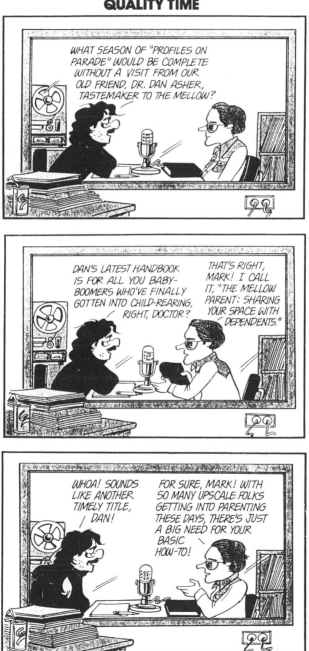

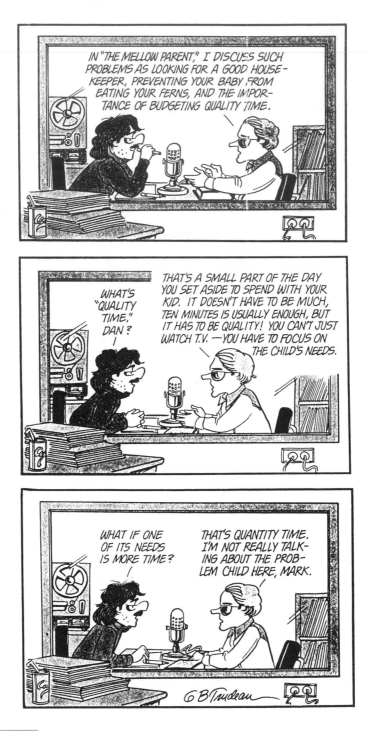

QUESTIONS

Thirty Questions That Parents Ask and Pediatricians Should Be Able to Answer

Listed below are questions frequently asked by parents. No one can have all the answers, but you should begin to learn some of them in your pediatric training. We have stratified the questions, with their answers, as a function of probable experience. If you have any questions about our answers, drop us a line.

Questions that a PL-1 should be able to answer:

1. If I chop up foods, such as hot dogs, very fine, is it safe to feed these to my 2-year-old?
   A. If they are chopped into very small pieces, they are safe; but it is important to remember that hot dog chunks are a common cause of aspiration in the 2-year-old. Another very dangerous food for any child under 3 years of age is peanuts. "Only a nut would feed a nut to a child." Instruct parents in the Heimlich maneuver.

2. Can shaking a baby or tossing him or her into the air playfully be harmful?
   A. Yes, both can be extremely harmful. Such play can injure the brain, neck, or spinal cord and has been known to produce retinal hemorrhages.

3. Is it true that it is harmful to swing or lift a child by holding his hands and pulling up on his arms?
   A. Yes, this can produce a "nursemaid's elbow"—which is a dislocation of the elbow.

4. My husband smokes in the house. Is this really a health danger to my young children?
   A. Absolutely. Smoking at home is known to aggravate asthma. There is a higher incidence of otitis media and other forms of respiratory illness among children living in a home with smokers. By the way, side-stream smoke also increases the non-smoking adult's risk for cancer. Get your husband to stop smoking or get rid of him.

5. I have a healthy 4-year-old. Should she receive the influenza vaccine?
   A. It is not necessary. The vaccine is advised for children with a variety of chronic illnesses.

6. Is it true that penicillin will cure the symptoms of a sore throat within 24 hours?
   A. Yes, but only if the symptoms are a result of an infection with the streptococcus microorganism. Without treatment, it will take 48 to 72 hours before symptoms subside.

7. Is it really possible for my son to have a streptococcal infection in his anal area?
   A. Definitely. It is characterized by pain and redness, usually without fever. Penicillin is the cure.

8. What is "croup"?

   A. Croup is the term applied to a condition that is characterized by a inspiratory noise called "stridor." It is often accompanied by a cough that sounds like the bark of a seal. Croup can be caused by infections or allergic swelling in the larnyx or "voice-box."

9. Is it safe to give my 10-month-old daughter swimming lessons?

   A. Not a good idea. She can swallow a great deal of water while learning and that may cause convulsions. She will not really learn to swim at this age and does not have sufficient judgment to avoid water dangers when left alone.

10. Can you recommend a good book for me, a new parent, on child health?

    A. Yes. The best book on this subject is entitled *Your Child's Health,* by Dr. Barton D. Schmitt and is published by Bantam Books and is available in paperback.

Questions that a PL-2 should be able to answer:

1. My 16-year-old daughter often eats several glasses of ice cubes each day. Is there something wrong with her?

   A. Your daughter suffers from a condition termed "pagophagia" or ice-eating. "Pagos" is the Greek word for "ice" and "phagia" in Greek means "to eat." Compulsive ice-eating is usually a sign of iron deficiency and can often be promptly cured with iron therapy.

2. Can the rash from poison ivy be spread by exposure to the fluid from popped blisters?

   A. No. Poison ivy results from a hypersensitivity reaction to the plant's resins. Transmission only occurs by direct contact with the plant or with the hands, clothing, or pets that have resin on them. The blister fluid does not contain the resin.

3. My daughter is almost 3 and still not toilet trained. What am I doing wrong?

   A. Nothing. Toilet training should not begin until your child is ready. Readiness means that your child has the neurologic capacity to control bodily functions, understands the concepts of toileting, knows the language of the toilet, and, most importantly, wants to be clean and dry. This process may start as early as 1 year of age. I suspect that your child will train herself very soon.

4. We have a kitten at home. Can a kitten or cat cause any health problems for my 2-year-old son?

   A. Yes, definitely yes. Diseases and parasites such as cat scratch fever, toxoplasmosis, and *Toxocara cati* can be spread from a cat or kitten. Cat dander is often responsible for asthma. Now that you have a child you don't need any other pet. Get rid of the cat.

5. Is it safe to allow my son to play football with his high school team?

   A. It depends on the status of his physical maturity relative to others his own age, the protective equipment available, and the concern of the coach for the emotional and physical welfare of the members of the team.

6. My 5-year-old periodically becomes hoarse. What should I do?

   A. Get some ear plugs for yourself. The episodes of hoarseness are probably a consequence of excessive screaming on your child's part. "Scremer's nodules"—actual thickening of the vocal cords—can result from overuse of the voice. If hoarseness persists, your child should be seen by an otolaryngologist.

7. My child has pink urine after eating beets. What does this mean?

   A. About 7% of the population will demonstrate "beeturia" after eating the equivalent of one beet. This is a genetic trait. Beeturia is also seen in a very high percentage of children and adults with iron deficiency anemia. This form of beeturia disappears with iron therapy. To be certain of the cause of your child's problem, a blood count should be obtained.

8. Is it appropriate for a young child to attend the funeral of his grandparent?

   A. If he wants to go, then you should let him. Never force a child, of any age, to attend a viewing or a funeral.

9. Does an exclusively breast-fed infant require supplemental iron?

   A. Not during the first 6 months of life. Studies have shown that the iron status of an exclusively breast-fed infant is as good as an infant receiving an iron-fortified formula at age 6 months. If breast milk remains the sole source of nutrition beyond 6 months of age, iron supplements are indicated, because studies have shown that about 15% of such infants will be iron deficient by 9 months of age.

10. What kind of shoes should I buy for my baby when she starts walking?

   A. The least expensive sneakers you can find. Shoes are only necessary for the protection of the feet from the dirt, glass, and manure of the streets and are not required to enhance the act of locomotion.

Questions that a PL-3 should be able to answer:

1. My 2-year-old is a finnicky eater and I'm not sure she's eating all the foods she needs. Should I supplement her diet with vitamins?

   A. No, they are unnecessary. Put a balanced meal before the child and she will take what she needs. Vitamins are only "fish-food" for a person eating a balanced diet. The excess vitamins you provide will appear in the child's urine, and when they are flushed down the toilet they will eventually reach the fish in the sea.

2. I'm a working mother with three young children. Not surprisingly, I often come home tired. Can you give me some advice to make returning home after a tough day better for all of us?

   A. There are no easy answers for a task that stumps even "superwoman." But these suggestions may help:

   - When you pick up your child from day care, bring a snack for the trip home.
   - Take turns with your spouse leaving work early, so one of you can pick up your child before you are both exhausted.

- Establish a homecoming routine that gives you recovery time. Tell your children that they will get your full attention after you have a chance to catch your breath and get dinner started.
- Reward your children for good behavior. Try a chart with gold stars or a special picture to color.
- Expect your school-age children to begin their homework after school and before you arrive.
- Reduce meal preparation during the week by cooking on weekends and freezing the servings until you need them.
- If you can afford it, hire a high school student as a mother's helper for that first hour at home.
- Involve the children with dinner chores, such as setting the table, clearing the table, and the like.
- Share the evening tasks with your spouse.
- If possible, take the family out to dinner occasionally to give everyone a break.

3. Should I give my child aspirin?

   A. No, except under a physician's direction for some very special circumstances, such as Kawasaki's disease or acute rheumatic fever.

4. Does it help to put butter on burns?

   A. The best thing to put on a burn immediately is ice. The ice will relieve the pain and reduce the damage done by the burn. Topical vitamin E is much better than butter in reducing the scarring and damage done by a small burn.

5. Can iron deficiency anemia produce any harm in a 1-year-old?

   A. Yes. Recent studies demonstrate that iron deficiency anemia results in cognitive delays in 1- and 2-year-olds that may not be correctable with iron therapy.

6. When can you begin giving a child an allowance?

   A. When you can afford it and when the child has some appreciation of the value of money and when you have agreed upon the fact that the allowance is dependent on the satisfactory performance of some responsibilities. This usually begins at age 8–9.

7. Can fruit juice cause stomach aches or diarrhea in my 6-year-old?

   A. Yes, if they consume large quantities of juice and if the juice contains non-absorbable sugars such as sorbitol. Apple juice, for example, contains large quantities of sorbitol.

8. Can a child have an ear infection without a fever?

   A. Yes. About one-half of episodes of otitis media are not associated with temperature elevation beyond 100.4°

9. Our 12-year-old son wants an All-Terrain vehicle. Are they safe?

   A. No. Don't buy it either for him or for you.

10. My teenage daughter says that kissing is good exercise. Is this true?

    A. Not if her goal is to lose weight. It is estimated that a single kiss burns up 9 calories and that by kissing three times a day for 1 year, she could lose 2.8 pounds.

R

RED CELL

Red Cell Distribution Width

Age-appropriate Values for RBC Distribution Width

AGE	NO. OF PATIENTS	RBC DISTRIBUTION WIDTH (MEAN ± SD)
1–6 mo	68	13.0 ± 1.5
7–12 mo	84	13.7 ± 0.9
13–24 mo	108	13.4 ± 1.0
2–3 yr	119	13.2 ± 0.8
4–5 yr	151	12.7 ± 0.9
6–8 yr	106	12.6 ± 0.8
9–11 yr	98	12.8 ± 1.0

Reference: Novak RW: Red blood cell distribution width in pediatric microcytic anemias. Pediatrics 80:251, 1987, with permission.

RENAL FAILURE

The FE_{Na} Test: Use in the Differential Diagnosis of Acute Renal Failure

The physician is frequently faced with the problem of distinguishing prerenal azotemia from acute tubular necrosis in patients with acute renal failure.

In the oliguric phase of these two conditions, the renal tubule handles sodium in distinctly different fashions. In prerenal azotemia, the renal tubule avidly reabsorbs the filtered sodium; in acute tubular necrosis, the reabsorption of sodium is restricted.

These observations provide the basis for a simple test for differentiating these two conditions—the "FE_{Na} test" (FE_{Na} is the excreted fraction of the filtered sodium).

The test is performed by measuring both sodium and creatinine in simultaneously collected samples of plasma and urine.

The FE_{Na} is calculated as follows:

$$\frac{\dfrac{[\text{Sodium}]\, U}{[\text{Sodium}]\, P}}{\dfrac{[\text{Creatinine}]\, U}{[\text{Creatinine P}]}} \times 100$$

U and P represent concentrations in urine and plasma, respectively.

In general, an FE_{Na} of less than 1 indicates prerenal azotemia, and an FE_{Na} of more than 3 indicates acute tubular necrosis.

Reference: Espinel CH: The FE_{Na} test: Use in the differential diagnosis of acute renal failure. JAMA 236:579, 1976.
From McMillan J, et al: The Whole Pediatrician Catalog. Philadelphia, W.B. Saunders, 1977, p 316, with permission.

RESPIRATORY DISTRESS

The Diagnosis of Newborns with Acute Respiratory Distress

The newborn with clinical signs of acute respiratory distress—central cyanosis, tachypnea (>60 breaths/min), tachycardia (>160 beats/min), retractions, grunting, and nasal flaring—demands immediate attention. A review of the maternal history, the age of onset of respiratory distress, a physical examination, and laboratory tests (particularly a chest x-ray) will greatly aid the clinician in assessing this problem further. The following differential diagnosis should be of use:

1. **Upper airway obstruction**

   Choanal atresia
   Masses (encephalocele, tumor)
   Macroglossia
   Nasal stiffness
   Cleft palate
   Laryngeal obstruction (paralysis, web, tumor, stenosis, atresia, malacia)
   Tracheal obstruction (mass, web, stenosis, atresia, malacia, cleft, vascular ring, goiter)

2. **Pulmonary**

   Hyaline membrane disease
   Transient tachypnea of the newborn
   Aspiration of meconium, gastric, or amniotic fluid
   Pneumonia
   Pneumothorax, pneumo-mediastinum
   Persistent pulmonary hypertension
   Tracheoesophageal fistula
   Pulmonary hemorrhage
   Hypoplasia or agenesis of the lungs
   Cystic disease (emphysema, cysts)
   Pleural effusions (e.g., chylothorax)
   Pulmonary sequestrations

3. **Cardiac**

   Cyanotic congenital heart disease
   Acyanotic congenital heart disease
   Arrhythmia (paroxysmal supraventricular tachycardia, block)
   Increased intravascular volume (iatrogenic fluid overload)
   High output failure (hyperthyroidism, arterial-venous malformation)
   Pneumopericardium
   Cardiomyopathy (infection, endocardial fibroelastosis, hypertrophic cardiomyopathy)

4. **Thoracic**

   Chest wall deformities (chondrodystrophies, rib deformities)
   Masses (tumors, cysts)

5. **Metabolic**

   Hypoglycemia
   Infant of a diabetic mother
   Inborn errors of metabolism

6. **Diaphragmatic**

   Hernia (foramen of Bochdalek)
   Paralysis (phrenic nerve)
   Eventration

7. **Neuromuscular**

CNS damage (trauma, hemorrhage)
Medication (maternal sedation,
   narcotic withdrawal)
Muscular weakness (e.g.,
   myasthenia gravis)
Congenital defects

8. **Infections**

Sepsis
Pneumonia (viral, bacterial)

9. **Hematologic/vascular**

Hyperviscosity, hypervolemia
Anemia
Hemoglobinopathy

10. **Other**

Asphyxia
Acidosis
Hypothermia
Hyperthermia

Reference: Schreiner RL, Bradburn NC. Newborns with acute respiratory distress: Diagnosis and management. Pediatrics in Review 9(9):279–285, 1988. Adapted from Table 2 of cited paper.

RESPIRATORY VIRUSES

Clinical Syndromes Produced by Respiratory Viruses

Upper respiratory tract infections and pneumonia are among the most frequently made diagnoses in pediatric clinics and emergency rooms, particularly during the winter months. All too frequently, these infections are lumped together as upper respiratory infections (URIs), viral syndrome, or "influenza-like" syndrome. Many viruses, aside from influenza, are capable of producing respiratory symptoms.

Clinical Syndromes Produced by Respiratory Viruses

VIRUSES	CORYZA	PHARYNGITIS	CROUP	FLU-LIKE ILLNESS	PLEURODYNIA	TRACHEO-BRONCHITIS	PNEUMONIA
Influenza A	●	●	●	●		●	●
Influenza B	●	●	●	●		●	●
Influenza C	●	●		●			
Parainfluenza (1–3)	●	●	●	●		●	●*
Respiratory syncytial	●	●				●*	●*
Coxsackie A	●	●					
Coxsackie B	●	●			●		
Echo	●	●	●		●		
Adenoviruses (1–7, 14, 21)	●	●		●		●	●
Rhinoviruses (>100)	●		●*			●*	●*
Coronaviruses	●						
Herpesviruses (1, 2)		●					
Epstein-Barr	●	●		●			

*In children only

The term influenza, incidentally, originated in Italy during the 15th century. A particularly severe epidemic of a respiratory viral syndrome at that time was attributed to the *influentia* (influence) of the stars and evil forces.

Reference: Rytel MW: Influenza and its complications. Recognition and prevention. Hospital Practice 22:102A–102V, 1987. Table adapted from cited reference.

The Clinical Manifestations of Respiratory Syncytial Virus

Respiratory syncytial virus (RSV) is an all too common cause of epidemic winter respiratory disease in infants, children, and adults. Its severity spans a wide spectrum ranging from a common cold to bronchiolitis (the most common presentation) to respiratory distress, apnea, cyanosis, and pneumonia. RSV is potentially most life-threatening in infants with other underlying conditions such as congenital heart disease (especially conditions with high pulmonary flow), bronchopulmonary dysplasia, other chronic irreversible pulmonary disorders (e.g., cystic fibrosis, pulmonary hemosiderosis, bronchiolitis obliterans, and idiopathic pulmonary hypertension), and all children on immunosuppressive regimens (e.g., transplantation patients, cancer patients treated with chemotherapy or radiation therapy, and patients on high-dose steroid regimens) or children with immunodeficiency syndromes (e.g., severe combined immune deficiency).

Although bronchiolitis is the most frequent presentation of an RSV infection, pneumonia is the most common admitting diagnosis for infants infected with RSV who require hospitalization. Factors that contribute to the severity of illness, in addition to those described above, include age, size of inoculum, and characteristics of an RSV infection:

Common characteristics ($>$75% of all cases)

Rhinorrhea
Cough
Airway hyperactivity
Hypoxemia
Air trapping (hyperinflated lungs on x-ray examination)

Uncommon Characteristics ($<$20% of all cases)

Prolonged fever (T $>$ 102° F)	Hepatosplenomegaly
Otitis media	Enlarged cardiac silhouette
Hoarseness	Hilar adenopathy
Pleural effusion	

The differential diagnosis for RSV pneumonia should include:

1. **Chlamydial pneumonia** as it occurs in the same age group and presents with air trapping and wheezing. The distinguishing point between these two diseases is that chlamydial disease is more prolonged and insidious than RSV.
2. Congenital anomalies of the respiratory tract
3. Foreign bodies

4. Reactive airway disease
5. Infection with other respiratory agents (e.g., influenza virus, parainfluenza viruses, adenovirus, pertussis (*Bordetella*), or mycoplasma).

Reference: Laufer DA, Edelson PJ: Respiratory syncytial virus infection and cardio-pulmonary disease. Pediatr Ann 16:644–653, 1987.

RETROPHARYNX

Retropharyngeal Abscess

The retropharyngeal space extends from the base of the skull to about the level of the second thoracic vertebra. Abscess in this space results from suppuration of the lymph nodes, which run in two parallel chains and drain the nasopharynx, adenoids, and posterior paranasal sinuses. During childhood these nodes are prominent, but they atrophy during adolescence. Though trauma and adjacent vertebral osteomyelitis can predispose to the development of retropharyngeal abscess, local respiratory tract infection is usually felt to be the initiating event. Extension of the infection may result in mediastinitis or asphyxia due to increasing pressure or rupture of the abscess.

Both aerobic and anaerobic bacteria may be isolated from retropharyngeal abscesses, and more than one organism is often found. The frequent isolation of *Staphylococcus aureus* and beta-lactamase-producing anaerobes warrants the use of antibiotics effective against penicillin-resistant oropharyngeal flora. Surgical drainage of the abscess is critical.

The 63 bacteria isolated from 17 children with retropharyngeal abscess are listed below:

Bacteria Isolated from Children with Retropharyngeal Abscess

ISOLATES	NO. OF ISOLATES
Aerobic and facultative	
Gram-positive cocci	
Viridans streptococci	11
Staphylococcus aureus	8
Beta-hemolytic *Streptococcus* Group A	6
Streptococcus pneumoniae	1
Streptococcus constellatus	1
Streptococcus morbillorum	1
Micrococcus	3
Gram-negative cocci	
Neisseria sp.	7
Gram-negative bacilli	
Eikenella corrodens	3
Haemophilus influenzae (nontypable)	3
Haemophilus parainfluenzae	1
Total no. of aerobes	45

Table continued on next page.

Bacteria Isolated from Children with Retropharyngeal Abscess (Cont.)

ISOLATES	NO. OF ISOLATES
Anaerobic	
Anaerobic cocci	
Peptostreptococcus species	3
Veilonella parvula	1
Microaerophilic streptoccus	1
Gram-positive bacilli	
Eubacterium lentum	2
Gram-negative bacilli	
Bacteroides melaningogenicus	7
Bacteroides capillosus	2
Bacteroides species	1
Fusobacterium species	1
Total no. of anaerobes	18

Reference: Asmar BI: Bacteriology of retropharyngeal abscess in children. Pediatr Infect Dis J 8:595–597, 1990.

RETT SYNDROME

The Diagnosis of Rett Syndrome

The diagnosis of Rett syndrome, a severe developmental disorder occurring in young girls, usually between 6 and 18 months of age, can be difficult in view of the fact that it is dependent on history and physical findings alone. There is no laboratory test to confirm the diagnosis. These children experience rapid decline in motor and cognitive function after a period of apparently normal development. In those children who have begun to speak, all meaningful communication is lost, including eye contact. The patients often experience interrupted sleep and periods of uncontrollable screaming. Prevalence is between 1/10,000 and 1/15,000.

The implications of this diagnosis are tragic for both the patient and family. The criteria that can be used to support or exclude the diagnosis are listed below:

1. **Necessary criteria**

    Normal prenatal and perinatal period
    Apparently normal development first 6 mo
    Normal head circumference at birth
    Deceleration of head growth between 5 mo and 4 yr
    Loss of purposeful hand skills between 6 mo and 30 mo; communication
        dysfunction; social withdrawal
    Stereotypic hand movements
    Gait apraxia and truncal ataxia between 1 to 4 yr
    Diagnosis tentative until 2 to 5 yr of age

2. **Supportive criteria**

Breathing dysfunction	Peripheral vasomotor disturbances
EEG abnormalities	Scoliosis
Seizures	Growth retardation
Spasticity	Hypotrophic small feet

3. **Exclusion Criteria**

Intrauterine growth retardation	Evidence of perinatally acquired
Organomegaly—signs of storage	brain damage
disease	Identifiable metabolic disorder
Retinopathy/optic atrophy	Evidence of serious CNS infection
Microcephaly at birth	or trauma

RHINITIS

Diagnosis and Natural History of Allergic Rhinitis

Allergic rhinitis, which is ranked by the National Center for Health Statistics as the sixth most prevalent chronic condition in the U.S., has its peak incidence in childhood and adolescence. It is an atopic hypersensitivity response to foreign allergens mediated by IgE antibodies, but not all persons with IgE antibody have clinical disease. The most common allergens are the following:

Grass pollens (late spring/early summer)
Tree pollens (early spring)
Weed pollens (late summer/autumn)
Animal danders
House-dust mites
Insects
Mold spores
Foods (uncommonly associated)

Symptoms include paroxysmal sneezing; watery, profuse rhinorrhea; nasal congestion (stuffy nose); itching of the nose and eyes; and lacrimation and ocular redness. Other symptoms that can occur are noisy breathing, snoring, hyposmia or anosmia, itchy palate or pharynx, throat clearing, and cough. Children may have "allergic shiners," a dark discoloration in the infraorbital regions secondary to obstruction of venous drainage. The key to diagnosis is the temporal correlation of symptoms with allergic exposure.

As with most allergies, avoidance of the offending allergens is the most effective treatment, which makes identification of the allergens an important component of the therapeutic strategy. However, many of the methods commonly used to diagnose allergies are only minimally helpful in managing allergic rhinitis, including early and late skin-test responses, measurement of IgE levels, and calculation of histamine release by basophils. The natural history of allergic rhinitis is presented in the schematic of sensitization (Phase 1) and clinical disease (Phase 2) shown on the following page:

Phase 1
Sensitization

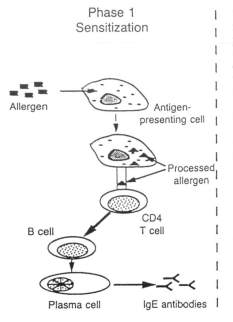

Simplified schematic representation of the natural history of allergic rhinitis. During phase 1 persons become sensitized to an allergen, and during phase 2 clinical disease develops. The overwhelming majority of patients have an early response on reexposure to allergen. The early response is dominated by activation of mast cells and release of mediators. After the early response, most patients have cellular infiltration of the nasal mucosa that causes late inflammatory events. These include the spontaneous recurrence of release of mediators (late-phase reaction), hyperresponsiveness to irritants, and increased responsiveness to allergen (priming). The circles indicate the heterogeneity of these late inflammatory events. The inflammation can resolve spontaneously, cause a complication, or potentially lead to an irreversible form of chronic rhinitis. (From Naclerio RM, N Engl J Med, 325: 861, 1991, with permission.)

Phase 2
Clinical Disease

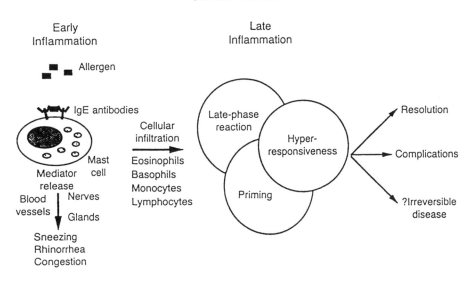

References: Naclerio RM: Allergic rhinitis. N Engl J Med 325:860–869, 1991.
Simons FER: Allergic rhinitis and associated disorders. In Oski FA, et al (eds): Principles and Practice of Pediatrics. Philadelphia, J.B. Lippincott, 1990, pp 219–223.

Persistent Rhinitis in the Newborn

Because neonates are often obligate nose breathers, nasal congestion and rhinorrhea may be a difficult problem. The causes of persistent rhinitis in the newborn are listed below along with the treatment of each type.

Rhinitis in the Newborn

ENTITY	CAUSE	TREATMENT
Transient idiopathic stuffy nose of the newborn	Unknown	Normal saline nosedrops may be instilled and then removed after a few minutes with cotton-tipped applicators or gentle suction on a rubber bulb syringe. If the congestion interferes with feeding, 2 drops of 0.125% phenylephrine (Neo-Synephrine) may be instilled in the nose just before meals for several days.
Chemical rhinitis	Due to overtreatment of idiopathic stuffy nose with topical nasoconstrictors	Discontinue nosedrops. Use oral decongestants for 2 days.
Pyogenic rhinitis	These infants have bacterial infection despite absence of purulent discharge. Diagnose via cultures of discharge	Same as for idiopathic stuffy nose.
Congenital syphilis	Maternal syphilis	Penicillin.
Hypothyroidism	Congenital hypothyroidism	Thyroid hormone replacement.
Choanal atresia	Congenital defect	Place oral airway immediately. Definitive surgery by otolaryngologist.
Nasal fracture	Birth trauma	Diagnose by examination for subluxation of the nasal septum causing occlusion of the nasal passages. Refer to otolaryngologist.

Reference: Simons FER: Allergic rhinitis and associated disorders. In Oski FA, et al (eds): Principles and Practice of Pediatrics. Philadelphia, J.B. Lippincott, 1990, pp 219–223.

RHYTHMIC BEHAVIORS

Rocking and Rolling—And Head Banging

Body rocking, head banging, and head rolling are three rhythmic behaviors that may show up in normal infants between 6 and 10 months of age and may last up to 18 months. Head banging is the most upsetting to parents, who often consult pediatricians because of concern about self-injury, as well as the disruption to the household, often in the middle of the night. Neighbors also have been known to urge intervention.

The average banger is a male (about 3 to 1), usually awake and in bed, usually banging against the headboard, and usually not crying or showing any evidence of temper. Some seem exceptionally relaxed and even blissful during the activity.

The most common positions for head banging were described by de Lissovoy and further discussed by Hoder and Cohen:

1. **The hands and knees position**, in which the child stands on hands and knees and rocks back and forth; on the forward motion the forehead or cranial cap is struck against the crib.
2. **The sitting position**, in which the child is braced or sitting against the side of the crib or the head board. The knees are drawn up or the legs may be straight out; the arms and hands serve to brace the body in motion. The motion is mainly a trunk movement, or it is limited to throwing the head repeatedly to the rear, striking the crib.
3. **The prone position**, in which the child is lying prone; the head is raised and then dropped on the pillow or mattress or brought down with considerable force.
4. **Multiple positions**, in which the child kneels, stands, or sits as he holds onto the bars or the railing of the crib while striking his forehead.
5. **The supine position**, in which , while supine, the child rolls either his head or his whole body from side to side with the head striking the sides of the crib.

In most cases these patterns of motor behavior are transient and resolve spontaneously. Parents should be reassured that no brain damage will result.

References: De Lissovoy: Head banging in early childhood. Child Dev 33:43–56, 1962.
Hoder EL, Cohen DJ: Repetitive behavior patterns of childhood. In Levine MD, et al (eds): Developmental-Behavioral Pediatrics. Philadelphia, W.B. Saunders, 1983, pp 612–614.

RICKETS

Origin of the Name

Most scholars believe that the term is derived from the Greek work "rachitis" (a disease of the spine), and hence the use of the medical synonym rachitis for "rickets." Professor H. A. Skinner felt the term originated from the Anglo-Saxon term "wricken" (to twist). A 17th century writer named John Aubrey added still another "twist" to this story when he wrote:

I will whilst 'tis in my mind insert this Remarque, viz., about 1620 one Ricketts of Newberye, a Practitioner in Physick, was excellent at the Curing of Children with swoln heads, and small legges; and the Disease being new, and without a name, He being so famous for the cure of it, they called the Disease the Ricketts . . . and now 'tis good sport to see how they vex their lexicons, and fetch it from the Greek.

At any rate, when trying to look erudite on the wards, be careful not to confuse the 17th century "Dr. Ricketts" with Howard Taylor Ricketts (1871–1910), the American pathologist who in 1906 discovered the etiology of Rocky Mountain spotted fever and other typhus-like diseases. These microorganisms are designated the genus *Rickettsia* and the family Rickettsiaceae in his honor.

Reference: Haubrich WS: Medical Meanings. New York, Harcourt Brace Jovanovich, 1984, pp 212–213.

The Three-Stage Chemical Evolution of Rickets

Rickets—or avitaminosis D—is a defect in the mineralization of the growing skeleton, including bone and the cartilage of the growth plate. The three stages of the chemical evolution of the disease are as follows:

Stage 1 (Intestinal Calcium Transport Decreased)

Serum calcium decreased   X-ray—normal
Serum phosphorus normal   Tetany may occur
Serum alkaline phosphatase normal

Stage 2 (Compensatory Hyperparathyroidism)

Serum calcium normal   Serum bicarbonate decreased
Serum phosphorus decreased   Serum chloride increased
Serum alkaline phosphatase   Aminoaciduria
  increased   X-ray—active rickets

Stage 3 (Parathyroid Response No Longer Sustains Normal Serum Calcium)

Serum calcium decreased   Serum chloride increased
Serum phosphorus decreased   Aminoaciduria
Serum alkaline phosphatase   X-ray—florid rickets
  increased   Tetany may occur
Serum bicarbonate decreased

References: Bergstrom W: Personal communication, 1991. Glorieux FH: Rickets: The continuing challenge. N Engl J Med 325:1875–1877, 1991.

Causes of Rickets

CAUSE	SOURCE OF DEFICIENCY
Diet	
Calcium deficiency	Low intake
High phytin content (e.g., soy formula)	Malabsorption
Inadequate sunlight and vitamin D supplementation	Malapsorption
Medications	
Antacids	Malabsorption
Furosemide	Excretion
Anticonvulsants (phenytoin or phenobarbital)	Malabsorption
Prematurity	
Inadequate calcium intake	Low intake
Inadequate phosphate intake	Low intake
Vitamin D deficiency	Malabsorption
Inadequate stores	
Increased requirement (suspected but not proved)	

Table continued on next page.

CAUSE	SOURCE OF DEFICIENCY
Disease	
Renal insufficiency	Malabsorption
Hepatic insufficiency	Malabsorption
Malabsorption	Malabsorption
Renal tubular dysfunction	
Phosphaturia	Excretion
Renal tubular acidosis with hypercalciuria	Excretion
Absent renal 1-hydroxylase	Malabsorption
Fanconi syndrome	Malabsorption, excretion
Primary or secondary to tubular damage in cystinosis, tyrosinosis, galactosemia, fructose intolerance, Wilson's disease, or poisoning with lead or other metals	
Hypophosphatasia (alkaline phosphatase deficiency)	Local effect on bone matrix
Calcitriol receptor dysfunction (genetic)	Malabsorption
Decreased affinity	
Ineffective nuclear translation	
Tumor(s)	Excretion

Reference: From Bergstrom WH: Twenty ways to get rickets in the 1990s. Contemp Pediatr December:92, 1991, with permission.

Children at High Risk for Rickets

Small premature infants
Urban breast-fed infants who do not receive supplemental vitamin D

Children with chronic renal insufficiency
Children with biliary atresia or liver disease

Reference: From Bergstrom WH: Twenty ways to get rickets in the 1990s. Contemp Pediatr December:93, 1991, with permission.

Causes of Calcitriol Deficiency*

Insufficient UV exposure and inadequate vitamin D supplementation
Malabsorption of supplemental vitamin D in steatorrhea (acholic or celiac)
Defective hepatic 25-hydroxylation

Defective renal 1-hydroxylation caused by:
Parenchymal hypoplasia or damage
Hereditary absence of 1-hydroxylase
Genetic defect in the calcitriol receptor[8]
Genetic defect in nuclear translation of the calcitriol-receptor complex[8]

*Calcitriol deficiency leads to inadequate calcium and phosphate reabsorption.
Reference: From Bergstrom WH: Twenty ways to get rickets in the 1990s. Contemp Pediatr December:98, 1991, with permission.

Radiographic Findings in Rickets

The radiographic signs of rickets are the same regardless of the disorder responsible for undermineralization.

Knees and wrists

Epiphyseal centers are indistinct or invisible

Metaphyseal zones of provisional calcification have faint, irregular outlines

Increased distance from the visible mineralized portion of the shafts to the epiphyseal centers is apparent

Ends of ulna and fibia are concave

Ends of bones are widened

In severe rickets, density of the bone shafts is reduced

Chest

Ends of ribs are expanded, cupped, indistinct, and appear farther than usual from the sternum

Proximal humeri show changes listed for knees and wrists but lesser in degree because linear growth is slower

When rickets heals

Supernormal amounts of mineral, visible as dense transverse bands, appear in the formerly deficient zones of provisional calcification

Dense lines may also appear in subperiosteal osteoid parallel to the bone shafts and can be misinterpreted as evidence of trauma

Reference: From Bergstrom WH: Twenty ways to get rickets in the 1990s. Contemp Pediatr December:100, 1991, with permission.

Diagnosis and Management of Rickets

CAUSE	DIAGNOSTIC TOOLS	MANAGEMENT
Calcium deficiency		
Low intake	History	Modify diet to include at least 500 mg/d of CA
Marginal intake + excess phytin	History	Modify diet
Extreme prematurity (birth weight $<$ 1,500 g)	History	Adjust intake to 200 mg/kg/d[1]
Steatorrhea	Stool fat Serum 25-OH-D_3 low	25-OH-D_3 (5–7 μg/kg/d) if serum level is low; supplement dietary Ca[12]
Anticonvulsants (phenobarbital or phenytoin)	History	Vitamin D 1,000–2,000 IU/d
Furosemide	Hypercalciuria (urine Ca/Cr $>$ 0.2)	
Renal tubular acidosis	Serum CO_2 low Urine pH 6.0 or above Hypercalciuria (urine Ca/Cr $>$ 0.2)	Base supplement: 3–10 mM/kg/d as $NaHCO_3$ or citrate
Vitamin D deficiency		
Insufficient UV light	History	400 IU/d of vitamin D
No vitamin D supplement	Low 25-OH-D_3	

Table continued on next page.

CAUSE	DIAGNOSTIC TOOLS	MANAGEMENT
Vitamin D deficiency *(Cont.)*		
Liver disease	Low 25-OH-D$_3$	25-OH-D 5–7 μg/kg/d[12]
Renal disorders may reduce calcitriol formation:	BUN or Cr high	Calcitriol 0.25–1.0 μg/d
Hypoplasia or parenchymal damage	Serum P usually high	CaCO$_3$ to restrict P absorption and supplement dietary Ca[13]
	Serum Ca low (may be normal in secondary hyperparathyroidism)	
	Alkaline phosphatase high	Restrict milk and protein sources to lower P load
Specific hydroxylase deficiency	Chemical results of Ca deficiency	Calcitriol 0.5–1.0 μg/d
	25-OH-D^3 normal	
	Calcitriol low	
Vitamin D present but ineffective		
Receptor defect	Phenotype (alopecia)	Calcitriol 10–30 μg/d
Nuclear translation defect	Chemical results of Ca deficiency	Parenteral Ca 1 g/d
	High calcitriol	
	Skin fibroblast cultures to differentiate receptor from nuclear translation defects	
Phosphorus deficiency		
Diet	Low serum P	Adjust formula or
(limited to very premature infants)	Radiographic signs of rickets	parenteral source to give 100 mg/kg/d
Antacid excess	History	Alternative gastric HCl
(aluminum hydroxide)	Low serum P	control (e.g., cimetidine)
Excessive phosphaturia from tubular dysfunction (calcitriol formation may also be deficient)	History	Supplement P and
	Low serum P	calcitriol[11] if low
Isolated, X-linked normocalciuric (common)	Urine Ca/Cr normal	Supplement P and
	Calcitriol normal	calcitriol
Isolated, recessive hypercalciuric (very rare[7])	History	Supplement P
	Urine Ca/Cr high	
	Calcitriol high	
With acidosis, glucosuria, and aminoaciduria alone (Fanconi syndrome) or the result of metal poisoning, fructose intolerance, tyrosinemia, galactosemia, cystinosis, or Wilson's disease	History	Supplement alkali, P and
	Urine and serum analysis (high serum chloride low serum bircarbonate)	calcitriol as indicated by serum analysis
Fanconi syndrome plus cerebral and eye defects (Lowe syndrome)	History	Same as for Fanconi
	Physical findings	syndrome
	Serum and urine analysis (same as for Fanconi syndrome)	
Tumors	Phosphaturia	Excision; if not feasible,
Mesenchymal[9]	Calcitriol *low* (mesenchymal	calcitriol and P
Sebaceous nevi[10]	tumors may be small	supplement
Neurofibromastosis	and cryptic)	

Key: BUN = blood urea nitrogen: CA = calcium; CaCO$_3$ = calcium carbonate: Cr = Creatinine; NaHCO$_3$ = sodium bicarbonate; P = phosphorus; 25-OH-D$_3$ = 25 hydroxyvitamin D; UV = ultraviolet.

Reference: From Bergstrom WH: Twenty ways to get rickets in the 1990s. Contemp Pediatr December:102–103, 1991, with permission.

S

SCROTUM

The Infant and Child with Acute Scrotum

The presentation of an infant or child with an enlarged, tender, and discolored scrotum is generally a call for alarm, both on the part of the patient and the physician. It is essential to diagnose quickly and correctly the patient with an acute scrotum to avoid irreversible testicular injury. This is particularly the case with the most common cause of acute scrotum in children, torsion of the testicle.

Many urologists recommend testicular radionucleotide scans and Doppler and scrotal ultrasound examinations to confirm the diagnosis of the acute scrotum. A simpler means to differentiate torsion from less threatening problems such as epididymitis and orchitis, however, is to test for the cremasteric reflex—the reflex is almost always absent in a patient with torsion (see also p. 304).

Causes of the Acute Scrotum

1. Testicular torsion
   a. Extravaginal torsion is found exclusively in neonates. It is caused by a twisting of the spermatic cord above the tunica vaginalis, thus cutting off the blood supply. Transillumination can be useful in distinguishing extravaginal torsion from hydrocele.
   b. Intravaginal torsion is a twisting of the testes within the tunica vaginalis. It can occur anytime in life but is most common in the prepubertal and postpubertal male.
2. Epididymitis
3. Torsion of testicular appendages yields localized tenderness at the upper pole of the testis or epididymis. A "blue-dot" sign is pathognomonic of this entity, representing the necrotic appendage beneath the skin.
4. Orchitis
5. Strangulated inguinal hernia
6. Idiopathic scrotal edema
7. Henoch-Schönlein purpura
8. Tumor
9. Trauma
10. Extrascrotal disease (e.g., intraabdominal sepsis and formation of a pyocele).

Reference: Hermann D: The pediatric acute scrotum. Pediatr Ann 18:198–204, 1989.

The Importance of the Cremasteric Reflex in Acute Scrotal Swelling in Children

The importance of accurate and rapid diagnosis of the acute scrotum cannot be overemphasized. There exists a wide variety of diagnostic modalities that have been reported to improve assessment and dictate which patient should undergo surgical exploration. The most valuable aid in differentiating testicular torsion (which requires rapid correction to avoid testicular damage) from other causes of acute scrotal swelling remains the presence or absence of the cremasteric reflex. (The testicles are suspended by the cremaster muscle [from the Greek *kremaster*, to hang]).

In a prospective study of 245 boys, from the newborn period to age 18; who presented with acute scrotal swelling, the presence of the cremasteric reflex (stroking the inner thigh to cause an elevation of the ipsilateral testis by contraction of the cremaster muscle) was the most reliable clinical finding in ruling out testicular torsion. The correlation between the presence of ipsilateral cremasteric reflex and the absence of testicular torsion was 100%. Absence of this reflex, therefore, should strongly increase your suspicion of torsion.

Cremasteric Reflex in Acute Scrotal Swelling

DIAGNOSIS	NO OF PTS	CREMASTERIC REFLEX	
		PRESENT	ABSENT
Testis torsion	56	0	56
Hydatid torsion	77	58	19
Epididymitis	47	31	16
Hernia/hydrocele	22	8	14
Trauma	22	19	3
Leukemia	5	0	5
Varicocele	4	4	0
Orchialgia	4	2	2
Idiopathic scrotal edema	3	1	2
Henoch-Schönlein purpura	3	1	2
Testis tumor	1	0	1
Insect bite	1	1	0
	245	125	120

Reference: Rabinavitz R: The importance of the cremasteric reflex in acute swelling in children. J Urol 132:89–90, 1984.

SEIZURES

Common Causes	Uncommon Causes	
Febrile seizures	CNS infection	CNS injury
Idiopathic seizures	Aseptic meningitis	Anoxic encephalopathy
	Bacterial meningitis	Child abuse
	Viral encephalitis	Concussion
		Hemorrhage
		Hypoglycemia

Rare Causes

CNS infection
  Congenital infection
  Parasitic infection
  Syphilis
  Tetanus
  Tuberculosis

Congenital CNS malformation
  Agenesis/dysgenesis
    Holoproscencephaly
    Porencephaly
  Hydrocephalus

Drugs/toxins
  Aminophylline
  Amphetamines
  Antihistamines
  Atropine
  Camphor
  Carbon monoxide
  Drug withdrawal
  Heavy metals
  Hexachlorophine
  Hydrocarbons
  Local anesthetics
  Narcotics
  Organophosphates
  Penicillin
  Pertussis toxoid
  Phencyclidine
  Scabicides
  Steroids
  Tricyclic antidepressants

Inborn errors of metabolism
  Aminoacidopathy
  Galactosemia
  Organic aciduria
  Storage disease

Metabolic
  Hypernatremia
  Hypocalcemia
  Hypomagnesemia
  Hyponatremia

Miscellaneous
  Arrhythmia
  Dysmorphogenic syndromes (many)
  Kernicterus
  Metachromatic leukodystrophy
  Pyridoxine deficiency

Miscellaneous *(Cont.)*
  Rett syndrome
  Reye's syndrome
  Subacute sclerosing
    panencephalitis

Neurocutaneous syndrome
  Incontinentia pigmenti
  Linear sebaceous nevus
  Neurofibromatosis
  Sturge-Weber disease
  Tuberous sclerosis

Seizure mimics
  Breathholding spells
  Hyperventilation
  Malingering
  Masturbation
  Migraine
  Myoclonus
  Narcolepsy
  Orthostatic hypotension
  Pallid infantile syncope
  Panic disorder
  Paroxysmal torticollis of infancy
  Pseudoseizures
  Sandifer's syndrome (gastro-
    esophageal reflux)
  Shivering on urination
  Shuddering attacks
  Sleep disorders
  Syncope
  Tics
  Vertigo

Systemic infection
  Roseola
  Shigella

Tumors

Vascular
  A-V malformation
  Embolic phenomenon
  Hemorrhage
  Hypertension
  Sickle-cell disease
  Thrombosis
  Vasculitis

Classification of Seizures and Epilepsy

Seizures and epilepsy are classified according to a scheme developed by the International League Against Epilepsy (ILAE). An abbreviated version of the classification is shown below:

Classification of Seizures and Epileptic Syndromes

Partial seizures
    Simple partial seizures (consciousness preserved)
        With motor signs (jacksonian, adversive)
        With somatosensory or special sensory symptoms
        With autonomic symptoms or signs
        With psychic symptoms
    Complex partial seizures (consciousness impaired)
        Simple partial onset followed by impaired consciousness
        Impaired consciousness at onset
    Secondarily generalized seizures
        Simple partial seizures evolving to generalized tonic-clonic seizures
    Complex partial seizures evolving to generalized tonic-clonic seizures
    Simple partial seizures evolving to complex partial seizures, then to
        generalized tonic-clonic seizures

Generalized-onset seizures
    Tonic-clonic seizures
    Absence seizures
    Atypical absence seizures
    Myoclonic seizures
    Tonic seizures
    Atonic seizures

Localization-related (focal) epilepsies
    Idiopathic
        Benign focal epilepsy of childhood
    Symptomatic
        Chronic progressive epilepsia
           partialis continua
        Temporal-lobe epilepsy
        Extratemporal epilepsy

Generalized epilepsy
    Idiopathic
        Benign neonatal convulsions
        Childhood absence epilepsy
        Juvenile myoclonic epilepsy
        Other generalized idiopathic
           epilepsy
    Cryptogenic or symptomatic
        West syndrome (infantile spasms)
        Early myoclonic encephalopathy
        Lennox-Gastaut syndrome
        Progressive myoclonic epilepsy

Special syndromes
    Febrile seizures

Reference: Scheuer ML, Pedley TA: The evaluation and treatment of seizures. N Engl J Med 323:1468–1474, 1990. Table reproduced from cited paper, with permission.

What Are the Criteria for Simple Febrile Seizure?

Age 6 months to 6 years
Generalized seizure (indicating involvement of both cerebral hemispheres) of less than 20 minutes duration
Occurs within 24 hours of fever onset

Normal results from neurologic and developmental examination
Negative family history of afebrile seizures

Reference: Schweich P: Emergency medicine except poisoning. In Oski FA, et al (eds): Principles and Practice of Pediatrics. Philadelphia, J.B. Lippincott, 1990, p 771.

To Treat or Not to Treat After a First Seizure?

Should the child receive antiepileptic drug therapy after a nonfebrile first seizure? This is a central and still controversial issue in the management of epilepsy. It begs the follow-up question, why treat seizures?

Seizures are treated mainly because of their psychosocial consequences. Children with epilepsy often have difficulty with interpersonal relationships and self-esteem, as well as vocational problems later in life. There are reports of slightly increased mortality in association with seizure disorders, but there is yet no proof that patients on medication have less mortality than untreated individuals. Because 25–41% of patients taking antiepileptic drugs have recurrent seizures, the effectiveness of antiepileptic drugs in preventing recurrence of seizures has also been questioned. Also, there is no evidence at this time that seizures beget further seizures.

So which children should be treated?

The decision to treat should be based on several factors, including:

> Age
> Type of seizure
> Frequency of seizures and time between
> Timing and circumstance of occurrence of seizures
> Risk of further occurrence
> Precipitating factors
> Risk of drug treatment (30% of patients have side-effects requiring
>   modification of therapy)
> Probable consequences of further seizures
> Probability of treatment success

The chance of having an additional seizure after the first is about 30% (range 16–62%), and the second seizure tends to occur within 12 months. In children with absence seizures, the occurrence is at the high end of the range. The chance of having an additional seizure after the second is 50–75%. Studies of predictors of seizure recurrence have reported that it is often possible to identify patients with a relatively low risk of seizure recurrence.

Although the final decision to treat or not to treat must be made individually for each patient, the following guidelines may be offered:

1. Treat a child who has experienced two or more tonic-clonic seizures.
2. Treat children who experience seizures that impair consciousness, such as absence and partial complex seizures, which tend to occur more often— sometimes daily—than the rare generalized tonic-clonic seizures and can impair function because of their frequency.

References: Scheuer ML, Pedley TA: The evaluation and treatment of seizures. N Engl J Med 323: 1468–1474, 1990.

Shinnar S, Berg AT, Moshe SL, et al: Risk of seizure recurrence following a first unprovoked seizure in childhood: A prospective study. Pediatrics 85:1067–1085, 1990.

van Donselaar CA, Geerts AT, Schimscheimer RJ: Idiopathic first seizure in adult life: Who should be treated? Br Med J 302:620–623, 1991.

Vining EPG, Freeman JM: Management of childhood seizures. In Asbury AK, et al: Diseases of the Nervous System. Philadelphia, W.B. Saunders, 1986, pp 1018–1032.

Hauser WA, Anderson VE, Loewenson RB, McRoberts SM: Seizure recurrence after a first unprovoked seizure. N Engl J Med 307:522–528, 1982.

SEXUALITY

Sexual Behavior in Children: What's Normal?

Questions frequently arise in the clinic surrounding the topics of sexuality and sexual behavior in children. More often than not, these questions reveal a great deal about the comfort level and value system parents attach to this developmental issue. To aid in this dialogue, listed below are the frequencies of a large variety of sexual behaviors noted among 880 preadolescent boys and girls (ages 2–12).

Frequency of Sexual Behaviors (Percent Endorsement)

NO.	ITEM (ABBREVIATEED)	OVERALL	2–6, BOYS	2–6, GIRLS	7–12, BOYS	7–12 GIRLS
10.	Puts mouth on sex parts	0.1	0.4	0.0	0.0	0.0
15.	Asks to engage in sex acts	0.4	1.2	0.0	0.0	0.6
7.	Masturbates with object	0.8	0.8	0.8	0.0	1.7
17.	Inserts objects in vagina/anus	0.9	0.0	2.8	0.0	0.6
9.	Imitates intercourse	1.1	0.8	0.4	2.4	1.1
14.	Sexual sounds	1.4	0.4	0.8	3.9	0.6
30.	French kisses	2.5	1.6	4.0	2.4	1.7
28.	Undresses other people	2.6	4.4	4.4	0.5	0.0
29.	Asks to watch explicit television	2.7	0.0	1.6	6.8	3.4
19.	Imitates sexual behavior with dolls	3.2	0.8	4.0	1.5	7.5
2.	Wants to be opposite sex	4.9	7.3	7.5	1.9	1.1
22.	Talks about sexual acts	5.7	2.4	2.8	9.2	10.3
1.	Dresses like opposite sex	5.8	6.0	9.5	3.4	2.9
8.	Touches others' sex parts	6.0	8.9	5.6	4.9	4.0
16.	Rubs body against people	6.7	8.5	8.3	4.4	4.6
31.	Hugs strange adults	7.3	6.5	14.3	2.4	4.0
32.	Shows sex parts to children	8.1	15.7	7.5	4.4	2.3
62.	Uses sexual words	8.8	4.8	1.2	19.9	12.1
33.	Overly aggressive, overly passive	10.4	8.1	17.5	6.3	8.6
27.	Talks flirtatiously	10.6	8.5	15.9	2.9	14.9
13.	Pretends to be opposite sex	13.0	16.9	20.6	2.9	8.0
4.	Masturbates with hand	15.3	22.6	16.3	11.2	8.6
21.	Looks at nude pictures	15.5	11.3	7.9	27.2	18.4
20.	Shows sex parts to adults	16.0	25.8	17.9	9.7	6.9
3.	Touches sex parts in public	19.7	35.5	19.0	15.5	2.9
34.	Interested in opposite sex	23.0	21.0	20.6	19.9	32.8
18.	Tries to look at people undressing	28.5	33.9	33.3	27.7	14.9
6.	Touches breasts	30.7	43.5	48.4	11.7	9.2
26.	Kisses nonfamily children	33.9	41.1	55.2	9.7	21.3
23.	Kisses nonfamily adults	36.2	41.1	52.4	18.9	26.4
25.	Sits with crotch exposed	36.4	35.1	59.1	15.5	29.9
24.	Undresses in front of others	41.2	49.6	61.9	21.4	23.0
11.	Touches sex parts at home	45.8	64.1	54.4	36.4	18.4
5.	Scratches crotch	52.2	58.1	67.9	40.8	34.5
35.	Boy-girl toys	53.9	63.3	71.4	30.6	42.5
	Additional items (Dec-Jan)					
42.	Touches animal sex parts	1.3	4.5	0.0	0.0	0.0
37.	Mouth on mother's breast	2.6	0.0	7.7	0.0	0.0

Table continued on next page.

Frequency of Sexual Behaviors (Percent Endorsement) (Cont.)

NO.	ITEM (ABBREVIATEED)	OVERALL	2–6, BOYS	2–6, GIRLS	7–12, BOYS	7–12 GIRLS
40.	Overly friendly with strange men	7.1	4.5	11.5	2.9	8.0
36.	Stands too close	11.6	6.8	15.4	14.7	8.0
41.	Shy about undressing	38.7	29.5	32.7	50.0	52.0
43.	Walks around nude	41.9	47.7	65.4	20.6	12.0
38.	Walks around in underwear	52.9	54.5	75.0	44.1	16.0
39.	Shy with strange men	64.5	63.6	80.8	47.1	56.0

Reference: Friedrich WN, et al: Normative sexual behavior in children. Pediatrics 88:456–464, 1991, with permission.

SHORT STATURE

Use of Bone Age Determination in the Diagnosis of Short Stature

The cause for short stature may often be determined by careful history and physical examination. Nutritional or emotional deprivation, chronic disease, or a history of short stature in other family members may provide an explanation for decreased height. Facial appearance may suggest a genetic or chromosomal abnormality. Organ enlargement may lead to a diagnosis of a storage disease.

Often, however, the diagnosis is not readily apparent. In these cases, it is helpful to begin with a comparison of skeletal maturation (bone age) to height age and chronologic age. The table lists the diagnoses that should be suggested by such a comparison, and the clinical features accompanying each diagnosis.

Comparison of Bone Age to Height Age and Chronologic Age

MEASUREMENT	DIAGNOSIS SUGGESTED	CLINICAL FEATURES
Bone age equal to or slightly behind chronologic age	Primordial short stature	Birth weight and length below normal for gestational age. Subsequent growth parallel to, but below, 3rd percentile. Normal onset and progression of puberty. Minor skeletal abnormalities. Includes genetic and chromosomal aberrations, e.g., Down's syndrome and Turner's syndrome. Short stature as adult.
	Familial short stature	Normal length and weight for first 1 to 2 years of life. Height falls below 3rd percentile at 5 to 10 years of age. Puberty not delayed. "Normal" adult height not attained.

Table continued on next page.

Comparison of Bone Age to Height Age and Chronologic Age (Cont.)

MEASUREMENT	DIAGNOSIS SUGGESTED	CLINICAL FEATURES
Bone age retarded in relation to chronologic age, but less retarded than height age	Constitutional short stature	Appropriate weight and length for gestational age at birth. Slow growth during childhood. Delayed onset of puberty. Other family members may remember similar growth pattern. Important to differentiate from hypothyroidism and growth hormone deficiency. Ultimately reach "normal" adult height.
	Metabolic disorders, e.g.: Hypophosphatemic rickets Hypophosphatasia Mucopolysaccharidoses Glycogen storage diseases Renal tubular acidosis Bartter's syndrome Vasopressin-resistant diabetes insipidus	Clinical and laboratory findings consistent with these disorders.
	Organic acidemias and acidurias Hemolytic anemias Disorders of mineral metabolism Immunoglobulin or white blood cell abnormality Others	Clinical and laboratory findings consistent with these disorders.
	Chronic disease, e.g.: Chronic infection Hepatic disease Pulmonary disease Renal disease Malabsorption Malignancy Collagen vascular disease Others	Clinical and laboratory findings consistent with the disease; initial clue may be increased erythrocyte sedimentation rate. May exhibit variable growth rate over several years.
Bone age equal to or advanced in comparison with height age	Familial short stature	See above.

Table continued on next page.

Comparison of Bone Age to Height Age and Chronologic Age (Cont.)

MEASUREMENT	DIAGNOSIS SUGGESTED	CLINICAL FEATURES
Bone age equal to or advanced in comparison with height age *(Cont.)*	Sexual precocity with androgen excess	Increased linear growth early in life with early closure of epiphyses. Clinical signs of androgen excess (facial, axillary, and pubic hair, penile or clitoral enlargement).
	Sexual precocity with estrogen excess	Early closure of epiphyses without prior augmentation of linear growth. Clinical signs of estrogen excess (breast enlargement, galactorrhea in females, and so on).
Bone age greatly decreased and less than or equal to height age	Hypothyroidism	Degree of growth retardation depends upon age of onset. Congenital hypothyroidism is associated with severe growth failure. In juvenile hypothyroidism, the growth retardation is more insidious. Delayed dental age.
	Cushing's syndrome (most often iatrogenic)	Truncal obesity, moon facies, violaceous striae, hirsutism, muscle weakness, hypertension.
	Hypopituitarism and growth hormone deficiency. Causes include: Congenital absence of pituitary Infection Reticuloendothelioses Vascular infarcts and anomalies Trauma Irradiation Surgical resection Malnutrition	Delayed dental age. Puberty often delayed. May have neurologic abnormalities.
	Maternal deprivation	May have impaired motor and intellectual development. May or may not be associated with malnutrition. May have growth hormone deficiency.

Reference: Gotlin RW, Mace JW: Diagnosis and management of short stature in childhood and adolescence. Curr Probl Pediatr 2:4, 1972.

SHWACHMAN'S SYNDROME

Pancreatic Insufficiency and Neutropenia

When Shwachman's syndrome was first described in 1964, the hallmarks of this rare entity were exocrine pancreatic insufficiency, bone marrow hypoplasia and associated neutropenia, metaphyseal chondroplasia, growth retardation, and recurrent soft tissue infections. Since that initial case report, many more manifestations of Shwachman's syndrome have been elaborated and described. These protean features of the disorder are listed in the table below.

The exact pathogenic basis for the hematologic and other features of this multisystem illness has yet to be determined, although some have hypothesized that the basic defect of the Shwachman syndrome may lie in the function of the microtubular and microfilament elements of many different cell types in the body. The relative contributions of impaired cellular motility, instead of neutropenia, to these patients' increased susceptibility toward infections is also unclear.

Features Associated with Shwachman's Syndrome

Exocrine pancreatic insufficiency	Neonatal problems
Steatorrhea	Poor feeding, respiratory
Growth retardation	distress
Skeletal abnormalities	Psychomotor retardation
Metaphyseal dyschondroplasia, delayed	Hypotonia
maturation, rib abnormalities, long	Hepatomegaly
bone tubulation, clinodactyly	Raised SGOT and SGPT
Narrow thorax	Renal tubular dysfunction
Hematologic abnormalities	Ichthyosis
Bone marow hypoplasia, neutropenia,	Dental abnormalities
thrombocytopenia, raised HbF,	Delayed puberty
lymphoproliferative and myelo-	Diabetes mellitus
proliferative neoplasia	Dysmorphic features
Recurrent infections	Endocardial fibrosis
Defective neutrophil mobility	Hirschsprung's disease

References: Shwachman H, Diamond LK, Oski FA, Khow KT: The syndrome of pancreatic insufficiency and bone marrrow dysfunction. J Pediatr 65:645, 1964.

Aggett PJ, Cavanagh NPC, Matthew DJ, et al: Shwachman's syndrome: A review of 21 cases. Arch Dis Child 55:331, 1980.

Anderson DC, et al: Quantitative and functional disorders of granulocytes. In Oski FA, et al (eds): Principles and Practice of Pediatrics. Philadelphia, J.B. Lippincott, 1990, p 1535.

SINUSES

The Paranasal Sinuses and the Mastoid Sinus

At what age does sinusitis become a diagnostic possibility?

It is useful to remember the ages at which the sinuses are pneumatized. Once a true sinus is present, the possibility of infection exists.

Sinuses present at birth	Anterior and posterior **ethmoid.**
	Maxillary antra.

| Two to four years | Pneumatization of **frontal** sinsuses begins—complete by 5 to 9 years of age. **Sphenoid** sinus becomes visible by age 3. |

The **mastoid antrum** is present at birth, and pneumatization of the temporal bone starts in early infancy. The **mastoid process** is not present at birth, but begins to grow during the first year. Pneumatization is a slow, irregular process, but is generally complete prior to adolescence.

Sinusitis is seen with increased frequency in patients with cyanotic heart disease, in leukemia and aplastic anemia while patients are neutropenic, in cystic fibrosis, and in patients with a history of nasal allergies.

Reference: McMillan JA, et al (eds): The Whole Pediatrician Catalog. Philadelphia, W.B. Saunders, 1977, pp 190–191, with permission.

SKIN SIGNS

Tache Cérébrale and Dermatographia

Diagnostic information can be obtained from stroking the skin. When the skin over the abdomen, back, or chest is gently stroked with the fingernail or a blunted point, two major responses may be elicited: (1) tache cérébrale and (2) dermatographia.

In tache cérébrale (cerebral spot), the stroking produces a red streak that is flanked by thin, pale margins. This sign develops within 30 seconds of stroking and persists for several minutes. It has been noted to be present in patients with scarlet fever, hydrocephalus, a variety of febrile illnesses, and, most particularly, in meningitis. It can be used as an early clue to the presence of meningitis, particularly in the neonatal period. The French name derives from the presence of the sign as a concomitant of several nervous (or "cerebral") diseases.

Dermatographia, meaning literally "writing on the skin," is the marking of the skin by rubbing with a blunted point at sufficient pressure. The stroking produces a white or pale line with red margins. This wheal is seen in patients with fair skin, in those with vasomotor instability, or in extreme form in patients with urticaria pigmentosa (Darier's sign). Dermatographism, the tendency to show dermatographia, is present in 2–5% of the population, but only a subgroup has symptomatic dermatographism, one of the physical urticarias.

Reference: Martin GI: The significance of tâche cérébrale in neonatal meningitis (letter). J Pediatr 87:322, 1975.

SLEEPING PATTERNS

Crying, Feeding, and Sleeping Patterns in Infants 1 to 12 Months of Age

What is normal crying time, feeding time, or sleeping time for infants? Mothers often are concerned or complain that their baby is abnormal. With the following guidelines you can either reassure them or be alerted to a possible problem.

Mothers who feel a need for additional help generally have babies that cry for more than 6 hours per day, take more than 6.0 hours to feed, and spend less than 7 hours sleeping.

Mean Times for Infant Activities

ACTIVITY	MEAN TIMES IN HOURS (WITH RANGES)			
	< 3 Mo	3–5 Mo	6–8 Mo	> 9 Mo
Crying	1.6 (0–5.0)	1.3 (0–9.5)	1.4 (0–3.0)	1.1 (0–3.5)
Feeding	3.1 (1.0–6.8)	2.4 (1.3–5.3)	2.0 (1.0–3.8)	2.1 (0.8–4.5)
Sleeping	15.2 (11.8–20.5)	14.3 (10.0–18.5)	13.5 (10.3–17.8)	13.4 (10.3–16.0)

Reference: Michelsson K, et al: Child Care Health Dev 16:99–111, 1990.

SNAKE BITE

Is This a Poisonous Snake Bite?

This question is posed to physicians in offices and emergency rooms several thousand times a year in this country. A correct and prompt answer is essential for proper treatment. Failure to use antivenom early when indicated can be fatal; its inappropriate employment for a bite by a harmless snake may be hazardous due to severe reactions.

The problem has two parts. First, was the bite due to a harmless or a poisonous snake? Second, if the snake was venomous, is envenomation present or likely? The question may be resolved by examination of the snake so that it may be put in the category of either a venomous or a nonvenomous variety and by examination of the patient to determine if venomation has occurred. Basic dependable guidelines for attaining both these goals will be outlined. They may be used by the amateur who has no knowledge of serpents at all. This discussion applies only to those snakes that are *native to the continental United States* and does not relate to foreign species introduced into this country as pets or exhibits.

Examination of the Snake

One should not attempt to identify the exact species, since this is often a challenge for even the genuine expert due to pitfalls involving confusing color variate (albinism and malanism) and deceptive patterns (atypical or absent). Undue delay may result by waiting to locate an available herpetologist in a nearby zoo, museum, or zoology department. One should instead inspect the snake and, from the guidelines provided, assign it to the harmless or harmful group. The problem is somewhat simplified since in the mainland United States there are only two families of indigenous poisonous serpents.

Crotalidae.   These are the pit vipers, which include all rattlesnakes, cotton-mouths (water moccasin), and copperheads (highland moccasin). One or more of this family has been found in all states, with the exception of Maine, Alaska, and Hawaii. The head is large and triangular. The neck is relatively slender, so that it is readily distinguishable from the thick, heavy body. The pupil is vertically elliptical. Pit organs (loreal pits) are pathognomonic of all members of this group. A pit is present on each side of the head, and it resembles an extra nostril. The pits are deep, readily visible between the eye and the nostril, and located just below a line connecting these two structures. One or two fangs are found on the upper jaw of all pit vipers. They are specialized hollow or grooved teeth, which are recurved and longer than the other teeth. It is through these that the venom is injected. In this family the fangs are movable and when not in use are folded up against the palate. A white membrane may cover the fang down to the tip. Normally there are two fangs in the upper jaw—one on each side of the maxilla— so the classic bite pattern shows two fang punctures. However, one or both may be broken off or shed, in which instance there may be only a single fang mark present or none at all. *No envenomation is possible if fangs are absent.* Reserve fangs are always present, so the missing fang is replaced soon. Rarely, one or two reserve fangs may be functioning along with the customary complement of one or two fangs. In such a circumstance the bite pattern will be atypical, demonstrating three or four fang punctures.

Herpetologists identify species by meticulous scale counts of the head, neck, body, and tail. For practical purposes one may observe the scales (scutes, shields, plates) on the ventral surface of the body just posterior to the anus (subcaudal scales). In this family the subcaudal scales are usually arranged in a single row, but exceptions occur in which the rows are double. In the majority of harmless snakes the subcaudal scales are double, but this is not infallible either since exceptions are found. Rattles, of course, are specific for rattlesnakes and are not present in the copperhead, cottonmouth, other venomous species, or harmless snakes. They break off because of wear and tear, or during ecdysis (molting), so the number is inconstant regardless of the age of the reptile. If all rattles have been lost or if the specimen is a baby that has not yet developed rattles, there will be a slight enlargement at the tip of the tail known as the button. Other poisonous snakes do not show a button, nor do nonvenomous species. Also, the end of the tail of a rattlesnake that has lost its rattles is short and blunt, whereas the tip of the tail of a harmless snake is usually gradually tapered.

Elapidae. This family is represented in this country only by the coral snake. Unlike the pit vipers the coral snake is restricted to the southern states and is generally not found north of Arizona, Arkansas, or the Carolinas. Compared to the rattlesnakes and moccasins, the head is narrow and the neck and body are slender, giving a cylindrical configuration which is quite different from the shape of the pit vipers. The pupil is circular, thus resembling that of our indigenous harmless varieties. Pit organs are not present. Two fangs are present—one on each side of the maxilla (unless one or both have been shed). They are erect, fixed, and smaller than those of the pit vipers. Subcaudal scales tend to be in a double row similar to those of nonvenomous snakes, but rarely may be in a single row in the coral snake. Both rattles and tail button are absent. The coral snake is an exception to the general rule of not trying species identification, since there are confusing imitators that are harmless. Fortunately the nonvenomous mimics are easy to differentiate from the potent coral snake. The coral snake has a black snout and broad body rings of red and black that are separated by a narrower band of yellow. The mnemonic "red next to yellow kills a fellow" is helpful to keep in mind. The harmless look-alikes (scarlet snake, scarlet king snake) show a grey or red snout and red and yellow rings that are separated by a black band. Here the mnemonic to remember is "red against black is venom lack."

Summary of Family Characteristics—Native Harmless Versus Native Venomous Snakes in the Continental United States

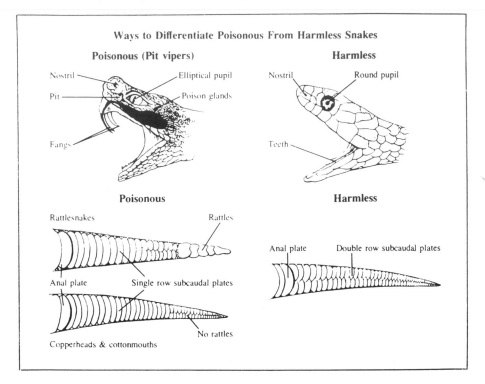

Nonvenomous Versus Venomous Characteristics of Continental U.S. Snakes

NONVENOMOUS		VENOMOUS
Oval	Head	Large and triangular (pit vipers); small and narrow (coral snake)
Round	Pupils	Vertically elliptical (pit vipers); round (coral snake)
Absent	Pit organs	Present in all pit vipers (copperhead, cottonmouth, rattlesnakes); absent in coral snake
Absent	Fangs	Present in all venomous species. Large, long, recurved teeth. Long and movable in pit vipers. Short, erect, and fixed in coral snake. Usually 2 (1 on each side upper jaw) unless shed or reserve fangs also in use
Double row usually, but exceptions	Subcaudal scales (anus to tip of tail)	Single row in pit vipers, but with exceptions; double row in coral snake, but exceptions
Absent	Rattles	Present in all rattlesnakes unless lost or undeveloped in baby. If missing a button, present at tip of tail. No rattles in other venomous species or in harmless snakes

Table continued on next page.

Nonvenomous Versus Venomous Characteristics
of Continental U.S. Snakes (Cont.)

NONVENOMOUS		VENOMOUS
Usually ends in gradual taper	Tip of tail	Short and blunt in rattlesnake if rattles lost
	Bite pattern (seldom perfect)	
Total of 6 with no fang marks; four rows maxillary teeth and 2 rows mandibular teeth	Number of rows	Total of 4 with 1–2 fang marks (rarely 3–4 if reserve fangs functional). Two rows with fang marks from maxillary teeth. Two rows without fang marks from mandibular teeth
Series scratches or tiny punctures (1–2 mm deep); pattern of mandibular teeth often imperfect	Appearance	Series scratches or tiny punctures (1–2 mm deep) plus fang marks. Fang marks recognizable as larger and deeper punctures than those from nonfang teeth. Mandibular teeth often indistinct

Examination of the Patient

This is to determine if envenomation has taken place. If it has occurred, immediate vigorous therapy is required. If the snake was not captured, presence or absence of envenomation will be the sole criterion available for deciding if the snake was harmless or poisonous. Verbal descriptions of escaped snakes are generally unreliable. The bite pattern is helpful and may be diagnostic as indicated earlier, but it does not indicate if envenomation has in fact occurred. Even though the victim has been struck by a venomous serpent, envenomation may not ensue. This is the result of various circumstances that influence the flow of venom, the amount of venom injected, and the toxicity of the venom. Evaluation of envenomation depends on the development of local and systemic symptoms and signs. The following are the usual clinical effects which may appear after injection of a sufficient amount of a potent venom.

Local Symptoms and Signs. The two P's (puncture and pain) and the two E's (edema and erythema) constitute the classic local reaction to deposition of a potent venom in the tissues. At least two should be present to substantiate the diagnosis.

I. **Puncture:** One or two fang marks are present (rarely three or four if reserve fangs in use). These punctures are larger and deeper than those from the other teeth. A wheal or vesicle may develop at the site. If at least one fang mark is not present, then envenomation could not have taken place. Bleeding is usually brisk.

II. **Pain:** Usually develops within 5 to 10 minutes of the strike. It may be delayed up to an hour under certain conditions and may be lacking with a coral snake bite. In a classic case of moderate to severe envenomation involving a pit viper, the pain appears promptly and is severe and unremitting.

III. **Edema:** Typically obvious within 5 to 10 minutes. It also may be delayed up to an hour or absent with a coral snake bite. The swelling may progress up the limb during the next 36 hours and eventually reach the trunk. The overlying skin becomes tense and shiny. The extent of the edema is one of the criteria used in the clinical grading of the severity of envenomation for assessing the amount of antivenom required and for monitoring the progress of the case.

IV. **Erythema:** Redness is ordinarily visible within 5 to 10 minutes. It may not appear for an hour and may be absent after a bite by a coral snake. Later, other types of discoloration develop with pit viper bites as hemorrhages occur in the tissues. Eventually some blueness usually follows unlike the typical reaction to a severe insect bite.

NOTE: Exceptions in the time of appearance and number of these four cardinal signs occur in some pit viper bites owing to variability of potency and amount of venom injected. Also in the event of a fortuitous strike directly into a vessel, there may be absence of local manifestations along with the rapid appearance of systemic signs. Local signs may be missing with coral snake bites owing to the predominance of neurotoxin over hemotoxin.

V. **Hemorrhage:** Petechiae and ecchymoses commonly occur, particularly with pit viper bites. Oozing from fang marks often continues for several hours. This is in contradistinction to the wounds from nonfang teeth, which cease bleeding promptly with both poisonous and nonpoisonous species.

VI. **Paresthesias:** Numbness and/or tingling frequently are noted at the bite site and around the mouth.

VII. **Late local signs:** Tissue necrosis and thrombosis may develop, with sloughing of tissues and gangrene of the extremities. This type of response is common with pit vipers but less so with coral snakes due to the difference in the venoms. Localized lymphadenopathy is a feature in some.

Systemic Symptoms and Signs. These are produced by the hematogenous or lymphogenous dissemination of the venom. Some of the toxins have enzymatic activity. Owing to the multiplicity of the effects of these diverse protein molecules, the clinical manifestations are numerous and protean. A consistent clinical picture may not be present.

I. **General:** Lassitude, weakness, fatigue, nonwhirling dizziness, diaphoresis, sialorrhea, and the sensation of a "full" or "thick" tongue.

II. **Pulmonic:** Edema, respiratory failure, and death.

III. **Cardiac:** Hypotension, congestive failure, cardiac arrest, and death.

IV. **Renal:** Hematuria, proteinuria, azotemia, and renal failure with death.

V. **Gastrointestinal:** Nausea, emesis, hematemesis, and melena.

VI. **Hematologic:** Alterations of the coagulation system, with petechiae, ecchymoses, bleeding into subcutaneous and muscle tissues, hemorrhages into viscera, and bloody effusions into serous cavities. Laboratory determinations may demonstrate prolonged prothrombin time, thrombocytopenia, fibrinolysis, and prolonged bleeding and clotting times. Epistaxis, hematuria, hematemesis, and melena are common with severe envenomation.

VII. **Central nervous system:** Headache, blurred vision, paresthesias, slurred speech, bulbar palsies, generalized convulsions, and paralyses of the extremities. Deep tendon reflexes are variable. The sensorium typically remains intact, with a lucid and oriented patient. Sometimes somnolence may be a feature, and occasionally euphoria is present if the individual has been dosed with the traditional snake bite remedy, whiskey. Disorientation and states bordering on delirium and mania may occur in some victims owing to the hysteria and snake phobia seen in some adults following exposure to a serpent.

VIII. **Death:** Fatalities are due to respiratory failure, cardiac decompensation, renal shutdown, hemorrhage, or irreversible shock.

The physician who has no knowledge of snakes can render an intelligent decision about a snake bite by following the guidelines given regarding inspection of the snake, observation of the bite pattern, and examination of the patient. Irrefutable proof of the poisonous nature of a snake native to the continental United States includes the presence of fangs, pit organs, rattles, and a vertically elliptical pupil. All of these are present in the pit vipers (rattlesnakes, copperheads, and cottonmouth moccasins). The coral snake lacks the pit organs and rattles and has a circular pupil. Otherwise, all indigenous snakes with a round pupil are harmless. Fang marks are diagnostic of a venomous species and are larger and deeper than the scratches or superficial punctures produced by the nonfang teeth. If the patient shows pain, puncture, edema, and erythema, envenomation has taken place. These local signs appear within an hour of the bite, and systemic signs develop later. Local manifestations may be absent with coral snake bite, in which case generalized signs and symptoms develop rapidly.

Specially prepared by Dr. William D. Alsever, Syracuse, New York. (From McMillan JA, et al (eds): The Whole Pediatrician Catalog, Vol. 2. Philadelphia, W.B. Saunders, 1979, with permission.)

References:
Conant R: A Field Guide to Reptile and Amphibians of Eastern and Central North America. New York, Houghton-Mifflin, 1975.
Dept. of the Navy, Bureau of Medicine and Surgery; Poisonous Snakes of the World: A Manual for Use by the U.S. Amphibious Forces. Washington, D.C., U.S. Government Printing Office, 1968.
Stickel, WH: Venomous Snakes of the United States and Treatment of their Bites. Wildlife leaflet 339. Washington, D.C., U.S. Department of the Interior, Fish and Wildlife Service, 1952.
Pope, CH, and Perkins, RM: Differences in the patterns of venomous and harmless snake bites. Arch Surg 49:331, 1944.
Parrish HM, et al: Snake bite: A pediatric problem. Clin Pediatr 4:237, 1965.
Snyder R: Snake bite seminar. Am J Dis Child 103:117, 1962.
Russell, FE, et al: Snake venom poisoning: Experiences with 550 cases. JAMA 233.341, 1975.
Glass TG Jr: Snake bite. Hosp Med Am J Dis Child, July, 1971, p 31.
Parrish HM, et al: Snake bite: Poisonous until proven otherwise. Patient Care, May 30, 1971, p 76.
Russell FE: Injuries by Venomous Animals. National Clearinghouse for Poison Control Centers, Bulletin for Jan–Feb, 1967. Washington, D.C., U.S. Department of Health Education and Welfare, 1967.
Arnold RE: What To Do about Bites and Stings of Venomous Animals. New York, Collier Books, 1973.

Other readings:
Auerbach PS, Geehr EC: Management of Wilderness and Environmental Emergencies, 2nd ed. St. Louis, C.V. Mosby, 1989.
Boyer Hassen L: Reptile and arthropod envenomations. Occup Med State Art Rev 6:447–461, 1991.
Kitchens CS: Envenomation by the Eastern coral snake: A study of 39 victims. JAMA 258:1615–1618, 1987.
Klauber LM: Rattlesnakes: Their Habits, Life Histories, and Influence on Mankind, abridged edition. Berkeley, CA, University of California Press, 1982.
Pennell TC: The management of snake and spider bite in the southeastern United States. Am Surgeon 53:198–204, 1987.

Russell FE, Banner W: Snake venom poisoning. In Rakel RE: Conn's Current Therapy. Philadelphia, W.B. Saunders, 1988, pp 1002–1005.

Stewart RM, et al: Antivenin and fasciotomy/debridement in the treatment of the severe rattlesnake bite. Am J Surgery 158:543–547, 1989.

Tu AT: Rattlesnake Venoms: Their Action and Treatment. New York, Marcel Dekker, 1982.

Wingert WA, Chan L: Rattlesnake bites in Southern California and rationale for recommended treatment. West J Med 148:37–44, 1988.

SODIUM: HYPERNATREMIA

Hypernatremia is defined here as a serum sodium level higher than 145 mEq/L.

Common Causes

Diarrhea
High environmental
    temperatures

Uncommon Causes

Nephrogenic diabetes insipidus
Postobstructive diuresis
Salt poisoning
Sickle-cell nephropathy

Rare Causes

Cushing's disease
Hypercalcemia
    nephropathy

SODIUM: HYPONATREMIA

Hyponatremia is defined here as a sodium level lower than 130 mEq/L.

Common Causes

Diarrhea
Excessive salt-free infusions
Syndrome of inappropriate
    ADH secretion (SIADH)
Water intoxication

Uncommon Causes

Acute renal failure
Chronic renal failure
Congestive heart failure
High environmental
    temperatures

Rare Causes

Adrenal insufficiency
Cirrhosis
Cystic fibrosis and excessive sweating

SPLENOMEGALY

Common Causes

Acute infections (bacterial, viral, rickettsial, protozoal, spirochetal, myobacterial)
Congenital hemolytic anemias
    Hemoglobinopathies
    Hereditary spherocytosis
    Thalassemia major; thalassemia intermedia

Uncommon Causes

Congestive splenomegaly
Cyanotic congenital heart disease
Hodgkin's disease
Juvenile rheumatoid arthritis

Leukemia
Lupus erythematosus
Non-Hodgkin's disease
Severe iron-deficiency

Rare Causes

Acquired autoimmune hemolytic anemia
Amyloidosis
Beckwith-Wiedemann syndrome
Brucellosis
Chronic granulomatous disease
Congenital erythropoietic prophyria
Dysgammaglobulinemia
Hemophagocytic syndromes
Histiocytosis
Hurler's syndrome and other
   mucopolysaccharide disorders

Malaria (in the United States)
Metastatic neuroblastoma
Myelofibrosis
Osteopetrosis
Sarcoidosis
Serum sickness
Splenic cyst or hemangioma
Storage disease (e.g. Gaucher's,
   Neimann-Pick)
Wolman's disease

THE SPOILED CHILD SYNDROME

The pediatrician is called upon to wear many hats. One of the more difficult roles is counselor to the parent concerned about a "spoiled" child. The concept demands differentiation between normal behavior patterns and the excessive self-centeredness that marks the spoiled child. The cause of the spoiled child syndrome is often not a lack of discipline by the parents, but a lack of consistent limit-setting.

Age-Related Normal Behavior Pattern

The Crying Infant. Brazelton's time-honored study of crying in infancy (*Pediatrics* 29:579–588, 1962) indicated that the average infant cried 2¼ hours per day for the first 7 weeks of life. Whether due to hunger, colic, or want of attention, the infant's cry represents a genuine need to which the parent ought to be encouraged to respond. After 3 to 4 months of age, a cry may become a manipulation demanding modification techniques on the part of the parent.

The Exploring Toddler. As the infant discovers his or her mobility, curiosity becomes infinite. The "search and destroy" or "baby taste test" activities can frighten or aggravate the most equanimitous parent. An understanding of this stage as a normal part in development will help the parent to "child proof" the home and to begin the process of setting limits for the child.

The Terrible Two's. As the child approaches 2 years of age, his sense of autonomy is beginning to emerge. This is often the time that conflicts between the parent and the newly assertive child begin. The characteristic independence and resistance to parental authority can be dampened by a variety of techniques. One way to avoid confrontation is to offer the child choices within the parent's limits. Thus, both the parent and the emerging individual maintain a sense of control.

As with most human behaviors, those of the normal child are on a continuum with those labelled disruptive or spoiled. The family environment, the presence of stressors, and the individual's inherent coping abilities can shift the balance. In the absence of childhood handicaps or family stresses, such as separation and divorce, parental alcoholism, or parental mental illness, there are certain behavior patterns that do not fit any but the "spoiled" category. In these cases, the parent needs both guidance and assurance that the setting of consistent limits and appropriate punishments for infractions can be effective.

Behavior Patterns Suggestive of True Spoiling

Trained Night Feeding.   Beal's 1969 study on night feeding concluded that by 4 months of age, 95% of infants should sleep through the night without a feeding. The older infant who continues to cry for a 2 A.M. meal is often the child of caring parents who have attended every cry with a breast or bottle. Failure to break the snacking cycle and use cuddling or a pacifier can lead to the development of spoiling.

Trained Night Crying.   As with trained night feeding, trained night crying represents the infant's training of the parent. The new parent in particular is loathe to leave a crying infant in bed. But here, as with other infant behaviors, the "need" has to be distinguished from the "want" if the parent desires rest. A helpful hint might be placing the infant in his or her crib while still awake with an assurance that 10 to 15 minutes of crying is part of the infant's own settling mechanism. Trained responsiveness from the parent can diminish the baby's own ability to achieve sleep.

Recurrent Temper Tantrums.   A tantrum is a "fit of bad temper" representing both anger and frustration. They generally surface in the toddler who is attempting to assert independence and can be a frightening spectacle for the parent. Tantrums, like limitations, are occasionally inevitable. If the tantrum is rewarded by the loosening of restrictions, it is apt to recur. Reassure the parents that though the desire to please their child may be strong, ignoring the tantrum will likely bring this behavior to an end without harming the child. With tantrums, as with other disruptive behaviors, a little anticipatory guidance can go a long way.

The Toddler Who Is Out of Control.   This is often a child whose parents have "tried everything" to modify the kicking, biting, refusals to eat, sleep, or toilet train. If the modifications have been inconsistent, so will be the responses. Instruction in the use of "time out" and the importance of its regular use should help the troubled parents. Remind the parents that the un-training of disruptive behaviors will not be miraculous and will require patience, but that with continued enforcement, they will be successful.

In summary, the parents of the unruly child need guidance and support. It is probably best not to label a child "spoiled" but to stress the normal behavior patterns of children at various ages and to offer solutions for avoiding or correcting disruptive behaviors. By emphasizing consistency and de-emphasizing worry you can help the parents learn the effectiveness of limits.

Reference: McIntosh BJ: Spoiled Child Syndrome. Pediatrics 83:108–115, 1989.

SPORTS

What Are the Guidelines for Disqualifying Conditions for Sports Participation?

In 1988 the American Academy of Pediatrics published new guidelines for participation in competitive sports, which are summarized in the tables below:

Classification of Athletic Events According to Probability for Contact and Degree of Strenuousness

CONTACT/ COLLISION	LIMITED CONTACT/IMPACT	NONCONTACT		
		Strenuous	Moderately Strenuous	Nonstrenuous
Boxing	Baseball	Aerobic dancing	Badminton	Archery
Field hockey	Basketball	Crew	Curling	Golf
Football	Bicycling	Fencing	Table tennis	Riflery
Ice hockey	Diving	Field		
Lacrosse	Field	Discus		
Martial arts	High jump	Javelin		
Rodeo	Pole vault	Shot put		
Soccer	Gymnastics	Running		
Wrestling	Horseback rising	Swimming		
	Skating	Tennis		
	Ice	Track		
	Roller	Weight lifting		
	Skiing			
	Cross-country			
	Downhill			
	Water			
	Softball			
	Squash, handball			
	Volleyball			

Reprinted with permission from *Pediatrics*, May 1988; 81:5. Copyright ©1988 American Academy of Pediatrics.

Recommendations for Participation in Competitive Sports

	CONTACT/ COLLISION	LIMITED CONTACT/ IMPACT	NONCONTACT		
			Strenuous	Moderately Strenuous	Nonstrenuous
Atlantoaxial instability * Swimming: no butterfly, breast stroke, or diving starts.	No	No	Yes*	Yes	Yes
Acute illness * Needs individual assessment, e.g., contagiousness to others, risk of worsening illness.	*	*	*	*	*
Cardiovascular					
Carditis	No	No	No	No	No
Hypertension					
Mild	Yes	Yes	Yes	Yes	Yes
Moderate	*	*	*	*	*
Severe	*	*	*	*	*
* Needs individual assessment.					

Table continued on next page.

Recommendations for Participation in Competitive Sports (Cont.)

	CONTACT/ COLLISION	LIMITED CONTACT/ IMPACT	NONCONTACT Strenuous	NONCONTACT Moderately Strenuous	NONCONTACT Nonstrenuous
Cardiovascular *(Cont.)*					
Congenital heart disease	†	†	†	†	†
† Patients with mild forms can be allowed a full range of physical activities; patients with moderate or severe forms, or who are postoperative, should be evaluated by a cardiologist before athletic participation.					
Eyes					
Absence or loss of function					
of one eye	*	*	*	*	*
Detached retina	†	†	†	†	†
* Availability of American Society for Testing and Materials (ASTM)-approved eye guards may allow competitor to participate in most sports, but this must be judged on an individual basis.					
† Consult ophthalmologist.					
Inguinal hernia	Yes	Yes	Yes	Yes	Yes
Kidney: Absence of one	No	Yes	Yes	Yes	Yes
Liver: Enlarged	No	No	Yes	Yes	Yes
Musculoskeletal disorders	*	*	*	*	*
* Needs individual assessment.					
Neurologic					
History of serious head or spine trauma, repeated concussions, or craniotomy	*	*	Yes	Yes	Yes
Convulsive disorder					
Well controlled	Yes	Yes	Yes	Yes	Yes
Poorly controlled	No	No	Yes†	Yes	Yes‡
* Needs individual assessment.					
† No swimming or weight lifting.					
‡ No archery or riflery.					
Ovary: Absence of one	Yes	Yes	Yes	Yes	Yes
Respiratory					
Pulmonary insufficiency	*	*	*	*	Yes
Asthma	Yes	Yes	Yes	Yes	Yes
* May be allowed to compete if oxygenation remains satisfactory during a graded stress test.					
Sickle cell trait	Yes	Yes	Yes	Yes	Yes
Skin: Boils, herpes, impetigo, scabies	*	*	Yes	Yes	Yes
* No gymnastics with mats, martial arts, wrestling, or contact sports until not contagious.					
Spleen: Enlarged	No	No	No	Yes	Yes
Testicle: Absence or undescended	Yes*	Yes*	Yes	Yes	Yes
* Certain sports may require protective cup.					

Reference: DuRant RH, et al: Findings from the preparticipation athletic examination and athletic injuries. Am J Dis Child 146:85–91, 1992.

Menarche and Menstruation in the Athlete

The Committee on Sports Medicine of the AAP has recommended that any medical evaluation of a female athlete should include a focus on menstrual history. Pubertal development appears to be delayed in thin athletes, especially ballet dancers and runners.

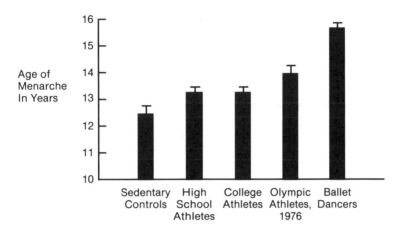

Exercise and age of menarche. Pubertal development appears to be delayed in thin athletes.

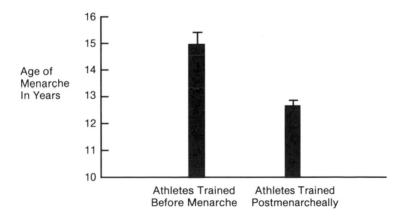

Athletes who began their training premenarcheally experienced a delay in menarche.

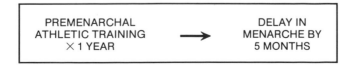

For each year of training before menarch, menarche is delayed by 5 months.

When should initiation of pubertal changes in an athlete be considered abnormal? The following guidelines are helpful:

1. If no pubertal changes occur by the chronologic age of 13 years (two standard deviations outside the normal variation), examination should be done to rule out thyroid abnormalities, prolactin-secreting adenomas, ovarian dysgenesis, and chromosomal abnormality.
2. If there is no period by the age of 16 with some pubertal growth, then a definite search must be made for anatomic causes of amenorrhea and mullerian agenesis.
3. The AAP Committee on Sports Medicine has recommended that a work-up be instituted if menarche is delayed by 1 year beyond the age of onset of menses of other female family members.
4. If the patient, her parents, or coach are anxious about late menarche or delayed puberty, a limited individualized work-up should be offered.

Some common causes of delayed menarche are listed below:

Some Common Causes of Delayed Menarche

Hypothalamic	**Ovarian**
Space-occupying lesions (e.g., cranio-pharyngioma, glioma)	Gonadal dysgenesis—chromosomal abnormalities
Functional disturbances of hypothalamic-pituitary axis (e.g., anorexia nervosa, emotional stress, athletics, eating disorders, drugs)	Tumors
	Polycystic ovaries
	Resistant ovary syndrome
Pituitary	**Uterine or vaginal**
Hypopituitarism—idiopathic	Absence of uterus (e.g., mullerian agenesis)
Prolactin-secreting adenomas	Complete or partial absence of vagina
	Imperforate hymen resulting in hematocolpos

Other
Congenital adrenal hyperplasia
Hypothyroidism or hyperthyroidism
Debilitating chronic disease (e.g., congenital heart disease, Crohn's disease, collagen disorders, renal failure)

References: From Gidwani GP: The athlete and menstruation. Adolescent Medicine State of the Art Reviews 2:27–45, 1991, with permission.
Frisch RE, Wishak G, Vincent L: Delayed menarche and amenorrhea in ballet dancers. N Engl J Med 303:17–19, 1980.

STOOL

Stool Frequency in Healthy Infants and Children

Knowledge of the normal range of bowel movements can help physicians and parents deal with concerns regarding both constipation and diarrhea. Although both of these entities are more a function of the state of stool hydration, the issue of frequency frequently enters into the thinking. Listed in the following table are some norms based on age:

Number of Stools Per Day

	PERCENTILES				
AGE	3	10	50	90	97
5 days–1 mo	0.9	1.3	2.7	5.1	6.0
1–5 mo	0.6	1.0	1.8	2.6	4.4
5–12 mo	0.8	1.1	1.8	2.8	3.8
1–3 yr	0.6	0.8	1.4	2.2	2.9
3–6 yr	0.4	0.6	1.1	1.6	2.1
Over 6 yr	0.4	0.7	1.0	1.4	1.9

Reference: Fontana M, et al: Bowel frequency in healthy children. Acta Paediatr Scand 78:682–684, 1989.

Stool Frequency in Infants as a Function of Feeding Style

Do breastfed infants have more stools than bottle-fed babies? On average, the answer is yes, but great individual variation exists according to different feedings, as is revealed by the numbers below from a study of 185 infants under 3 months of age.

Stool Frequency

	PERCENTILES				
TYPE OF FEEDING	3	10	50	90	97
Human milk	0.8	1.1	2.9	5.5	6.1
Formula	0.8	0.9	2.0	2.8	3.9
Human milk + formula	0.8	0.8	2.3	3.6	5.7

Reference: Fontana M, et al: Bowel frequency in healthy children. Acta Paediatr Scand 78:862–684, 1989.

The Floating Stool

There is a persistent myth that it is the fat content that buoys the floating stool. We thought this myth had been deflated in the early 1970s in a series of poetic testaments in *The New England Journal of Medicine*. The following sample gives ample argument to the fact that it's the air in stool that keeps it afloat, not the fat.

Floaters and Sinkers

To the Editor: The recent article "Floating Stools—Flatus versus Fat." inspired me to embrace the Muse as follows:

> While safe's the stool that comes a sinker,
> The floater's apt to be a stinker.

> So it's not fat but, rather, flatus
> Imparts the elevated status.

Freehold, NJ   Joseph D. Teller

References: Teller JD: Floaters and sinkers. N Engl J Med 287:52, 1972, with permission. Levitt MD, Duane WC: Floating stools—flatus versus fat. N Engl J Med 386:973, 1972.

STRABISMUS

Strabismus, or squint, is a result of one of the three major pathologic processes:

1. An imbalance in the ocular muscles of the two eyes as a result of maldevelopment or innervation.
2. A difference in the refraction of the two eyes.
3. A visual defect in one eye.

Strabismus may be either paralytic or nonparalytic. Nonparalytic strabismus is seen frequently in infants during the first 6 months of life. After this age strabismus requires an explanation and treatment in order to avoid amblyopia. A paralytic squint is abnormal at any age.

When the squint is of the nonparalytic type (concomitant), all muscles move the eye normally, but they do not work in conjunction with each other. The two eyes are in the same position relative to each other, whatever the direction of gaze. The nonparalytic squint is not associated with diplopia. In young infants the presence of strabismus can easily be confirmed by shining a light at the eyes from directly in front of the patient. The reflection of the light should normally be in the center of the pupil or at a corresponding point on both corneas.

When the squint is of the paralytic type (nonconcomitant) owing to muscle paralysis, the eyes are straight except when moved in the direction of the paralyzed muscle. If full ocular movements are elicited in one eye when the other is covered, then a paralytic strabismus can be excluded.

Nonparalytic squint is seen in children with hydrocephalus, cerebral palsy, retinoblastoma, corneal opacities, and refractive errors.

Paralytic squint should suggest the presence of a brain stem lesion and increased intracranial pressure.

Reference: From McMillan JA, et al (eds): The Whole Pediatrician Catalog. Philadelphia, W.B. Saunders, 1977, p 12, with permission.

STRIDOR

Common Causes

Allergic reaction
Croup
Foreign body aspiration
Hypertrophied tonsils/adenoids
Peritonsillar abscess
Postinstrumentation edema

Retropharyngeal abscess
Secretions
Spasmotic croup
Subglottic stenosis (congenital, postintubation)
Vocal cord nodules

Uncommon Causes

Corrosive ingestion
Epiglottitis
Granuloma (postintubation/tracheostomy)
Laryngeal trauma

Tracheitis (bacterial)
Vocal cord paralysis (congenital postsurgical)
Vocal cord polyps

Rare Causes

Angioneurotic edema
Congenital goiter
Cricoarytenoid arthritis (JRA)
Diphtheria
Ectopic thyroid
Esophageal foreign body
External tracheal compression
    Hemorrhage
    Infection
    Tumor
Farber's disease
Glossoptosis
Hemangioma
Hypoplastic larynx

Internal laryngocele
Laryngeal papilloma
Larangeal tumors
Laryngismus stridulus (rickets)
Marcoglossia
Opitz-Frias syndrome
Pierre Robin syndrome
Post-tracheostomy stricture
Psychogenic stridor
Tetany
Thyroglossal duct cyst
Tracheoesophageal fistula
Tracheo-laryngo-esophageal cleft
Vascular ring

Stymied by Stridor?

Stridor is a harsh, high pitched sound made during breathing, especially inspiration. It is always indicative of a pathologic problem. Think in anatomic terms and you will usually find the cause.

Stridor at the Epiglottis

Congenital anomalies:	Aryepiglottic cyst
	Dermoid cyst
	Thyroglossal duct cyst
	Lingual thyroid
	Flabby epiglottis
Inflammatory disease:	Epiglottitis: bacterial origin, allergic origin

Stridor at the Larynx and Subglottic Region

Congenital anomalies:	Hemangioma or lymphangioma
	Unilateral or bilateral vocal cord paralysis
	Laryngeal and/or subglottic stenosis
	Laryngomalacia
	Laryngeal cyst
	Papilloma
Trauma:	Birth injury
	Postlaryngoscopy
	Postlaryngeal catheterization
Inflammatory disease:	Laryngitis
	Laryngeal abscess
	Subglottic edema (of allergic origin)
Foreign body:	Radiopaque or radiolucent
Metabolic disorders:	Laryngismus stridulus (rickets)

Stridor from the Trachea

Congenital anomalies:	Hemangioma or lymphangioma
	Tracheomalacia
	Cartilage ring abnormalities ("segmental malacia")
Foreign body:	Radiopaque or radiolucent
Postoperative:	After tracheal intubation
	Stricture after tracheostomy
	Narrowing at the level of tracheoesophageal fistula

Stridor from Causes Originating Outside the Respiratory Tract

Congenital anomalies:	Vascular ring or anomalous innominate artery
	Esophageal atresia
	Tracheoesophageal fistula
	Aberrant or ectopic thyroid tissue
	Congenital goiter
	Carcinoma of thyroid
Inflammatory origin:	Retropharyngeal abscess
	Retroesophageal abscess
Foreign body:	Within the esophagus
Postoperative:	After tracheoesophageal fistula closure
	After mid-mediastinal surgery

Reference: Grünebaum M: Respiratory Stridor—a challenge for the paediatric radiologist. Clin Radiol 24:485, 1973.

STROKE

Stroke in Children and Teenagers

The incidence of stroke in children and adolescents is extremely low; this is largely due to the rare occurrence of significant atherosclerosis in these age groups. When strokes do occur in children and teenagers, they are often severe and frequently associated with seizure disorders, motor deficits, and death. Persistent aphasia, on the other hand, which is a common feature of stroke in adults, rarely accompanies stroke in children. When confronted with a child presenting with signs and symptoms of a cerebrovascular accident, the clinician needs to consider three important factors before applying the differential diagnosis that appears below: (1) the patient's age, (2) the presence of other or underlying medical conditions, and (3) the clinical presentation of the stroke.

1. Strokes *not* associated with underlying systemic disease

    a. **Acute hemiplegia of childhood** (acute infantile hemiplegia) refers to the sudden onset of hemiparesis that is not associated with intracranial hemorrhage. Of these cases 60% present with severe, generalized seizures and coma. The neurologic examination is remarkable for weakness. Although

there exists a large number of pathologic entities that can cause acute hemiplegia of childhood, we shall divide them into five major processes:
  i. Occlusive vascular disease at the base of the brain associated with telangiectasia of the basal ganglia (Moyamoya syndrome)
  ii. Occlusive vascular disease at the base of the brain without telangiectasia.
  iii. Narrowing of the origin of the internal carotid artery
  iv. Distal branch occlusion of the intracranial arteries
  v. Corkscrew pattern in small terminal arteries

  b. **Intracranial hemorrhage** is strongly suggested by the sudden onset of a neurologic deficit in association with headache, somnolence, and nuchal rigidity. The CT scan of the head is usually diagnostic.
  i. **Arteriovenous malformations** are the most common cause of sub-arachnoid hemorrhage in children. They may or may not be associated with a neurologic deficit; a history of seizures may exist.
  ii. **Aneurysms** are rare in infants but are more common as age increases. The initial episode of aneurysmal hemorrhage may not be associated with focal neurologic signs, but subsequent episodes often yield significant deficits. Aneurysmal hemorrhages may rarely present as frequent headaches or cranial nerve palsies. Polycystic kidney disease and coarctation of the aorta are predisposing factors to aneurysms.

2. Strokes associated with underlying systemic diseases
  a. **Congenital heart disease** (particularly cyanotic heart disease)
  i. Stroke may occur to a *right to left shunt* that allows emboli to bypass the lungs and enter the arterial circulation of the brain.
  ii. During surgical procedures requiring *cardiac bypass*, air emboli, foreign material, and thrombi can yield neurologic deficits.
  iii. **Venous thrombi**
  iv. **Polycythemia**

  b. **Purulent venous thrombosis** (secondary to pyogenic infections of the mastoids, paranasal sinuses, scalp, or face)
  i. **Lateral sinus thrombosis** can present with increased intracranial pressure and abducens (cranial nerve VI) paralysis
  ii. **Saggital sinus thrombosis** can present with increased intracranial pressure and evolving neurologic signs.
  iii. **Cavernous sinus thrombosis** is classically associated with proptosis, vascular engorgement of the bulbar conjunctivae, retinal hemorrhages, and extraoccular muscle palsies.

  c. **Trauma**
  i. **Direct injury to the head**
  ii. **Injury to the neck** with intraoral damage (e.g., a traumatic injury to the posterior pharyngeal wall) can yield a dissecting aneurysm of the carotid vessels. With traumatic injuries to the head and neck, there is typically a latent period of 2 to 24 hours, followed by the onset of hemiparesis in association with somnolence and increased intracranial pressure; this latency period is probably because the trauma causes an intimal tear in a major artery, followed by dissecting aneurysm formation and thrombosis of the vessel.

d. **Sickle cell anemia:** Acute hemiparesis is a complication of older children and adolescents with sickle cell disease, most likely secondary to thrombosis in the capillaries and venules of the white matter. Vasoocclusive crises of the cerebral vessels have also been theorized to contribute to the incidence of stroke in these children. Arterial thrombi in major vessels and intracranial hemorrhage occur rarely.

e. **Homocystinuria:** This is an autosomal recessive defect in methionine metabolism that manifests itself as mental retardation, dislocation of the lenses, and tall stature. The defect also affects platelet function, which can yield an arterial or venous occlusion. Further, homocystine deficiency causes endothelial damage and leads to increased platelet consumption.

f. **Rare causes of stroke in children**
   i. Hematologic
      (a) Thrombotic thrombocytopenic purpura and other consumption coagulopathies
      (b) Thrombocytosis
      (c) Polycythemia
   ii. Cardiac disorders
      (a) Arrythmias
      (b) Bacterial endocarditis
      (c) Atrial myxoma
   iii. Rheumatologic disorder
      (a) Vasculitis (e.g., periarteritis nodosa, giant cell arteritis, Takayasu's arteritis)
      (b) Systemic lupus erythematosis
   iv. Migraine
      (a) Hemiplegic migraine
      (b) Basilar artery migraine
      (c) Alternating hemiplegia of childhood
   v. Viral infections (e.g., coxsackie A-9 encephalitis)
   vi. Neurocutaneous disorders
      (a) Neurofibromatosis
      (b) Sturge-Weber syndrome
      (c) Tuberous sclerosis
   vii. Metastatic neoplasms
      (a) Rhabdomyosarcoma
      (b) Neuroblastoma
      (c) Primary brain tumors
   viii. Atherosclerotic disease
      (a) Progeria
      (b) Hypercholesterolemias
      (c) Hyperlipidemias
   ix. High-dose radiation to head and neck yielding occlusion or stenosis of the internal carotid arteries (usually occurs 2 to 22 years after the course of radiotherapy)
   x. Necrotizing angiitis associated with intravenous methaamphetamine abuse.

Reference: Golden GS: Strokes in children and adolescents. Stroke 9:169–171, 1978.

SUDDEN DEATH

Sudden Death Among Young People

Although an uncommon phenomenon among children and young adults, sudden death is a startling and complex problem that presents itself with a frequency of 1.3 to 8.5 per 100,000 patient years.[1,2] One-third to one-half of these deaths are secondary to cardiac disease. Congenital cardiac disease is a more common cause of sudden death during infancy and early childhood. Hypertrophic cardiomyopathy and precocious atherosclerosis are more frequent causes of sudden death among adolescents and young adults.

Common Causes of Sudden Death in Young Persons

Noncardiac causes	**Occult "unexpected cardiac causes"**
Toxic substance abuse	Conduction-system abnormality
Abdominal hemorrhage	Heart block (primary or secondary)
Cerebral hemorrhage	Sinus-node dysfunction (primary or secondary)
Pulmonary disease or abnormality	Ventricular tachyarrhythmia
	Myocardial tumor
Pre-existing "known and clinical	Right ventricular dysplasia
diagnosable cardiac causes"	QT prolongation syndrome
Myocarditis	Primary arrhythmia
Hypertrophic cardiomyopathy	Wolff-Parkinson-White syndrome
Mitral-valve prolapse	Coronary arteritis or precocious atherosclerosis
Major congenital heart lesions	Intramural coronary artery
Aortic stenosis	Anomolous origin of left coronary artery
Tetralogy of Fallot	from pulmonary trunk
Ebstein's anomaly	Aberrant origin from "wrong" sinus
Pulmonary vascular	of Valsalva
obstruction (primary	Dissecting aortic aneurysm as a result
or secondary)	of Marfan's disease
Cystic medial necrosis	

References: 1. Liberthson RR, et al: Case records of the Massachusetts General Hospital (Case No. 22-1989). N Engl J Med 320:1475–1483, 1989.
2. Driscoll DJ, Edward WD: Sudden unexpected death in children and adolescents. J Am Coll Cardiol 5(Suppl):118B–121B, 1985.
3. Kennedy HL, Whitlock JA, Buckingham TA: Sudden death in young persons—an urban study (abstract) J Am Coll Cardiol 3:485, 1984.

SUNLIGHT

Sun Exposure: To Have or Have Not

We have entered a new era. Fewer and fewer people covet the once sought after "healthy glow" of a summer tan. As reports surface about the risks of a blistering burn before the third decade, more parents want advice about sun exposure. As a pediatrician, be prepared to answer questions about summer sun intensity and keep a mental list of the diseases and drugs that predispose young (and old) skin to photosensitivity.

Advise parents that the sun is at its maximum intensity between the hours of 11 A.M. and 3 P.M. and offer this handy rule of thumb: "When your shadow is shorter than you are tall, the sun is more likely to burn you than at other times, so seek protection with proper clothing, shade, sun screens or other means" (Lancet 1:44, 1990).

Diseases Exacerbated or Precipitated by Sunlight

Viral
  Herpes simplex
  Certain viral exanthems
Genetic and metabolic
  Xeroderma pigmentosum
  Albinism
  Vitiligo
  Darier's disease (pseudoxanthoma
    elasticum)
  Bloom's syndrome
  Rothmund-Thompson Syndrome
  Certain porphyrias
  Hartnup's disease
  Phenylketonuria

Collagen vascular
  Systemic lupus erythematosus
  Discoid lupus erythematosus
  Dermatomyositis
Miscellaneous
  Solar urticaria
  Hydroa aestivale (Hutchinson's
    summer prurigo) and
    vacciniforme
  Photosensitive eczema
  Polymorphous light eruption

Drugs Predisposing to Sunburn or Photoreaction

Antibiotics
  Sulfonamides
  Tetracyclines
  Nalidixic acid
  Griseofulvin
Acne preparations
  Retinoids (topical and systemic)
Antiepileptics
  Hydantoin
  Trimethadione
  Barbiturates

Other
  Certain chemotherapeutic agents
  Antimalarials
  Phenothiazines
  Coal tars
  Psoralens
  Chlorothiazide diuretics

Reference: Hebert AA, Esterly NB: When the sun takes its toll. Contemp Peds June: 16–21, 1985.

SWEAT TEST

The False Positive Sweat Test

A sweat chloride value in excess of 60 mEq/L is generally considered diagnostic of cystic fibrosis. In adults, the normal range may be somewhat higher, i.e., 60–80 mEq/L. But even when the sweat test has been carefully performed (and this is not always the case), other causes of an elevated sweat chloride must be carefully considered before making a diagnosis. These other causes include:

Adrenal insufficiency, untreated	Hypothyroidism
Ectodermal dysplasia	Mucopolysaccharidoses
Hereditary nephrogenic diabetes insipidus	Malnutrition
Glucose-6-phosphatase deficiency	Fucosidosis
Pupillatonia, hyporeflexia, and segmental hypohydrosis with autonomic dysfunction	

False-negative sweat chloride results may be caused by edema.

A diagnosis of cystic fibrosis should not be made on the basis of a positive sweat test alone. At least one of the following four criteria must also be present:

1. Documented family history of cystic fibrosis
2. Chronic pulmonary disease
3. Pancreatic insufficiency
4. A genotype consistent with the diagnosis.

SYNCOPE

The Work-up of Syncopal Episodes

The symptom of syncope has been defined as the reversible, atraumatic loss of consciousness and is usually associated with an inability to stand upright. This reaction can be due to some underlying impairment in cardiac output resulting in diminished cerebral perfusion. Careful evaluation of the patient presenting with syncopal episodes is clearly warranted, because that person may be at risk for injury, toward himself or others, especially if engaged in some activity such as driving, playing sports, crossing the street, and so on. Furthermore, patients who are having syncopal attacks secondary to some form of cardiac impairment are at risk for serious arrhythmias and sudden death.

1. **The Etiology of Syncope**

    a. *Vascular/reflex*

    Vasodepressor, orthostatic hypotension, cough, micturition, swallow, migraine, Takayasu disease, hyperventilation, carotid sinus, pregnancy, anemia, volume loss.

    b. *Psychologic*

    Hysteria, hyperventilation, fearful or threatening stimuli

    c. *Cardiac*

    Obstruction, arrhythmia, heart block, myocarditis, cardiomyopathy, mitral valve prolapse, pericardial effusion, prolonged QT syndrome, coronary anomaly, pulmonary artery hypertension, right ventricular dysplasia

    d. *Neurologic*

    Epilepsy, vertigo, central autonomic insufficiency (e.g., Riley-Day syndrome and Shy-Drager syndrome)

e. *Metabolic*

Low values for glucose, clacium, magnesium, or pO_2; abnormal values for sodium, potassium, or chloride

f. *Drugs*

Tricyclic antidepressants, antihypertensives, diuretics, barbiturates, phenothiazines, nitrates, cocaine, and other drugs of abuse.

2. **The Prodrome in Vasovagal Syncope**

(Vascular/reflex/psychologic categories of diagnosis account for the vast majority of syncopal episodes in both children and adults)

a. *Physiologic factors*
Hunger
Fatigue
Illness
Hot, crowded rooms
Pain
Anxiety
Perceived threat
Sight of blood

b. *Symptoms*
Pallor/clammy skin
Sweating
Dilated pupils
Blurred vision
Nausea/epigastric distress
Lightheadedness
Dizziness
Weakness

3. **The Reflex of Physiology in Syncopal Episodes**

a. Recall the following important equations in cardiac physiology:
   i. Heart rate × stroke volume = cardiac output
   ii. Cardiac output × total peripheral resistance = blood pressure
   iii. Heart rate × stroke volume × total peripheral resistance = blood pressure

b. Factors that determine heart rate:
   Vagal tone (inhibitory)
   Catecholamines (stimulant)
   Sympathetic tone (stimulant)

c. Factors that determine stroke volume:
   Circulating blood volume
   Venous return (e.g., muscle tone, respiratory motion, tissue pressure, pregnancy)
   Sympathetic tone

d. Factors that determine total peripheral resistance:
   Baroreceptor tone (e.g., carotid sinus, aortic arch)
   Arteriolar tone (as determined by electrolyte balance, catecholamines, and autonomic tone)
   Drugs

4. **Primary Workup for Patient with Syncope**

Although the etiology of syncope may frequently be revealed from an accurate history, a number of laboratory tests are available when the history alone is not sufficient. The following table (Table 1) summarizes the primary workup of these patients:

Table 1. Primary Work-up for Patient with Syncope*

	ATHLETE WITH SYNCOPE	PATIENT WITH CARDIAC SYNCOPE	PATIENT ON DRUGS	PATIENT WITH NEUROLOGIC/ PSYCHOLOGIC PROBLEMS	PATIENT WITH RECURRENT SYNCOPE OR SYNCOPE OF UNDETERMINED ORIGIN	PATIENT WITH REFLEX SYNCOPE
History	X	X	X	X	X	X
Physical examination	X	X	X	X	X	X
ECG	X	X	X	X	X	X
Laboratory: CBC, electrolytes, glucose, Ca^{2+}, Mg^{2+}	X	X	X	X	X	X
Holter monitor	XX	XX		XX	XX	
Hyperventilation test				XX		XX
Serum bicarbonate				XX		
EEG				XX	XX	
Carotid sinus massage						XX
Telemetry		XX				
Echocardiogram		XX				
Stress test	XX	XX			XX	
Intracardiac electro- physiology study	XX				XX	
Specific laboratory serum for drugs			XX			

* X indicates test, technique, or procedure that should be used in all patients with syncope. This is the initial screen to help sort the patients into one of the six general categories (column heads). XX indicates additional testing that may be required based on the results of the initial screen.

As described by Branch, "fainting spells share the common mechanism of transient inadequacy of cerebral perfusion due to inappropriate vasodilatation with pooling of blood in the extremities. They share common characteristics of being brief, usually without adverse consequences, and usually occurring while the patient is standing, sometimes while sitting, and rarely if ever while recumbent. Diagnostic clues are provided by the setting, the onset, the patient's appearance, and the recovery (Table 2)."

Table 2. Differentiating Vasovagal Syncope from Seizure from Cardiac Syncope

	VASOVAGAL SYNCOPE	SEIZURE	CARDIAC SYNCOPE
Onset	Prodromal weakness, nausea, diaphoresis, lasting seconds to minutes	Sudden onset, or brief aura: deja vu, olfactory, gustatory, visual, etc.	Sudden onset or preceded by cardiac symptoms: chest tightness, dyspnea, diaphoresis, palpitations

Table continued on next page.

Table 2. Differentiating Vasovagal Syncope from Seizure from Cardiac Syncope (Cont.)

	VASOVAGAL SYNCOPE	SEIZURE	CARDIAC SYNCOPE
Typical settings	Emotional upset, prolonged standing, uncomfortable surroundings, or on first arising with full bladder	Any setting, including sleep, sometimes blinking lights, monotonous music	Any setting, often without warning
Occurrence	Only when upright	Any position	Any position
Appearance	Pallor, weak pulse	Cyanosis, stertorous breathing	Pallor, variable pulse
Residiuum	Rapid recovery but may recur on standing, occasional brief clonic movements, or urinary incontinence	Prolonged recovery with postictal state, Todd's paresis	Recovery may be rapid or prolonged; if cardiac arrest: seizure-like activity, signs of cerebral hypoxia

From Branch WT (ed): Office Practice of Medicine, 2nd ed. Philadelphia, W.B. Saunders, 1987, with permission.

References: Ruckman RN: Cardiac causes of syncope. Pediatrics in Review 9(4):101–108, 1978.
Kapoor WN, et al: A prospective evaluation and follow-up of patients with syncope. N Engl J Med 309:197–204, 1983.
Branch WT: Approach to syncope. J Gen Intern Med 1:49–58, 1986.

SYNDROMES AND EPONYMS

Despite mounting opposition in some quarters, the use of eponymic names for syndromes, diseases, signs, et al. is likely to continue during all our lifetimes. The date and source of the originally published or reported description connected to the eponym (not always the first published description) are interesting, both for old (e.g., Pott's, 1779) and new (e.g., Kawasaki, 1974) syndromes and diseases. Listed below is a sampling:

Addison's disease.
Addison T: Anaemia. Disease of the supra-renal capsules. London Hosp Gaz 43:517–518, 1849.

Budd-Chiari syndrome.
Budd G: On diseases of the liver. London, Churchill, 1945.
Chiari H: Erhahrungen über Infarktbildungen in der Leber des Menschen. Zschr Heilk 19:475–512, 1898.

Calvé-Legg-Perthes syndrome.
Calvé F: Sur une forme particulière de coxalgie greffée. Sur les déformations caractéristiques de l'extremité supérieure du fémur. Rev Chir, Paris 42:54–84, 1910.
Legg AT: On obscure affection of the hip-joint. Boston Med & SJ 162:202–204, 1910.

Perthes GC: Über Arthritis deformans juvenilis. Deut Zschr Chir 107:111–159, 1910.

Cockayne's syndrome.
Cockayne EA: Dwarfism with retinal atrophy and deafness. Arch Dis Child, London 11:1–8, 1936.

Down's syndrome.
Down JL: Marriages of consanguinity in relation to degeneration of race. London Hosp Clin Lect Rep 3:224–236, 1866.
Down JL: Observations on an ethnic classification of idiots. London Hosp Clin Lect Rep 3:259–262, 1866.

Ebstein's anomaly.
Ebstein W: Ueber einen sehr seltenen Fall von Insufficienz der Valvula tricuspidalis bedingt durch eine angeborene hochgradige Missbildung derselben. Arch Anat Physiol, Leipzig, 1866, pp 238–253.

Ehlers-Danlos syndrome.
Ehlers E: Cutis laxa, Neigung zu Haemorrhagien in der Haut, Lockerung mehrerer Artikulationen. (Case for diagnosis.) Derm Zschr 8:173–174, 1901.
Danlos H: Un cas de cutis laxa avec tumeurs par contusion chronique de coudes et des genoux (xanthome juvénile pseudo-diabétique de MM. Hallopeau et Macé de Lépinay). Bull Soc Fr Derm Syph 19:70–72, 1908.

Tetralogy of Fallot.
Fallot EL: Contribution à l'anatomie pathologique de la maladie bleue (cyanose cardioque). Marseille Méd 24:77–93, 138–158, 270–286, 341–354, 403–420, 1888.

Fitz-Hugh and Curtis syndrome.
Fitz-Hugh T Jr: Acute gonococcic peritonitis of the right upper quadrant in women. JAMA 102:2094–2096, 1934.
Curtis AH: A cause of adhesions in the right upper quadrant. JAMA 94:1221–1222, 1930.

Goodpasture's syndrome.
Goodpasture EW: The significance of certain pulmonary lesions in relation to the etiology of influenza. Am J Med Sc 158:863–870, 1919.

Guillain-Barré syndrome.
Guillain G, Barré J, Strohl A: Sur un syndrome de radiculo-névrite avec hyperalbuminose du liquide céphalo-rachidien sans réaction cellulaire. Remarques sur les caractères cliniques et graphiques des réflexes tendineux. Bull Soc Méd Hôp Paris 40:1462–1470, 1916.

Hodgkin's disease.
Hodgkin T: On some morbid appearances of the absorbent glands and spleen. Med Chir Tr, London 17:68–114, 1832.

Kawasaki disease.
Kawasaki T, Kosaki F, Okawa S, et al: A new infantile acute febrile mucocutaneous lymph node syndrome (MLNS) prevailing in Japan. Pediatrics 54:271, 1974.

Klinefelter's syndrome.
Klinefelter HF Jr, Reifenstein EC Jr, Albright F: Syndrome characterized by gynecomastia, aspermatogenesis without A-leydigism, and increased excretion of follicle-stimulating hormone. J Clin Endocr 2:615–627, 1942.

de Lange syndrome.
Lange C de: Sur un type nouveau de dégénération (Typus amstelodamesis). Arch Méd Enf, Paris 36:713–719, 1933.
Lange C de: Congenital hypertrophy of the muscles, extrapyramidal motor disturbances and mental deficiency. A clinical entity. Am J Dis Child 48:243–268, 1934.

Marfan's syndrome.
Marfan AB: Un case de déformation congénitale des quatre, membres plus prononcée aux extremités, characterisée par l'allongement des os avec un certain degré d'amincissement. Bull Soc Méd Hôp, Paris 13:220–226, 1896.
Achard C: Arachnodactylie. Bull Soc Méd Hôp, Paris 19:834–843, 1902.

Meckel's diverticulum.
Meckel: Ueber die Divertikel am Darmkanal. Arch Physiol, Halle 9:421–453, 1809.

Ménière's syndrome.
Ménière P: Sur une forme particuliére de surdité grave dépendant d'une lésion de l'oreille interne. Gaz Med, Paris 16:29, 1861.

Mibelli's disease.
Mibelli V: Di una nuova forma de cheratosi "angiocheratoma." Gior Ital Mal Vener 30:285–301, 1889.

Münchausen's syndrome.
Asher R: Münchausen's syndrome. Lancet i:339–341, 1951.

Niemann-Pick disease.
Niemann AA: Ein unbekanntes Krankheitsbild. Jb Kinderh 79:1–10, 1914.
Pick L: Der Morbus Gaucher und die ihm änlichen Krankheiten (die lipoidzellige Splenohepatomegalie Typus Niemann und die diabetische Lipoid-zellenhypoplasie der Milz). Erg Inn Med Kinderh 29:519–627, 1926.

Pott's disease.
Pott P: Remarks on that kind of palsy of the lower limbs which is frequently found to accompany a curvature of the spine and is supposed to be caused by it, together with its method of cure. London, Johnson, 1779.

Reye's syndrome.
Reye RD, Morgan G, Baral J: Encephalopathy and fatty degeneration of the viscera. Lancet ii:749–752, 1963.

Riley-Day syndrome.
Riley CM, Day RL, et al: Central autonomic dysfunction with defective lacrimation. Report of five cases. Pediatrics 3:468–478, 1949.

Pierre Robin syndrome.
Robin P: La glossoptose, un grave danger pour nos enfants. Paris, 1929.

Schönlein-Henoch purpura.
Henoch H: Uber den Zusammenhang von Purpura und Intestinalstörungen. Berlin Klin Wschr 5:417–519, 1868.
Schönlein JL: Allemeine und specielle Pathologie und Therapie. Würzburg, Etlinger, 1832.

Stevens-Johnson syndrome.
Stevens AM, Johnson FC: A new eruptive fever associated with stomatitis and ophthalmia. Report of two cases in children. Am J Dis Child 24:526–533, 1922.

Whipple's disease.
Whipple GH: A hitherto undescribed disease characterized anatomically by deposits of fat and fatty acids in the intestinal and mesenteric lymphatic tissues. Bull Johns Hopkins Hosp 18:382–391, 1907.

Wilson's disease.
Wilson SAK: Progressive lenticular degeneration: A familial nervous disease associated with cirrhosis of the liver. Brain 34:295–509, 1912.

Wolff-Parkinson-White syndrome.
Wolff L, Parkinson J, White PD: bundle-branch block with short P-R interval in healthy young people prone to paroxysmal tachycardia. Am Heart J 5:685–704, 1930.

Reference: Jablonski S: Illustrated Dictionary of Eponymic Syndromes and Diseases. Philadelphia, W.B. Saunders, 1969.

Who Was Down?

John Langdon Down was born near Plymouth, England on November 18, 1828. He enrolled as a medical student at the London Hospital in 1853 and obtained a doctorate in 1859, after receiving the university gold medal for physiology. In the same year—1859—he was appointed medical superintendent of the Eastwood Asylum for idiots, at Redhill, Surrey, England, a post he held for 10 years and where he wrote a paper titled "Observations on an ethnic classification of idiots." He noted that many of his patients had similar clinical features and described them as follows:

> The face is flat and broad and destitute of prominence. Cheeks are roundish and extended laterally. The eyes are obliquely placed and the internal canthi more than normally distant from one another. The palpebral fissure is very narrow. The lips are large and thick with transverse fissures. The tongue is long, thick and much roughened. The nose is small.

He stated that "Their resemblance to each other was such that, when placed side by side, it is difficult to believe that they are not the children of the same parents.

Down's work at Eastwood brought him much recognition, and in 1869 he was able to establish an institution at Redhill, Surrey for mentally retarded children of the wealthy. He named it Normansfield after his friend, Norman Wilkinson. At Normansfield, Down wrote his monograph titled *Mental Affections of Childhood and Youth*, published in 1887, which contained the classic description of Down's syndrome. He also mentioned adrenogenital dystrophy, which subsequently gained recognition as Frölich's syndrome. Down worked at Normansfield until his death in 1896.

For about 100 years the term "mongolism" was used as the primary descriptive name for Down's syndrome, with the eponyms "Down's" and "Langdon-Down's" used as alternatives, the hyphenated form having been preferred by Down in his later life. However, controversy eventually arose because some regarded the reference to the Mongol ethnic group as insulting, and in 1965 representatives of the Mongolian People's Republic in the World Health Organization approached the Director General and petitioned him to abandon the term "mongolism." Their request was accepted, and the eponym Down's syndrome was adopted.

References: Beighton P, Beighton G: The Man Behind the Syndrome. Heidelberg, Springer-Verlag, 1986, pp 40–41.

Down JLH: Marriages of consanguinity in relation to degeneration of race. London Hosp Clin Lect Rep 3:224, 1866.

Down JLH: Observations on an ethnic classification of idiots. London Hosp Clin Lect Rep 3:259, 1866.

SYPHILIS

Approaching Congenital Syphilis

The diagnosis of congenital syphilis, like the diagnosis of many congenital infections, is often confounded by the absence of symptoms or signs in the newborn, as well as by the difficulty in interpreting neonatal serologic responses to infection. The abrupt rise in the number of reported cases of congenital syphilis in the late 1980s, however, has increased the need for guidelines that will insure the detection and appropriate management of newborns with this treatable disease. The tables and figures below represent the recommended approach for surveillance, diagnosis, evaluation, and treatment of congenital syphilis.

Congenital syphilis may be missed if serologic tests are not performed for both the mother and her infant at the time of delivery. Even when these tests are performed, some infants are not identified as having syphilis probably because the infection is very recent and there has been insufficient time for an antibody response to develop. Some infants with congenital syphilis of later onset do not present with a typical rash; therefore, at least in areas where the disease is prevalent, serologic tests for syphilis should be included in the evaluation of all febrile infants, even those with negative results on serologic testing at birth.

Table 1. Surveillance Case Definition for Congenital Syphilis

For reporting purposes, congenital syphilis includes cases of congenitally acquired syphilis in infants and children, as well as syphilitic stillbirths.

1. **Confirmed.** A confirmed case of congential syphilis is a case in which *Treponema pallidum* is identified by darkfield microscopy, fluorescent antibody, or other specific stains in specimens from lesions, placenta, umbilical cord, or autopsy material.

Table continued on next page.

Table 1. Surveillance Case Definition for Congenital Syphilis (Cont.)

2. **Presumptive.** A presumptive case of congenital syphilis is either of the following:

   a. Any case in which the infant's mother had untreated or inadequately treated* syphilis at delivery, regardless of findings in the infant

   b. Any case in which the infant or child is reactive to a treponemal test for syphilis and in which any **one** of the following is present:
      i. Any evidence of congenital syphilis on physical examination (Table II)
      ii. Any evidence of congenital syphilis on a long bone radiograph
      iii. Reactivity to a CSF VDRL test[†]
      iv. Elevated CSF cell count or protein (without other cause)[†]
      v. Quantitative nontreponemal serologic titer that is fourfold higher than the mother's (both specimens drawn at birth)
      vi. Reactive test for FTA-ABS 19S-IgM antibody[†]

3. **Syphilitic stillbirth.** A syphilitic stillbirth is defined as a fetal death in which the mother had untreated or inadequately treated syphilis at delivery of a fetus after a 20-week gestation or of a fetus weighing more than 500 gm.

Modified from Centers for Disease Control. MMWR 38:825–829, 1989.

* Inadequate treatment consists of any nonpenicillin therapy or penicillin given less than 30 days before delivery.

† It may be difficult to distinguish between congenital and acquired syphilis after infancy. Signs may not be obvious and stigmata may not yet have developed. Abnormal values of CSF VDRL test cell count, and protein, as well as IgM antibodies, may be found in either congenital or acquired syphilis. Findings on long bone radiographs may help to indicate congenital syphilis. The diagnosis may ultimately be based on maternal history and clinical judgment; the possibility of sexual abuse also needs to be considered.

Table 2. Evaluation for Early Congenital Syphilis

1. Maternal history, including results of serologic testing and treatment

2. Thorough physical examination

3. Long-bone radiographs
   a. Diaphyseal periostitis
   b. Osteochondritis
   c. Wimberger sign

4. Nontreponemal antibody titer
   a. VDRL test (simultaneous quantitative serum titer for mother and neonate)

5. Treponemal antibody titer
   FTA-ABS test
   FTA-ABS on 19S-IgM fraction of serum (CDC)

6. CSF analysis
   a. Cell count
   b. Protein level determination
   c. VDRL test

7. Other tests as clinically indicated
   a. Chest radiography
   b. Complete blood cell count
      i. Leukemoid reaction with or without monocytosis or lymphocytosis
      ii. Coombs negative hemolytic anemia
   c. Platelet count
      i. Thrombocytopenia
   d. Liver function tests
   e. Urinalysis

8. HIV antibody test

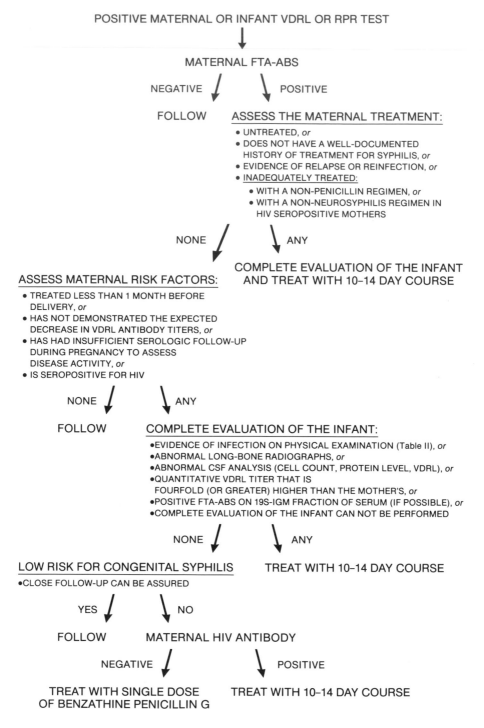

POSITIVE MATERNAL OR INFANT VDRL OR RPR TEST

MATERNAL FTA-ABS

NEGATIVE

POSITIVE

FOLLOW

ASSESS THE MATERNAL TREATMENT:
- UNTREATED, *or*
- DOES NOT HAVE A WELL-DOCUMENTED HISTORY OF TREATMENT FOR SYPHILIS, *or*
- EVIDENCE OF RELAPSE OR REINFECTION, *or*
- INADEQUATELY TREATED:
  - WITH A NON-PENICILLIN REGIMEN, *or*
  - WITH A NON-NEUROSYPHILIS REGIMEN IN HIV SEROPOSITIVE MOTHERS

NONE

ANY

COMPLETE EVALUATION OF THE INFANT AND TREAT WITH 10–14 DAY COURSE

ASSESS MATERNAL RISK FACTORS:
- TREATED LESS THAN 1 MONTH BEFORE DELIVERY, *or*
- HAS NOT DEMONSTRATED THE EXPECTED DECREASE IN VDRL ANTIBODY TITERS, *or*
- HAS HAD INSUFFICIENT SEROLOGIC FOLLOW-UP DURING PREGNANCY TO ASSESS DISEASE ACTIVITY, *or*
- IS SEROPOSITIVE FOR HIV

NONE

ANY

FOLLOW

COMPLETE EVALUATION OF THE INFANT:
- EVIDENCE OF INFECTION ON PHYSICAL EXAMINATION (Table II), *or*
- ABNORMAL LONG-BONE RADIOGRAPHS, *or*
- ABNORMAL CSF ANALYSIS (CELL COUNT, PROTEIN LEVEL, VDRL), *or*
- QUANTITATIVE VDRL TITER THAT IS FOURFOLD (OR GREATER) HIGHER THAN THE MOTHER'S, *or*
- POSITIVE FTA-ABS ON 19S-IGM FRACTION OF SERUM (IF POSSIBLE), *or*
- COMPLETE EVALUATION OF THE INFANT CAN NOT BE PERFORMED

NONE

ANY

LOW RISK FOR CONGENITAL SYPHILIS
- CLOSE FOLLOW-UP CAN BE ASSURED

TREAT WITH 10–14 DAY COURSE

YES

NO

FOLLOW

MATERNAL HIV ANTIBODY

NEGATIVE

POSITIVE

TREAT WITH SINGLE DOSE OF BENZATHINE PENICILLIN G

TREAT WITH 10–14 DAY COURSE

Figure 1. Algorithm for management of newborn infant born to mother with positive nontreponemal (VDRL or rapid plasma reagin) test result.

*Table 3. Recommended Antimicrobial Treatment Regimens for Infants
Born to Mothers with Positive VDRL Test Result*

1. For confirmed or presumptive congenital syphilis (**either** item A **or** item B)

    a. Crystalline penicillin G, 100,000 to 150,000 units/kg/day administered intravenously in divided doses every 8–12 hours for 10–14 days

    b. Procaine pencillin G, 50,000 units/kg/day administered once daily intramuscularly for 10–14 days

2. Recommended only for infants at low risk for congenital syphilis who were born to HIV-seronegative mothers adequately treated for syphilis and in whom close follow-up cannot be ensured.

    a. Benzathine penicillin G, 50,000 units/kg (administered intramuscularly as one-time dose)

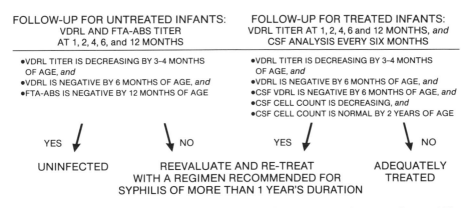

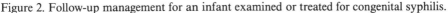

FOLLOW-UP FOR UNTREATED INFANTS: VDRL AND FTA-ABS TITER AT 1, 2, 4, 6, and 12 MONTHS	FOLLOW-UP FOR TREATED INFANTS: VDRL TITER AT 1, 2, 4, 6 and 12 MONTHS, *and* CSF ANALYSIS EVERY SIX MONTHS
•VDRL TITER IS DECREASING BY 3–4 MONTHS OF AGE, *and* •VDRL IS NEGATIVE BY 6 MONTHS OF AGE, *and* •FTA-ABS IS NEGATIVE BY 12 MONTHS OF AGE	•VDRL TITER IS DECREASING BY 3–4 MONTHS OF AGE, *and* •VDRL IS NEGATIVE BY 6 MONTHS OF AGE, *and* •CSF VDRL IS NEGATIVE BY 6 MONTHS OF AGE, *and* •CSF CELL COUNT IS DECREASING, *and* •CSF CELL COUNT IS NORMAL BY 2 YEARS OF AGE

YES ↓   ↓ NO   YES ↓   ↓ NO

UNINFECTED   REEVALUATE AND RE-TREAT WITH A REGIMEN RECOMMENDED FOR SYPHILIS OF MORE THAN 1 YEAR'S DURATION   ADEQUATELY TREATED

Figure 2. Follow-up management for an infant examined or treated for congenital syphilis.

References: Ikeda MK, Jenson HB: Evaluation and treatment of congenital syphilis. J Pediatr 117:843–852, 1990.

Dorfman DH, Glaser JH: Congenital syphilis presenting in infants after the newborn period. N Engl J Med 323: 1299–1302, 1990.

MY HEART LEAPS UP

My heart leaps up when I behold
   A rainbow in the sky:
So was it when my life began;
So is it now I am a man;
So be it when I shall grow old,
   Or let me die!
The Child is father of the Man;
And I could wish my days to be
Bound each to each by natural piety.

William Wordsworth

T

TEETH

Eruption of Deciduous Teeth

The eruption of the first tooth in an infant is accompanied by parental pride in the fact that yet another milestone is reached. The figure below indicates the age and the order in which deciduous teeth erupt. The dot represents the mean age, whereas the wavy line demonstrates normal variation. Exceptions to the sequence of eruption are uncommon. Late eruption is unlikely to be of significance; however, it has been associated with both hypothyroidism and rickets.

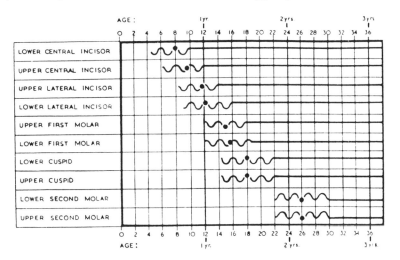

Reference: MacKeith R, Wood C: Digestion and absorption. In Infant Feeding and Feeding Difficulties. London, J. & A. Churchill, 1971, p 19, with permission.

TENNIS ELBOW

Tennis Elbow in Breastfeeding Mothers

Lateral epicondylitis or tennis elbow has been described in a variety of patients. It is classically seen when a person engages in repetitive, similar movements of the forearm extensor muscles, e.g., the continuous and monotonous swinging of tennis racket. The pain of lateral epicondylitis is particularly exacerbated by putting tension on the origin of the forearm extensor muscle, such as the active dorsiflexion of the wrist while grasping an object. Tennis elbow has also been reported to be secondary to infections, trauma, arthritis, and peripheral neuropathy. Recently, however, a new etiology of lateral epicondylitis has been noted—among breastfeeding mothers who used hand-operated breast pumps improperly. The figure below demonstrates improper and proper body mechanics while using a piston style breast pump in order to avoid this new entity: breast pump-induced tennis elbow.

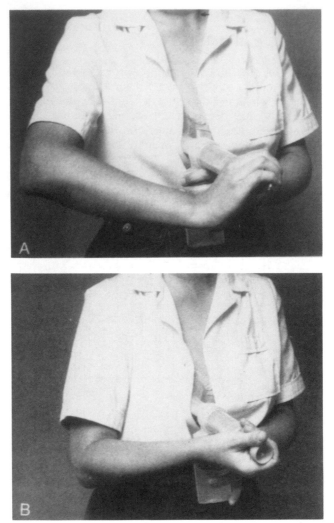

A, Subject demonstrating improper body mechanics while using a piston style breast pump. Note the flexion and abduction at the shoulder, pronation of the forearm, and dorsiflexion at the wrist resulting in the prominent bulge of the contralateral sternocleido-mastoid muscle (arrow) compensating to maintain proper body alignment. **B,** Subject demonstrating proper body mechanics with shoulder adducted and lying comfortably against the body, forearm in supination, and wrist slightly flexed.

Reference: Williams JM, Auerbach KG, Jacobi A: Lateral epicondylitis (tennis elbow) in breastfeeding mothers. Clin Pediatr 28:42–43, 1989.

TERMINOLOGY

What Is Meant By "Usually"?

We all too often use words that lack precision. We, ourselves, may not have a clear idea of what we mean let alone our listener.

A group of 51 individuals, highly skilled or professional workers, were asked to quantitate a number of inherently imprecise terms. Listed below are the words and what the readers believed to be the occurrence rate signified by the terms. The mean value as well as two standard deviations from the mean are provided so that you can appreciate how diverse are the interpretations of these commonly used words.

Imprecise Terminology

TERM	OCCURENCE RATE	
	Mean	*± 2 S.D. (%)*
Always	100%	—
Almost always	89%	75–100
Usually	71%	35–100
Frequently	68%	42–93
Often	59%	28–92
Occasionally	20%	0–42
Infrequently	12%	0–28
Rarely	55%	0–17
Never	0%	—

Since nothing is ever "never" or "always" you can see the problems you *usually* create in interpretation every time you use these imprecise worlds.

Reference: Toogood JH: What do we mean by "usually" (letter)? Lancet i:1094, 1980.

THALASSEMIAS

Classification of the Thalassemias

The thalassemias are a group of inherited blood disorders in which production of one or more of the hemoglobin polypeptide chains is diminished. The resultant erythrocytes produced in these disorders have a low intracellular hemoglobin content, or hypochromia, and are smaller in size than normal red blood cells (i.e., microcytosis). Further, the polypeptide globin chains that are produced in the patient with thalassemia are unstable and aggregate within the red blood cell, yielding membrane damage and early destruction both in the bone marrow and the peripheral circulation.

Classification of the thalassemias is based upon the type of globin chain, which is either absent or produced in diminished amounts.

Clinical Features of Thalassemias

TYPE	CLINICAL FEATURES
Alpha-thalassemia Type	
Silent carrier	No clinical stigmata
Thalassemia trait (heterozygous)	Mild anemia; hypochromic and microcytic red cells
Hemoglobin H disease	Splenomegaly; moderate-to-severe hemolytic anemia; mild jaundice
Hydrops fetalis (homozygous)	Death in utero
Beta-thalassemia Type	
Silent carrier	No clinical stigmata
β-thalassemia trait or minor (heterozygous)	Mild anemia; hypochromic and microcytic red cells; elevated HGA$_2$ and/or HGF
Thalassemia intermedia	Splenomegaly and severe anemia. Skeletal deformities, frequent fractures and arthritis are complications.
β-thalassemia major	Severe anemia incompatible with life unless regular blood transfusions are given.

Reference: Festa RS: Modern management of thalassemia. Pediatr Ann 14:597–606, 1985.

Complications of β-Thalassemia Major

β-thalassemia major or Cooley's anemia is one of the most serious of the thalassemias. Patients with this disease can only survive with frequent blood transfusions, careful attention to iron balance, and supportive therapy. The complications of β-thalassemia major result mainly from (1) excessive hematopoesis; (2) chronic hemolysis; and (3) iron overload with resultant organ damage.

1. **Complications due to excessive hematopoesis**
   a. Marked bone marrow hypertrophy and cortical thinning
   b. Bony changes, particularly in the craniofacial area ("rodent facies") secondary to maxillary overgrowth, protrusion of teeth, separation of the orbits, flattening of the nasal bridge, and malar prominence. These bony changes may yield:
      i. Chronic sinusitis
      ii. Impaired hearing
   c. Pathologic fractures (particularly in weight-bearing bones)
   d. Lymphadenopathy
   e. Hepatosplenomegaly

2. **Complications due to chronic hemolysis**
   a. Gallstones
   b. Leg ulcers (usually seen in late adolescence and early adulthood)

3. **Complications due to iron overload as a result of chronic transfusion therapy** (all tissues are affected by this iron overload, but the liver, spleen, and pancreas retain iron in the highest concentrations)
   a. Cardiac disease
      i. Pericarditis
      ii. Atrial and ventricular arrhythmias
      iii. Congestive heart failure
   b. Hepatic disease (hepatic fibrosis)

4. **Growth and endocrine dysfunction**
   a. Growth failure: Although children with thalassemia major on a chronic transfusion program grow normally until the age of 12, their growth velocity diminishes thereafter, and they fail to exhibit a pubescent growth spurt. Growth hormone levels are usually normal or elevated. The growth failure is probably secondary to chronic disease and iron overload.
   b. Delayed or incomplete sexual maturation
   c. Acquired hypothyroidism, hypoparathyroidism, and diabetes mellitus due to hemochromatosis.

Incidentally, Thomas Cooley, the Detroit pediatrician who first described thalassemia major in 1927, required only a microscope and his patients' peripheral smears to describe a disease that influenced the fields of hematology, human heredity, and population genetics.

References: Festa RS: Modern management of thalassemia. Pediatr Ann 14:597–606, 1985.
Zuelzer WW: Thomas Cooley. In Pediatric Profiles. St. Louis, C.V. Mosby, 1957, pp 135–143.

THEOPHYLLINE

Factors That Alter Theophylline Clearance in Children

Theophylline remains the most commonly used drug for treating children with asthma in the U.S. Despite improved formulations of theophylline that provide a sustained release of the xanthine derivative, and the ability to measure serum theophylline levels, many children are extremely variable in their absorption, metabolism, and clearance of the drug.

Theophylline has a theoretical bioavailability of 100%, and its metabolism and clearance are controlled principally by the liver, where 90% of the drug is metabolized and then excreted in the urine. Any disease or condition affecting the metabolic machinery of the liver, therefore, will play a significant role in altering a patient's metabolism and absorption of theophylline.

Factors Affecting Theophylline Metabolism

Facters that reduce clearance:
1. Liver disease
2. Congestive heart failure; cor pulmonale
3. Prolonged fever, particularly from viral infection
4. Macrolide antibiotics such as erythromycin and troleandomycin
5. Cimetidine
6. Age less than 1 year
7. Influenza vaccine
8. Acute hypoxemia
9. High carbohydrate/low protein diet
10. Propranolol
11. Furosemide

Table continued on next page.

Factors Affecting Theophylline Metabolism (Cont.)

Factors that increase clearance

1. Tobacco or marijuana smoking
2. Charcoal broiled foods (consumed in large quantities over a long period of time)
3. Phenobarbital
4. Phenytoin

5. Isoproterenol
6. High protein/low carbohydrate diet
7. Pregnancy
8. Rifampin
9. Tegretol

References: Adapted from Tinkelman DG: Theophylline—use and misuse in pediatric asthma. Hosp Prac 23:179–184, 1988.

Hen J: Office evaluation and management of pediatric asthma. Pediatr Ann 15:111–124, 1986.

THROMBOCYTOSIS

Significance of Thrombocytosis

In these days of automated cell counters, platelet counts are often determined whether we ask for them or not. As is often the case with unrequested and unnecessary laboratory studies, "abnormal" results are frequently reported. It turns out that platelet counts that previously would have been considered to be abnormally elevated are not particularly unusual among healthy pediatric patients. The figure below represents the distribution of platelet counts obtained from 805 ambulatory pediatric patients. Although the largest number of patients had platelet counts between 200,000 and 400,000/mm^3, 12.9% of the children had counts of greater than 500,000/mm^3, and 2% were greater than 700,000/mm^3. Children with elevated platelet counts were most often completely healthy, but some had evidence of viral or bacterial infection, and they tended to be younger than the children with "normal" counts.

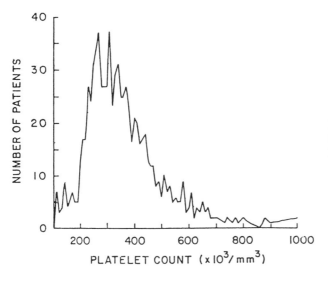

Distribution of platelet counts in 805 ambulatory pediatric patients.

Although "elevated" platelet counts among healthy children may be normal, extreme thrombocytosis is usually associated with a recognizable disease state. Among 94 children with platelet counts greater than 900,000/mm³, only one child was completely healthy. Recognized conditions associated with extreme thrombocytosis include the following:

Infection of any kind
Recovery from chemotherapy
Iron deficiency
Splenectomy
Malignancies
Respiratory distress

Inflammatory diseases such as Kawasaki
  disease, juvenile rheumatoid arthritis,
  and anaphylactoid purpura
Recent surgery
Metabolic diseases
Nephrotic syndrome

References: Heath HW, Pearson HA: Thrombocytosis in pediatric outpatients. J Pediatr 114:805–807, 1989.

Chan KW, Kaikov Y, Wadsworth LD: Thrombocytosis in childhood: A survey of 94 patients. Pediatrics 84:1064–1067, 1989.

Thrombocytosis in Childhood

With the increased availability of electronic cell counting, increased platelet counts are being noted more frequently. Listed below are the major causes of platelet counts in excess of 900,000/mm³.

Infection
Both viral and bacterial infections, particularly of the central nervous system.

Hematologic
Conditions in this group include consequences of chemotherapy, iron deficiency anemia, chronic myelogenous leukemia, and the early postsplenectomy state.

Respiratory
Respiratory distress syndrome, with or without bronchopulmonary dysplasia; severe respiratory obstruction.

Tissue damage or response to surgery
Trauma, postoperative response

Collagen vascular disease
Juvenile rheumatoid arthritis
Wegener granulomatosis
Anaphylactoid purpura

Metabolic diseases
When complicated with acidosis and dehydration

Nephrotic syndrome
An increase in platelet count can be viewed in many circumstances as an acute phase reactant.

Thrombocytosis, infants and children, is rarely associated with thrombotic consequences and requires no therapy.

Reference: Chan KW, et al: Thrombocytosis in childhood: A survey of 94 patients. Pediatrics 84:1064–1067, 1989.

TICK

Tick-Related Infection

Ticks are small, but they are large enough to carry with them many even smaller microorganisms that they inject into unsuspecting human hosts. Most of us are familiar with the clinical characteristics of the tick-borne infections in our own locale, but we may not appreciate the importance of these diseases in patients who have traveled prior to their illness. It is important, first, to remember to think of tick-related infection, and then to consider tick activity in the area, the geographic distribution of ticks known to carry specific pathogens, sites of tick exposure, and signs and symptoms at presentation related to the time of exposure. The incubation period for most of the infections carried by ticks is 3 to 5 days to 2 weeks.

If you have trouble remembering the regional and clinical characteristics of tick-borne infection, the following table may help.

Tick-borne Diseases in Children

DISEASE	ORGANISM	VECTOR	RESERVOIR	GEOGRAPHIC DISTRIBUTION	TYPE OF ILLNESS
Babesiosis	*Babesia microti*	*Ixodes dammini*	Rodents	Coastal area, islands of Massachusetts, Rhode Island, New York	Malaria-like, fever, anemia, renal failure
Lyme disease	*Borrelia burgdorferi*	*Ixodes dammini, Ixodes pacificus, Amblyomma americanum*	Migratory birds	Northeast, Midwest and Western United States[a]	Fever, rash (ECM), headache, myalgias, multiple stages
Tularemia	*Francisella tularensis*	*Dermacentor andersoni, Dermacentor variabilis, Amblyomma americanum*	Rabbits, dogs, rodents[b]	Southern, Southeastern and Midwest United States	Fever, lymphadenopathy, pneumonia
Rocky Mountain spotted fever	*Rickettsia rickettsii*	*Dermacentor andersoni, Dermacentor variabilis, Amblyomma americanum, Haemaphysalis leporis-palustris*	Dogs, cats, rodents, rabbits	Western hemisphere, especially Southeastern United States	Fever, headache, myalgias, rash, toxicity
Erhlichiosis	*Erhlichia canis*	*Rhipicephalus sanguineus*	Dogs	Southern, Southeastern, Midwest United States	Fever, chills, myalgias, hematologic abnormalities, similar to RMSF
	Erhlichia sennetsu	*Rhipichephalus sanguineus*	Dogs, rodents	Japan	
Relapsing fever	*Borrelia duttonii, Borrelia hermsii, Borrelia turicatae*	*Ornithodoros moubata*	Rodents, opossums, squirrels, armadillos	Western Mountains, Southern Plains, United States	Fever, chills, headache, myalgia, relapsing course
Queensland tick typhus	*Rickettsia australis*	Ixodid ticks	Rodents, dogs marsupials	Eastern Australia	Similar to RMSF, usually milder
Fievre boutonneuse	*Rickettsia conorii*	Ixodid ticks	Dogs, rodents	Worldwide	Similar to RMSF, usually milder

[a] Recent evidence for widespread disease in United States.
[b] Animals become ill with infection.

Table continued on next page.

Tick-borne Diseases in Children (Cont.)

DISEASE	ORGANISM	VECTOR	RESERVOIR	GEOGRAPHIC DISTRIBUTION	TYPE OF ILLNESS
Asian tick typhus	*Rickettsia siberica*	Ixodid ticks	Dogs, rodents	Central Asia, Russia	Similar to RMSF, usually milder; regional lymphadenopathy
Q fever	*Coxiella burnetti*	All endemic species[c]	Cattle, sheep, goats	Worldwide	Fever, headache, pneumonia
Colorado tick fever	Orbivirus	*Dermacentor andersoni*	Rodents, deer	Rocky Mountain states, Western Canada and Northern Sierras	Fever, headache, malaise, myalgias, leukopenia
Tick-borne encephalitis	Flavivirus	*Ixodes persulcatus, Ixodes ricinus*	Cattle, sheep, goats, rodents	Central Asia, Eastern Europe, Russia	Fever, headache, encephalitis, photophobia, hyperesthesias
Tick-bite granuloma		*All species*			Local reaction, granuloma, complement-mediated
Tick paralysis		*Dermacentor andersoni, Dermacentor variabilis*			Toxin-mediated, neurologic syndrome, ataxia, areflexia, ascending flaccid paralysis, mild fever

[c]Infection usually acquired by inhalation from animals; ticks important in animal transmission.
ECM, erythema chronicum migrans.

Because the diagnosis of most of these infections depends upon serologic testing, which often must be performed in a reference laboratory, empiric antibiotic therapy is often required. Most of the tick-related infections can be treated with tetracycline or chloramphenicol; however, amoxicillin or penicillin are the appropriate alternatives to tetracycline in the child younger than 8 or 9 years with suspected Lyme disease.

Reference: Jacobs RF: Tick exposure and related infections. Pediatr Infect Dis J 7:612–614, 1988.

TORTICOLLIS

Common Causes

Congenital, muscular, or vertebral anomalies

Uncommon Causes

Cervical adenopathy
Congenital nystagmus
Drug-induced (e.g., phenothiazines, haloperidol, metoclopramide, trimethobenzamide)
Paroxysmal

Pharyngitis
Retropharyngeal abscess
Secondary to reflux esophagitis (Sandifer's syndrome)
Superior oblique muscle weakness

Rare Causes

Calcification of intervertebral disks
Dystonia musculorum deformans
Eosinophilic granuloma of cervical
  vertebrae
Fibromyositis
Hepatolenticular degeneration
Juvenile rheumatoid arthritis
Kernicterus

Osteomyelitis of the cervical vertebrae
Pneumonia of an upper lobe
Posterior fossa tumor
Spasmus nutans
Spinal tumor
Subluxation or dislocation of cervical
  vertebrae

TOURETTE'S SYNDROME

Tics can occur commonly during childhood. Several studies estimate that about 3% of all children exhibit tics at some time. These symptoms are most commonly transient, however, and present as excessive blinking or grimacing. Less common are transient nonspecific vocalizations (e.g., clearing of the throat, sniffing, or frequent coughing).

There are occasions when the symptoms may become more chronic and persistent. When limited to motor symptoms, the condition is called **multiple chronic motor tic disorder.** In the child between ages 2 and 14 presenting with both vocal and motor symptoms that wax and wane in severity over time and have been present for more than a year, the term **Gilles de la Tourette's** or **Tourette syndrome** (TS) is used. Its etiology, unfortunately, remains poorly understood. The types of tics seen in this fascinating syndrome are listed below:

The Symptoms

1. **Motor tics**
   Blinking
   Grimacing
   Shrugging
   Mouth-opening
   Head-jerking
   Tongue movements

   Extending or flexing neck
   Jerking of trunk
   Jerking of extremities
   Tensing of abdominal muscles
   Kicking
   Lip-licking

2. **Vocal tics**
   Sniffing
   Coughing
   Clearing of the throat
   Hissing
   Barking
   Honking
   Snorting
   Squeaking

   Burping
   Repetition of letters
   Repetition of words or phrases
   Involuntary cursing (coprolalia)*
   Clicking
   Whistling
   Spitting
   Shrieking

*Although Georges Gilles de la Tourette's original 1885 description (Arch Neur, Paris, 9:19–42, 158–200, 1885) stressed coprolalia as a cardinal feature, subsequent studies have noted a 20 to 35% incidence rate of this symptom among patients with Tourette syndrome. Its absence, therefore, does not contradict the diagnosis.

3. **Complex symptoms**

Squatting	Repetitive sniffing
Jumping	Obscene gestures (copropraxia)
Twirling	Head-banging
Repetitive touching of objects and people	Self-injury (biting, scratching)

Diagnosis and Treatment

A careful history and physical are warranted, because between 21% and 54% of children with TS have symptoms of attention deficit disorder (ADD). Further, there exists a strong relationship between ADD patients treated with stimulant medications such as methylphenidate (Ritalin) and the subsequent development or exacerbation of tics.

It should be stressed that all of the medications suggested for Tourette syndrome provide only symptomatic relief and are not curative. Further, no evidence exists to suggest that early therapy with these medications has any effect on the long-term prognosis of tic disorders. Many Tourette syndrome patients have symptoms mild enough not to require pharmacologic intervention. In light of the side-effects from the medications listed, many physicians prefer not to use them.

1. **Agents available**

Haloperidol	Clonidine
Pimozide	Clonazepam
Fluphenazine	

2. **Potential side-effects of neuroleptic drugs**

Acute dystonic reactions	Tardive dyskinesia
Parkinsonian symptoms	Increased appetite
Anticholinergic symptoms	Depression
Sedation	Cognitive blunting
	School phobias

References: Barabas G: Tourette's syndrome: An overview. Pediatr Ann 17:391–393, 1988.

Erenberg G: Pharmacologic therapy of tics in childhood. Pediatr Ann 17:395–403, 1988.

Golden GS: The relationship between stimulant medication and tics. Pediatr Ann 17:405–408, 1988.

TRACHEOESOPHAGEAL FISTULA

Tracheoesophageal fistula (TEF) and esophageal atresia are the two types of esophageal malformations causing upper intestinal obstruction. TEF is the failure of the trachea and esophagus to divide linearly during embryogenesis. Esophageal atresia is the developmental occlusion of the esophagus in a localized segment of lumen. Both may present at birth with aspiration and both may occur as an isolated finding.

The diagnosis of tracheoesophageal fistula may be suggested by a variety of clinical observations. The five types of fistula are depicted below, along with the symptoms and signs that typically accompany them.

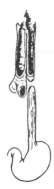

Type A
Symptoms and Signs:

Excessive mucus, aspiration
of saliva.
Scaphoid abdomen.
No gas in bowel on x-ray.
Cannot pass catheter into
stomach.
Gradually increasing respi-
ratory distress.
Polyhydramnios.

Type B
Symptoms and Signs:

Polyhydramnios.
Coughing, choking and
pneumonia from birth.
Scaphoid abdomen.
No gas in bowel on x-ray.

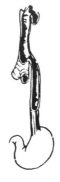

Type C
Symptoms and Signs:

Most common (80% of
cases).
Excessive mucus.
Gradually increasing respi-
ratory distress.
Polyhydramnios frequent
but not severe.
Gas in bowel on x-ray.

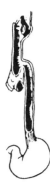

Type D
Symptoms and Signs:

Coughing, choking, and
pneumonia from birth.
Gas in bowel on x-ray.

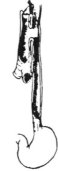

Type E
Symptoms and Signs:

Difficult to diagnose.
Coughing or cyanosis with
feeding.
Chronic aspiration pneu-
monia.

The differential diagnosis includes pharyngeal muscle weakness, vascular rings, and esophageal diverticula.

Discovery of a tracheoesophageal fistula should alert the physician to the possibility that other congenital anomalies may be present. Anomalies that have been found to be associated include:

Vertebral   Anal   Cardiac   Renal   Limb

Reference: Koops BL, Battaglia FC: The newborn infant. In Kempe CH, Silver HK, O'Brien D (eds): Current Pediatric Diagnosis and Treatment. Los Altos, California, Lange Medical Publications, 1984, p 84, with permission.

U

UMBILICUS

Abnormalities of the Pediatric Umbilicus

During both the prenatal and neonatal periods, the umbilicus is a site of many embryologic and structural changes (Fig. 1). Consequently, there exists a wide variety of umbilical abnormalities that require accurate diagnosis and, potentially, subsequent treatment. These abnormalities can be divided in terms of congenital anomalies, infections, signs of remote or underlying disorders, and rare causes of malignancy. We use an anatomic approach to delineate these disorders.

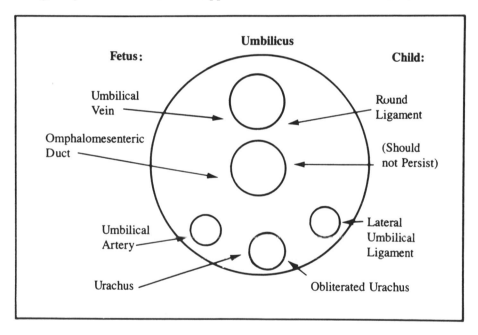

FIGURE 1. Relationship of umbilical structures in the fetus to those in the infant. *Left,* The left umbilical vein and both umbilical arteries persist; *Above,* Cross-section of the cord. Structures may be compared between the fetus and the child.

1. Anatomical Disorders of the Cord and Umbilicus

    a. **Single umbilical artery**
        i. Found in 0.5 to 0.9% of all births, the single umbilical artery is more common in whites than blacks; it is also more common in females and has been associated with infants of diabetic mothers, certain trisomy anomalies, and with thalidomide use during pregnancy.

    ii. There is a reported incidence of congenital anomalies associated with the single umbilical artery, including renal, cardiovascular, pulmonary, genitourinary, cerebrospinal, musculoskeletal, facial, and occular abnormalities. The work-up of a single umbilical artery, therefore, should include a thorough physical examination, especially for dysmorphism, parental counseling, good follow-up for identification of problems that may not be obvious at birth, and special screening studies (e.g., for cardiac or renal anomalies) as indicated.

  b. **Umbilical dysmorphism**
    i. Aarskog syndrome: short stature with facial, digital, and genital malformations and a prominent, protruding central portion of the umbilicus surrounded by a deep ovid depression.
    ii. Reiger syndrome: goniodysgenesis, hypodontia, and a broad prominent umbilicus with redundant umbilical skin.
    iii. Robinow syndrome: fetal face, short forearms with brachydactyly, genital hypoplasia, moderate dwarfing, and an abnormally high positioned, broad, and poorly epithelialized umbilicus
    iv. Beckwith-Wiedemann syndrome: macroglossia, gigantism, hyperinsulinemia and frequently associated with omphalocele.

  c. **Disorders of the umbilical stump**
    i. Omphalitis is an infection of the stump, which is frequently followed by sepsis.
    ii. Persistent omphalomesenteric remnants or ectopic viscera in a retained stalk (usually the stump atrophies and separates 12–14 days after birth; a stalk still present at 3 to 4 weeks should be surgically explored and excised).
    iii. Umbilical or pyogenic granuloma (these should be ablated with silver nitrate)

  d. **Incomplete obliteration of the omphalomesenteric duct** (Fig. 2)
  All of these entities require surgical evaluation and repair.
    i. Umbilical polyp
    ii. Umbilical sinus
    iii. Omphalomesenteric cyst (cysts are usually not diagnosed unless they undergo torsion, become infected, or enlarge when distended by secretions)
    iv. Fibrotic bands between the umbilicus and intestine
    v. Meckel's diverticulum
    vi. Omphalomesenteric fistula (persistant vitelline duct)

  e. **Incomplete obliteration of the allantois** (Fig. 3)
  These entities require surgical repair.
    i. Urachal sinus
    ii. Urachal cyst
    iii. Urachal diverticulum
    iv. Patent urachus

  f. **Abnormalities of the umbilical ring**
  Embryologically, the umbilical ring must constrict and close after the intestine has migrated into the abdominal cavity.
    i. Umbilical hernia (over 85% will close without surgical repair).

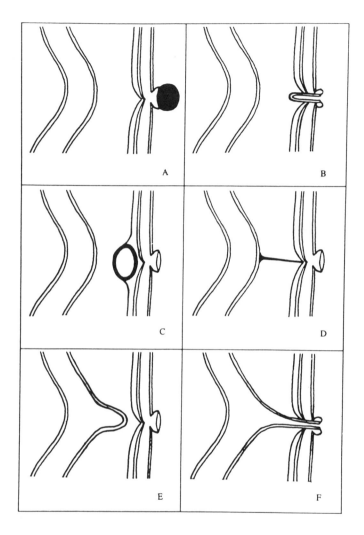

FIGURE 2. **Omphalomesenteric anomalies:** *A,* an umbilical polyp; *B,* umbilical sinus; *C,* an omphalomesenteric cyst, *D,* fibrotic bands between the umbilicus; *E,* Meckel's diverticulum; *F,* an omphalomesenteric fistula.

    ii. Gastroschisis is a defect in the abdominal wall of an extraumbilical location. It may represent a rupture, *in utero,* of an umbilical hernia at a weak point. Gastroschisis requires surgical treatment and closure to return the abdominal contents to their proper space.

   iii. Omphalocele results from a failure of the intestine to return from the vitelline duct to the abdomen. The omphalocele is covered by a thin, membranous sac, which encloses the intestine and often the liver with the cord arising from it. Risks include infection, dehydration, and hypothermia, and surgical closure is indicated. Both omphalocele and gastroschisis have a high association with other congenital anomalies (e.g., gastrointestinal, cardiac, renal, and chromosomal).

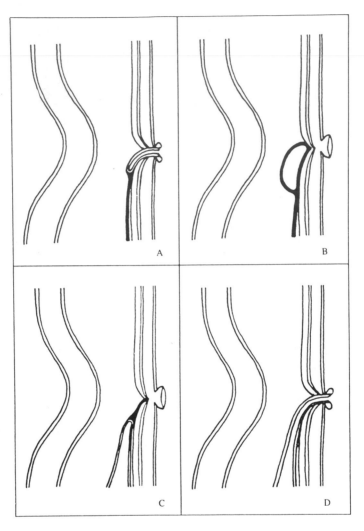

FIGURE 3. **Urachal anomalies::** *A,* urachal sinus; *B,* cyst; *C,* diverticulum; *D,* patent urachus.

2. Other Disorders of the Umbilicus
   a. **Umbilical tumors**
      i. Primary sarcoma
      ii. Primary hemangiomas
      iii. Arteriovenous malformations
   b. **Intraabdominal hemorrhage** can present with a bluish discoloration of an umbilical hernia (Hoffstater's sign)
   c. Acute pancreatitis can be heralded by periumbilical bruising (Cullen's sign).

References: Adapted from Black CT: Disorders of the pediatric umbilicus. Resident and Staff Physician 35:64–84, 1989, with permission.
Sapien RE, Hodge D: Evaluation of the umbilicus. J Am Acad Fam Phys 4:671–674, 1991.

UPPER AIRWAY OBSTRUCTION

Infectious Causes of Upper Airway Obstruction: Distinguishing the Features of Viral Croup, Epiglottitis, and Bacterial Tracheitis

The child presenting to the clinic or emergency room with upper airway obstruction demands immediate attention. There exist many causes of acute upper airway obstruction, including foreign bodies, diphtheria, infectious mononucleosis, and measles. More chronic or recurrent causes of stridor and upper airway obstruction include vascular rings, congenital heart disease, tracheal stenosis from previous intubation, severe allergic reactions leading to laryngospasm, and recurrent angioneurotic edema. The most common causes of potentially life-threatening upper airway obstruction, however, are infectious in origin: (1) viral laryngotracheobronchitis or croup; (2) epiglottitis; and (3) bacterial tracheitis. A prompt diagnosis, obviously, requires a sound knowledge of their distinguishing features in order to assure proper medical management.

Clinical Features of Viral Croup, Epiglottitis, and Bacterial Tracheitis

CLINICAL FEATURE	VIRAL CROUP	EPIGLOTTITIS	BACTERIAL TRACHEITIS
Site of airway obstruction	Infraglottis	Supraglottis	Infraglottis
Patient age			
Peak	2 yrs	3–6 yrs	2 yrs
Range	8 mo–5 yr	17 mo–adult	1 mo–9 yr
Sex	M > F (2:1)	M = F	M = F
Duration of illness prior to admission (hours)	12–78 hrs	2–48 hrs	24–96 hrs
Prodrome	Viral URI	Uncommon	Viral URI
Clinical features on presentation			
Stridor	Common	Uncommon	Common
Barking cough	>60%	Uncommon	>50%
Temperature (°C)	37.8	38.6	39.2
Hoarseness	20%	Uncommon	None
Retractions	Common	Uncommon	Varied
Wheezing	5%	None	10%
Cyanosis	10%	20%	10%
Dysphagia	None	10%	None
Drooling	None	10%	None
Appearance	Lying down, non-toxic	Sitting up, toxic	Varied
Season	Late spring; late fall	Year round	Year round
Progression	Slow	Rapid	Varied: slow–rapid
WBC range	5–11,000	16–22,000	8–20,000
PMN range (%)	40–80	60–95	40–80
Mean bands (%)	7	30	30

Table continued on next page.

Clinical Features of Viral Croup, Epiglottitis, and Bacterial Tracheitis (Cont.)

CLINICAL FEATURE	VIRAL CROUP	EPIGLOTTITIS	BACTERIAL TRACHEITIS
X-ray findings			
Subglottic narrowing (%)	90–100	None	60–100
Enlarged epiglottis (%)	None	100	Rare
Infiltrate on admission (%)	10	<30	>50
Infiltrate during admission (%)	Common	<30	100
Response to racemic epinephrine (%)	95	0	0
Positive tracheal cultures (%)			
Bacteria	0	70 (epiglottis)	100
Viral	100	0	50
Positive blood cultures (bacteria) (%)	0	90	0
Hospitalization (%)	10	100	100
Respiratory arrest	Rare	Increased risk	25%
Treatment (%)			
Intubation	3	99	65
Tracheostomy	<1	1	30
Mean duration of hospitalization (days)	7	5	21
Recurrence	5%	Rare	Rare
Etiologic agents	Parainfluenza type 1, 2, 3; respiratory syncytial virus; rhinovirus	*Haemophilus influenzae,* type b; β-hemolytic streptococci	*S. aureus; Haemophilus influenzae,* type b; streptococcus, group A; β- and hemolytic streptococci; *Neisseria; E. coli;* others

Reference: Adapted from Hen J: Current management of upper airway obstruction. Pediatr Ann 15:274–294, 1986.

URINALYSIS

Dangers of the Dipstick

The urine dipstick is an extremely quick and convenient method of screening for pH, protein, glucose, hemoglobin, ketones, bilirubin, and urobilinogen. The dipstick is a screening test, however, and its limitations must be kept in mind. The situations in which false positive and false negative results may be obtained are listed below:

pH. This determination is not altered except when the pH of the urine is acutally altered by drugs.

Protein. A highly alkaline urine may cause a false positive dipstick for protein.

The alternative test used for detecting protein other than albumin involves denaturing the protein with heat or sulfosalicylic acid to produce turbidity. A false positive result in this alternate test may be produced by:

Buniodyl	Radiographic agents such as
Chlorpromazine	iopanoic acid, iodopyracet,
Promazine	and iophenoxic acid
Carinamide	Sulfamethoxazole
Cephaloridine	Thymol
Cephalothin	Tolbutamide

Glucose. The dipstick technique for glucose may be falsely positive in the presence of bleach in the collecting vessel and vaginal powders containing glucose.

Ascorbic acid may produce a false negative result by retarding color development.

The Clinitest method may be used to quantitate the urinary glucose; however, other reducing agents may produce a false positive result. These include:

Sugars: galactose, lactose,	Homogentisic acid
levulose, maltose,	Glucuronic acid
or pentose	Bleach

Drugs that produce a false positive Clinitest result include:

Acetanalide	Cinchophen
p-aminosalicylic acid	Diatrizoate
Antipyrine	Isoniazid
Cephaloridine	Levodopa
Cephalithin	Nalidixic acid
Chloramphenicol	Oxytetracycline
Chlortetracycline	Tetracycline

Hemoglobin. A false positive test may be produced by myoglobin or the presence of oxidizing agents such as ascorbic acid.

Ketones. Aspirin may cause ketonemia in children, but the presence of aspirin in a ketonuric urine may produce a false negative dipstick.

False positive tests for ketones may be seen in the presence of:

Levodopa
Paraldehyde in the presence of ethanol
Phenformin

Bilirubin. False positives may be seen in the presence of:

Porphobilinigen	Chlorpromazine
Skatole	Phenazopyridine
Indole	Phenothiazines
Large quantities of bilirubin	Sulfadiazine
p-aminosalicylic acid	Sulfamethoxazole
Antipyrene	Sulfanilamide
Apronalide	Sulfonamides
Bromsulfophthalein	

Reference: Adapted from McMillan JA, et al (eds): The Whole Pediatrician Catalog, Vol. 2. Philadelphia, W.B. Saunders, 1979, pp 248–250, with permission.

URINE OUTPUT

Urine Output Measurement in Premature Infants

Lest we forget, urine, like water, does evaporate. This is especially true in the setting of the neonatal intensive care unit. A recent study of the rate and degree of fluid evaporation from disposable diapers under radiant warmers or in infant isolettes showed that evaporation was a function of time and was inversely related to the volume of fluid added to the diaper. Considering the importance of accurate determination of urine output for assessment of hydration status, renal function and nutrient retention in the premature and term neonate, the moral of this tale is clear: adhesive urine bags and frequent diaper inspection are imperative in the care of the low birth weight infant.

Reference: Cooke RJ, et al: Urine output measurement in premature infants. Pediatrics 83:116–118, 1989.

URINARY TRACT

Delayed Urination in the Newborn

One of the kindest acts a neonate can perform for his pediatrician is to urinate early in life. Ninety-nine to 100% of all normal infants urinate at least once by 48 hours of age. Approximately 23% will void first in the delivery room, and the act may not be reported to the nursery.

Failure to urinate by the first 1 to 2 days of life may be due to obstruction of urine flow or to inability to form urine. Causes of obstruction include

Imperforate prepuce	Neurogenic bladder
Urethral strictures	"Megacystic syndrome"
Urethral diverticulum	Ureterocele
Hypertrophy of the	Renal tumors
verumontanum	Cystic kidneys

Inability to form urine may result from

Postnatal intravascular hypovolemia
Restriction of oral fluids
Bilateral renal agenesis
Cortical necrosis
Tubular necrosis
Bilateral renal vein thrombosis
Congenital nephrotic syndrome
Congenital pyelonephritis
Congenital nephritis

Nonspecific symptoms or signs such as excessive crying, irritability, poor feeding, pallor, emesis, mottled skin, or weak pulse may suggest the development of uremia.

The physical examination may be more useful in establishing a specific diagnosis.

Physical Examination Following Delayed Urination

PALPATION OR PERCUSSION OF DISTENDED BLADDER	NO KIDNEYS PALPABLE	PALPABLE RENAL MASS
↓	↓	↓
Obstruction of urine flow	Bilateral renal agenesis	Renal vein thrombosis
↓	These infants are usually	Infantile polycystic
Examine meatus for	males and tend to have	kidneys
patency and look	lowset ears, epicanthal	
for epispadias or	folds, and a flattened	Hydronephrosis
hypospadias	nose	
		Cystic dysplasia
A urethral diverticulum may		
give rise to a bulge along		
the dorsum of the penis		Neoplasm

Reference: Moore ES, Galvez MD: Delayed micturition in the newborn period. J Pediatr 80:867, 1972

Urinary Tract

It is tempting to omit a urine culture in young infants being evaluated for a source of fever, although it is well recognized that urinary tract infections in such infants are associated with nonspecific signs and symptoms. In their evaluation of 100 infants 5 days to 8 months of age, all of whom had been discharged from the nursery in good health, Ginsburg and McCracken found the following characteristics:

- 75% of all infants with UTIs were less than 90 days of age.
- 75% of those infants with UTIs who were younger than 3 months were male.
- 95% of the male infants with UTI were uncircumcised.
- Fever, irritability, vomiting, and diarrhea were the only symptoms in over 90% of infants.
- Although bacteria could be visualized in 81% of stained urine samples, over 50% of the urine samples had less than 10 WBCs per high power field when examined microscopically.
- 25% of the infants had positive blood cultures, but all but one of the bacteremic infants were less than 3 months of age.
- 45% of girls and only 7% of boys with UTI were found to have radiologically detected abnormalities.

Reference: Ginsberg CM, McCracken GH: Urinary tract infections in young infants. Pediatrics 69:409, 1982.

Every night and every morn
Some to misery are born.
Every morn and every night
Some are born to sweet delight.
Some are born to sweet delight,
Some are born to endless night.

William Blake
From *Auguries of Innocence*

V

VAGINAL BLEEDING

Abnormal Vaginal Bleeding in Adolescents

Pediatricians caring for adolescent females frequently see patients with the presenting complaint of vaginal bleeding. Skill in defining the cause of this source of bleeding is vital in order to differentiate benign processes from those that are potentially deleterious. By convention, abnormal vaginal bleeding is excessive in duration and quantity, occurs more frequently than once every 20 days, or is associated with anemia. While the overwhelming majority of such abnormal vaginal bleeding during the teenage years is caused by dysfunctional uterine bleeding, a condition most likely secondary to an immature hypothalamic-pituitary-gonadal axis, careful analysis and evaluation are indicated. Listed below are some entities that should be considered before applying the label of dysfunctional uterine bleeding to such a patient.

1. **Vagina**
    a. Foreign bodies (usually heralded by a foul-smelling, bloody discharge)
    b. Lacerations
    c. Adolescents whose mothers were prescribed diethylstilbestrol (DES) during *their* pregnancy in order to suppress spontaneous abortions

2. **Cervix** (over 1 million teenagers a year become pregnant)
    a. Spontaneous abortion
    b. Incomplete abortion
    c. Threatened abortion
    d. Ectopic pregnancy
    e. Molar pregnancy
    f. Submucosal myomas

3. **Ovaries**
    a. Functional ovarian cysts (follicular or corpus luteal)
    b. Tumors
    c. Polycystic ovary disease

4. **Hypothalamic-pituitary** (e.g., prolactinomas)

5. **Adrenals**
    a. Addison's disease (adrenal insufficiency)
    b. Congenital adrenal hyperplasia

6. **Thyroid**
    a. Hypothyroidism
    b. Hyperthyroidism

7. **Sexually transmitted diseases**
    a. Vaginitis (e.g., *Trichomonas vaginalis* infection)
    b. Cervicitis (e.g., *Chlamydia trachomatis* or *Neisseria gonorrhoeae* infections)
    c. Uterus and salpinx (e.g., pelvic inflammatory disease)

8. **Endometriosis**

369

9. **Medications**
   a. Complications of contraceptives
      i. Oral contraceptive pill
      ii. Intrauterine devices
   b. Anticoagulants
   c. Gonadal and adrenal steroids
   d. Reserpine phenothiazines
   e. Monamine oxidase inhibitors
   f. Morphine
   g. Anticholinergics

10. **Hypothalamic-pituitary-gonadal dysfunction**
    a. Chronic illness
    b. Emotional stress, eating disorders, crash diets, obesity, exercise (all of the aforementioned are more commonly associated with amenorrhea than excessive bleeding).

11. **Bleeding disorders**
    a. Hereditary or acquired thrombocytopenia
    b. Hereditary or acquired platelet function defect
    c. Von Willebrand's disease
    d. Factor XIII or IX deficiency

12. **Dysfunctional uterine bleeding** (which is defined as abnormal vaginal bleeding that occurs in the absence of pregnancy, infection, neoplasms, or any other pathologic entity or disease).

References: Anderson MM, Irwin CE, Snyder DL: Abnormal vaginal bleeding in adolescents. Pediatr Ann 15:697–707, 1986.
Cowan BD, Morrison JC: Management of abnormal genital bleeding in girls and women. N Engl J Med 324:1710–1715, 1991.

VAS DEFERENS

Unilateral Absence of the Vas Deferens: A Useful Clinical Sign

The vas deferens of an adolescent male is easily palpated during a routine physical examination. The unilateral absence of the vas deferens, on the other hand, is associated with a 79% likelihood of finding a missing ipsilateral functioning renal unit. Such an association makes the absence of the vas deferens a significant anomaly, and examination for the presence of the ipsilateral renal unit (e.g., intravenous pyelogram) is mandatory.

Reference: Donohue RE, Fauver HE: Unilateral absence of the vas deferens. A useful clinical sign. JAMA 261:1180–1182, 1989.

VESICLES

Vesicular and Vesiculopustular Eruptions in the Newborn

There exists a large differential diagnosis for the newborn infant presenting with vesicular or vesiculopustular lesions. The first distinguishing factor the physician must ascertain is whether the lesions are caused by an infectious or noninfectious etiology. This can typically be done rather quickly and inexpensively with the following diagnostic tests:

1. Gram stain
2. Potassium hydroxide (KOH) preparation
3. Tzanck smear
4. Bacterial culture
5. VDRL of the mother and infant
6. Viral culture
7. Fungal culture
8. If necessary, a skin biopsy

Given the potential for sepsis, one should assume an infectious etiology in the newborn presenting with vesicular or vesiculopustular lesions and treat appropriately before the culture results are known. A differential diagnosis is presented below, separated in terms of infectious and noninfectious etiologies.

1. **Infectious vesicular and vesiculopustular lesions**
    a. Herpes simplex (vesicles are on an erythematous base and are usually 1 to 3 mm in diameter, arranged either in clusters or singly; bullae, macular exanthems, purpura, and zosteriform eruptions have also been reported).
    b. Congenital varicella
    c. Varicella-zoster (grouped vesicles on an erythematous base arranged in a dermatomal or segmental pattern).
    d. Congenital cutaneous candidiasis (lesions are typically erythematous macules that progress over the course of 1 to 3 days through papular, vesicular, and pustular stages, followed by superficial desquamation. Yellow vesicles have also been reported).
    e. *Staphylococcal aureus* infection can cause bullae, erosions, or diffuse superficial desquamation (i.e., the staphylococcal scalded skin syndrome).
    f. Congenital syphilis can yield vesicles and bullae (typically on the palms and soles but any location is possible).

2. **Noninfectious vesicular and vesiculopustular lesions**
    a. Erythema toxicum neonatorum (erythematous macules with a central vesicle or pustule, primarily on the trunk). A Wright's stain of the vesicle or pustular contents revealing sheets of eosinophils is diagnostic.
    b. Transient neonatal pustular melanosis (vesicopustules, collarettes of scale, and hyperpigmented macules may be noted on the neck and trunk. The vesicles and pustules resolve 48 hours after birth, leaving only scaly lesions or hyperpigmented macules.
    c. Heat rash or miliaria (usually a papular, vesicular or pustular rash). Frequently seen in the neonate who has been excessively warmed.
    d. Letterer-Siwe disease (infantile form of histiocytosis X). Infants characteristically present with scalp eruptions similar to that of seborrheic dermatitis. Purpura, ulcers, vesicles, and pustules have also been reported. Biopsy is usually diagnostic. Multiorgan involvement is common.
    e. Congenital self-healing reticulohistiocytosis (possibly a variant of Letterer-Siwe disease). Infants may present with vesicles but more typically display erythematous or blue papules and nodules.
    f. Urticaria pigmentosa (lesions are classically tan or reddish-brown papules, macules or nodules that appear urticaric with rubbing, [Darier's sign]). The skin biopsy reveals a perivascular and epidermal mast cell proliferation. These lesions can yield vesicles and bullae during the newborn period.
    g. Bullous mastocytosis (lesions are classically large bullae or erosions; vesicles are seen rarely).

h. Epidermolysis bullosa (a heterogeneous group of inherited skin disorders yielding easy blistering, with bullae and erosions, of the skin). Gentle rubbing, or Nicolsky's sign, can produce such lesions.
i. Dermatitis herpetiformis (vesicles and hemorrhagic crusts, particularly on the extremities).
j. Pemphigus vulgaris (blisters)
k. Herpes gestationis (blisters)
l. Incontinentia pigmenti (also known as Bloch-Sulzberger syndrome, melanoblastosis cutis linearis sive systematisata, melanosis corii degenerativa, and Absoe-Hansen's disease). It typically presents with erythema or vesicles or both at birth and often looks like erythema toxicum neonatorum. Seen almost exclusively in females, it is believed to be x-linked dominant and lethal in males. The lesions may be scattered but are more frequently linear in pattern. Neurologic, ocular, and dental anomalies are frequently present.
m. Incontinentia pigmenti achromians or hypomelanosis of Ito.

Reference: Rothman KF, et al: Case records of the Massachusetts General Hospital (Case #21-1989). New Engl J Med 320:1399–1410, 1989.

VERTIGO AND SYNCOPE

Vertigo (dizziness) and syncope (lightheadedness, fainting) may be difficult symptoms for a child to distinguish between with certainty. Many entities that are traditionally thought to cause syncope may also cause vertigo. Syncope will therefore be discussed as a subheading of causes of vertigo.

Common Causes

Benign paroxysmal vertigo
Drugs
  Alcohol
  Anticonvulsants
  Antihypertensives
  Aspirin
  Dilantin
  Gentamicin
  Narcotics
  Sedatives
  Streptomycin
Ear disease
  External canal impaction
    Cerumen
    Foreign body
  Inner ear disease
    Cholesteotoma (with extension)
    Fistula
    Mastoiditis (with extension)
    Suppurative labyrinthitis

Ear disease *(Cont.)*
  Inner ear disease *(Cont.)*
    Vestibular neuronitis
    Viral (acute) labyrinthitis
  Middle ear disease
    Chronic suppurative otitis (with extension)
    Hemotympanum (basilar skull fracture)
    Otitis media (rare as isolated finding)
    Serous otitis media
    Tympanic membrane perforation
Headache
  Basilar artery migraine complex
  Migraine
Hyperventilation syndrome
Seizure
  Aura/recovery phase
  Reflex seizure
Visual impairment

Uncommon Causes

Central nervous system
    infection
  Abscess
  Encephalitis
  Meningitis
Hypotension

Trauma
  Basilar skull fracture
  Cerebellar lesion/hemorrhage
  Labyrinthine trauma
  Postconcussion syndrome

Rare Causes

Adrenal insufficiency
Anemia
Arnold-Chiari malformation
Benign positional vertigo
Brain stem ischemia
Breath-holding spells
Central nervous system tumors
  Acoustic neuroma
  Brain stem glioma
  Cerebellar glioma
  Ependymoma
  Medulloblastoma
Demyelinating disease
  Multiple sclerosis
Endocrine disorders
  Adrenal insufficiency
  Diabetes mellitus
  Thyrotoxicosis
Hypertension
Hypoglycemia
Increased intracranial
  pressure
Ménière's syndrome
Pellagra
Psychosomatic illness
Ramsay Hunt syndrome

Syncope (many causes previously discussed)
  Cardiovascular etiologies
    Arrhythmia
      Atrioventricular block
      Cardioauditory syndrome
      Emery-Dreifuss muscular dystrophy
      Mitral valve prolapse
      Paroxysmal atrial tachycardia
      Paroxysmal ventricular tachycardia
      Prolonged QT syndrome
      Sick-sinus syndrome
    Cardiac anomalies
      Aortic stenosis
      Pulmonary stenosis
      Tetrology of Fallot
      Transposition
      Truncus arteriosus
    Carotid sinus syncope
    Dysautonomia (Riley-Day syndrome)
    Idiopathic hypertrophic subaortic stenosis
    Left atrial myxoma
    Myocardial infarction
    Orthostatic hypotension
    Pulmonary hypertension
    Vasovagal stimulation
Vestibulocerebellar ataxia

VISION

The Visual Acuity of Normal Children

A friend of yours tells you that her 1 year old child has been examined by her pediatrician and is said to have "perfect 20/20" vision. Your child, who is also 1, has 20/200 vision. Who should get a new physician?

Visual acuity at birth is poorer than at any other time of life and only gradually improves to the 20/20 range at the time of entrance to kindergarten. The accompanying table indicates the expected average acuity of preschool children. An acuity of 5/200 should not be misinterpreted to mean that the newborn is practically blind. Just stick your tongue out at a newborn and see what he does back to you!

Visual Acuity

AGE	AVERAGE UNCORRECTED ACUITY
Birth	5/200
1 year	20/200
2 years	20/40
3 years	20/30
4 years	20/25
5 years	20/20

Reference: McCrary JA: "E-game" visual acuity test for preschool children. JAMA 208:1195, 1969.

VULNERABLE CHILD SYNDROME

Parents of a child who was expected to die, or parents of an only child, or parents who have experienced the death of a child often react in a manner that produces a disturbance in the psychosexual development of their offspring. Learn to recognize the circumstances that produce "the vulnerable child" syndrome and its manifestations. The psychosexual disturbance manifests itself most commonly in the following ways:

1. **Difficulty with separation.** Child may be briefly entrusted to the care of grandparents, but baby sitters are rarely used. In extreme instances, mother and child never separate. Sleep problems are common. The child frequently sleeps with parents or in parents' room. Mother or father wakes frequently during the night to check on the status of the child.

2. **Infantilization.** Parents are unable to set disciplinary limits. Parent is overprotective, overindulgent, and oversolicitous. Child is overly dependent, disobedient, irritable, argumentative, and uncooperative. Children may be physically abusive to parents. Feeding problems are common.

3. **Bodily overconcerns.** Hypochondriacal complaints, recurrent abdominal pain, headaches, and infantile fears are prominent. School absence is common. Mothers express concern about minor respiratory infections, stool habits, "poor color," circles under the eyes, and blueness when crying.

4. **School underachievement.** Unspoken agreement that the child is only safe with mother may produce separation anxiety that results in poor school performance.

Predisposing Factors in the Production of the Vulnerable Child

1. Child is first-born to older parents who had resigned themselves to being childless.

2. Parents cannot have additional children as a result of a hysterectomy or other sterilization procedure.

3. The patient was born with congenital anomaly.

4. The patient was born prematurely.

5. The patient has an acquired handicap, e.g., epilepsy.

6. The child has had a truly life-threatening illness, such as erythroblastosis, nephrosis, or severe asthma.

7. During pregnancy the mother was told that the fetus might die.

8. Mother had a postpartum depression.

9. Mother has ambivalent feelings about child, such as instances where child was born out of wedlock.

10. Parents have unresolved grief reaction as a result of loss of another child.

11. A hereditary disorder is present in the family, such as cystic fibrosis or muscular dystrophy.

12. There is a psychological need on the part of the parents to find something physically wrong with the child in order to displace unacceptable feelings about the patient. Child is frequently brought to physicians because of parents' suspicion of leukemia, brain tumor, rheumatic fever, or other serious illness.

13. Separation of infant from his or her mother for phototherapy.

Treatment

1. Recognize the circumstances that may produce a vulnerable child and try to reassure parents about the health of the infant or child before symptoms appear.

2. Make authoritative statements about the child's well-being based on a thoughtful, cumulative history, physical examination, and pertinent measurements and laboratory findings.

3. Point out to the parents and get them to accept the reasons for their unnecessary concern, the child's responsive behavior, and the mutual reinforcement that is present.

Do not produce the syndrome yourself with comments such as "I thought for sure he was going to die," or "If she hadn't gotten here when she did we wouldn't have been able to save her," or "You are very lucky parents that we saved your child."

Reference: Green M, Solnit AJ: Reactions to the threatened loss of a child; A vulnerable child syndrome. Pediatrics 34:58, 1964.

Adapted from McMillan JA, et al (eds): The Whole Pediatrician Catalog. Philadelphia, W.B. Saunders, 1977, pp 51–52, with permission.

W

WALKERS

The AMA has summarized the epidemiology of walker injuries as follows:

1. Between 70% and 80% of infants will use a walker, mostly between ages 5 and 12 months; twice as many boys use walkers as girls.
2. Of infants who use walkers, 30% to 40% will have an accident.
3. Most walker accidents are minor and relatively few result in contact with a physician.
4. The most common types of accident involve falling down stairs, tipping over, and finger entrapment. Other injuries result from infants pulling objects down onto themselves.
5. Of infants seen in emergency departments for a walker injury, almost all *serious* trauma results from falling down stairs. Over 90% of all stairwell injuries among infants less than 12 months of age are related to use of walkers. Closed head injury is the most common serious walker injury, followed by fractures (skull, arm, clavicle) and other trauma, such as burns, dental injuries, and lacerations.
6. Of infants with serious injury, about one third stop walker use immediately, one third stop use within 2 months (usually because infants begin walking on their own), and one third are still using a walker 2 months after the injury.
7. Most walker injuries occur in the home with one or both parents present. Of injuries involving stairs, about half occur in houses *with* stairwell gates.
8. Although the occurrence of trauma is unrelated to the age at first use, a number of siblings, and parents' occupations, it is related to the amount of time spent in the walker. Fewer than 30% who spend less than 2 hours a day in a walker suffer a nonserious fall, compared with approximately 55% of infants who spend more than 2 hours per day in a walker.
9. The types of walkers involved in serious injury are fairly evenly divided between the X-frame, in which the steel support bars form an X, and the circular frame, in which the support bars go up in a straight vertical pattern to reach the upper tray.

Approximately one million walkers are sold in the U.S. each year. Although relatively rare, serious trauma does occasionally occur and physicians should counsel parents about the use of walkers, especially near stairwells.

There is no evidence that walkers promote bipedal ambulation.

Reference: AMA Board of Trustees: Use of infant walkers. Am J Dis Child 145:933–934, 1991.

WHEEZING

Common Causes

Aspiration
    Direct (e.g., defective swallow,
        neuromuscular disease)
    Indirect (gastroesophageal reflux,
        emesis)
Asthma
Atopic disease
Bronchiectasis
Bronchiolitis
Bronchitis
Foreign-body aspiration
Pneumonitis

Uncommon Causes

Bronchopulmonary dysplasia
Congestive heart failure
Cystic fibrosis
Hypersensitivity pneumonitis
    Allergic bronchopulmonary
        aspergillosis
Mediastinal mass/adenopathy
Pulmonary edema
Tracheobronchomalacia

Rare Causes

α1-Antitrypsin deficiency
Angioneurotic edema
Carcinoid syndrome
Factitious wheezing
Lobar emphysema
Neoplasm/tumor
Psychogenic airway obstruction
Pulmonary hemosiderosis

Pulmonary sequestration
Pulmonary vasculitis
Sarcoidosis
Tracheobronchostenosis
Tracheoesophageal fistula
Vascular ring/sling
Visceral larva migrans

WOUND CARE

In their zest to achieve antisepsis and ensure good wound healing, pediatricians and nurses may be creating the cosmetic surgery cases for tomorrow. Routine wound care in the acute setting usually consists of a 1:1 dilution of hydrogen peroxide and stock povidone iodine. Both of these solutions are extremely toxic to exposed fibroblasts and are, therefore, counterproductive agents as often used.

Recommendations regarding the use of these antiseptics include:

- A 1:100 dulution of hydrogen peroxide (greater strength may be used on already mature granulation tissue).

- A 1:1000 (1 ml/L) dilution of povidone iodine. This is problematic, because although fibroblast toxicity is minimized, so is bactericidal effect. The answer is to paint the perimeter of the wound but not the wound itself.

- Avoid antibiotic solutions in wounds in the acute stages due to recognized cytotoxicity.

Reference: Oberg MS, Lindsey D: Do not put hydrogen peroxide or povidone iodine into wounds. Am J Dis Child 141:27–28, 1987.

Put Sugar, Not Salt, in Their Wounds

It may seem counterintuitive, but granulated sugar has proven to be one of the safest, least expensive, and most "universal" antimicrobial treatments for infected wounds and superficial lesions. The success of sucrose solution as an antimicrobial depends on its water activity (a_w), which defines the water requirements for growth of a given microorganism.

Studies demonstrated in *The Lancet* showed that *195 g of sugar in 100 g of water* (a_w = 0.858) completely inhibited growth of *Staphylococcus aureus*. *S. aureus* (a_w = 0.86) happens to have the lowest a_w of common bacterial pathogens, including streptococci, *Klebsiella, E. coli, Corynebacterium, C. perfringens* and other clostridia, and *Pseudomonas*.

The limiting factor in this extraordinarily available and effective method of wound care is that application of solution to a wound causes an osmotic change in surrounding tissue. The osmotic pressure change results in dilution of the sucrose solution, necessitating the addition of more granulated sugar. This seems a small inconvenience given the ubiquity of sucrose. When preparing your next First Aid Kit, do not forget the sugar!

Reference: Chirife J, et al: Scientific basis for the use of granulated sugar in treatment of infected wounds (letter). Lancet i:560–561, 1982.

X

X-RAYS

It is doubtful that any resident or physician can imagine a single work day in the hospital without ordering an x-ray of some kind. One of the most frequent concerns parents have when consenting to a radiologic procedure has to do with the amount of radiation exposure a particular x-ray yields. Listed below are the range of radiation doses generated in a variety of medical procedures and "nonmedical" activities:

Range of Radiation Doses Received in Various Medical and Nonmedical Activities

TYPE OF RADIATION	DOSE (RAD, REM; VERY APPROXIMATE)*	LENGTH OF EXPOSURE	WHERE RECEIVED
Medical			
Chest film, newborn	0.004	Msec	Skin entrance dose; exit dose lower
CT, contiguous slices, child	2–5	Sec	Scanned volume
Lateral of lumbosacral spine, adult	0.5	Sec	Skin entrance dose; exit dose much lower
Cardiac catheterization	10–100	Hr	Skin entrance dose; exit dose much lower
Curative radiotherapy	7,000	Wk	Tumor and adjacent structures
Nonmedical			
Natural background at sea level	0.08	Yr	Whole body
Some professional jet pilots and flight crews, from cosmic rays	1	Yr	Whole body
Residents of certain areas of India with radioactive soil	3	Yr	Whole body
Radiation workers, current permitted dose	5	Permitted/yr	Radiation badge (usually worn on neck)
Dose at which half of population dies, nuclear warfare	450	Min	Whole body

*To convert to grays, divide by 100.

Reference: Kirkpatrick JA, Griscom NT: Imaging procedures for children. In Behrman R (ed): Nelson's Textbook of Pediatrics, 14th ed. Philadelphia, W.B. Saunders. 1992, p 262, with permission.

381

Y

YELLOW NAILS

Disorders of nail pigmentation have been associated with numerous conditions. The term *chromonychia* refers to an abnormality in color of the substance or surface of the nail plate and/or subungual tissues. Practically the entire color spectrum is represented in abnormalities of the nails, but this section will focus only on yellow nails. White nails (leukonychia) are the most common variant.

The nail should be studied with the fingers relaxed and not pressed against a surface, which can alter the hemodynamics and give a false appearance. The fingertip should then be blanched to try to differentiate between discoloration of the nail plate and the vascular bed. If a tropical agent is suspected as the cause, try removing it by scraping or by rubbing with a solvent.

The causes of staining include contact with exogenous agents, cosmetics, other topical applications, tobacco, trauma, physical agents, and fungal and bacterial infections.

Nails can provide an extended historical record of abnormalities of skin pigment that might otherwise go unnoticed.

Causes of Yellow Nails

TOPICAL/CONTACT	
Cosmetics	External agents *(Cont.)*
Chloroxine (+ aluminum)	Diquat
Formaldehyde in hardeners	Epoxy systems
Formaldehyde-phenol resins	Hydrofluoric acid
Hair dyes	Nitric acid and derivatives
Nail lacquers	Picric acid
Resorcinol in nail varnish	Tetryl
	Tobacco
Dermatoses	Weed and insect poisons
Fogo selvagem (wildfire pemphigus)	Yellow dyes, paints, polishes, and stains
Psoriasis	
Onychomycosis	Therapeutic agents
Yeast infection (dermatophytes	Amphotericin B
and nondermatophytes)	Dinitrochlorobenzene
	Fluorescein
External agents	
Chromium salts (yellow ochre color)	Trauma
Coal tar derivatives	Caustic soda
Dichromates	Hematoma in resolution
Dinitrophenol	Thermal injury

Table continued on next page.

Causes of Yellow Nails (Cont.)

HEREDITARY/SYSTEMIC

Aplasia cutis with dystrophic nails	Macular amyloidosis with familial nail
Beta carotene	dystrophy
Chronic pulmonary disease	Pachyonychia congenita
Diabetes mellitus	Peripheral vascular disease
D-penicillamine	Porphyria cutanea tarda
Familial amyloidosis with poly-	Progeria
neuropathy	Rifampin ingestion
Hyperbilirubinemia	Tetracycline ingestion
Incontinentia pigmenti (slightly yellow)	Yellow nail syndrome and lymphedema

Reference: Baran R, Dawber RPR: Diseases of the Nails and Their Management. Oxford, Blackwell Scientific Publications, 1984, pp 63–73.

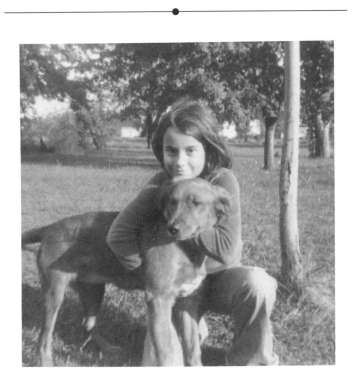

Z

ZOONOSES

Diseases You Can Acquire from Pets and Animals

Everyone knows that dogs are "man's best friend"—that is, unless you own a cat. Indeed, pets are a valuable addition to the family and can enrich a child's life with affection, companionship, and a sense of responsibility. But as wonderful as pets are, they present a potential risk to the health of humans, particularly children. Listed below are the more common zoonoses and the animals with which they are associated:

Potential Host Distribution of Selected Zoonoses

Column groupings: **DOMESTIC ANIMALS** = Horses, Cattle, Sheep, Goats, Swine, Dogs, Cats, Lab rodents, Poultry, Invertebrates. **WILD ANIMALS** = Fish, Amphibians, Reptiles, Birds and **MAMMALS** (Rodents, Primates, Carnivores, Ungulates, Others).

	Horses	Cattle	Sheep	Goats	Swine	Dogs	Cats	Lab rodents	Poultry	Invertebrates	Fish	Amphibians	Reptiles	Birds	Rodents	Primates	Carnivores	Ungulates	Others
Viral Diseases																			
Arbovirus encephalitis	X	X	X	X	X				X	X			X	X	X			X	X
Cat-scratch disease (virus suspected)							X										X		
Lymphocytic choriomeningitis						X		X							X				
Newcastle									X					X					
Rabies	X	X	X	X	X	X	X	X							X	X	X	X	X
Vesicular stomatitis	X	X			X					X									
Yellow Fever										X					X	X			X
Rickettsial Diseases																			
Q fever		X	X	X											X	X			
Rocky Mountain spotted fever		X	X					X		X					X				
Spirochetal Diseases																			
Leptospirosis	X	X	X	X	X	X	X	X							X	X	X	X	X
Rat-bite fever						X		X							X		X		
Bacterial Disease																			
Anthrax	X	X	X	X	X	X	X	X	X	X					X	X	X	X	X
Brucellosis	X	X	X	X	X	X	X	X	X	X					X		X	X	X
Erysipelas					X				X	X	X				X	X			

Table continued on next page.

Potential Host Distribution of Selected Zoonoses (Cont.)

	DOMESTIC ANIMALS									WILD ANIMALS					MAMMALS				
	Horses	Cattle	Sheep	Goats	Swine	Dogs	Cats	Lab rodents	Poultry	Invertebrates	Fish	Amphibians	Reptiles	Birds	Rodents	Primates	Carnivores	Ungulates	Others
Bacterial Disease *(Cont.)*																			
Hemorrhagic septicemia	X	X	X	X	X	X	X	X	X										
Listeriosis	X	X	X	X	X	X			X						X	X	X		
Melioidosis	X	X	X	X	X	X	X	X							X				
Plague			X	X		X	X	X							X	X	X		X
Pseudotuberculosis			X	X	X	X		X	X										
Psittacosis									X						X				
Salmonellosis	X	X	X	X	X	X	X	X	X	X	X	X	X	X	X	X	X	X	X
Scarlet fever		X			X														
Septic sore throat		X																	
Staphylococcosis		X																	
Tetanus	X											X							
Tuberculosis	X	X	X	X	X	X	X	X	X			X			X		X	X	X
Tularemia		X	X	X	X	X	X								X	X	X	X	X
Vibriosis		X	X	X															
Fungal Diseases																			
Actinomycosis	X	X	X	X	X	X	X								X		X	X	X
Aspergillosis	X	X	X	X	X			X	X						X				
Coccidioidomycosis	X	X	X	X	X	X									X	X	X	X	
Cryptococcosis	X	X	X	X	X	X	X					X			X		X	X	X
Epizootic lymphangitis	X																		
Histoplasmosis	X	X	X	X	X	X	X	X	X						X	X	X		X
Nocardiosis	X	X	X	X	X	X	X								X				X
North American blastomycosis	X					X													
Rhinosporidiosis	X	X																	
Ringworm	X	X	X	X	X	X	X	X	X						X	X	X	X	X
Sporotrichosis	X	X				X			X										
Streptothricosis	X	X	X	X		X												X	
Protozoan																			
Amebiasis																X			
Balantidiasis					X											X			
Leishmaniasis						X									X		X		
Plasmodium (malaria)																X			
Sarcocystis	X	X	X	X					X						X				X
Toxoplasmosis		X				X	X	X							X	X	X		X
Trypanosomiasis	X	X	X	X	X	X	X	X		X								X	X

From Fowler ME: Curr Probl Pediatr 4:3, 1974, with permission.

References: Fowler ME: Diseases of children acquired from nondomestic animals. Current Problems in Pediatrics 4:10, 1974.
Goscienski PJ: Zoonoses. Pediatr Infect Dis 2:69–81, 1983.

INDEX